Elements of Psychophysical Theory

OXFORD PSYCHOLOGY SERIES

EDITORS
DONALD E. BROADBENT
JAMES L. MCGAUGH
NICHOLAS J. MACKINTOSH
MICHAEL I. POSNER
ENDEL TULVING
LAWRENCE WEISKRANTZ

Elements of
Psychophysical Theory

JEAN-CLAUDE FALMAGNE

Professor of Psychology
New York University

OXFORD PSYCHOLOGY SERIES NO. 6

CLARENDON PRESS · OXFORD
OXFORD UNIVERSITY PRESS · NEW YORK
1985

Oxford University Press

Oxford   London   New York   Toronto
Delhi   Bombay   Calcutta   Madras   Karachi
Kuala Lumpur   Singapore   Hong Kong   Tokyo
Nairobi   Dar es Salaam   Cape Town
Melbourne   Auckland

and associated companies in
Beirut   Berlin   Ibadan   Mexico City   Nicosia

Published by Oxford University Press, Inc.,
200 Madison Avenue, New York, New York 10016

Library of Congress Cataloging in Publication Data

Falmagne, Jean-Claude.
  Elements of psychophysical theory.
  (Oxford psychology series; no. 6)
  Includes index.
  1. Psychophysics.   2. Psychometrics.   3. Psychology—Mathematical models.
I. Title.   II. Series.
BF237.F25   1984   152.1   85-3087
ISBN 0-19-503493-7

Printed in Great Britain at the University Press, Oxford

Preface

This book is intended as a self-contained graduate text for a two-semester course discussing the basic concepts of measurement and psychophysics. The level of the material is geared to students in experimental psychology with a relatively modest background in mathematics (e.g., two semesters of undergraduate calculus), but well motivated and prepared to work hard. In a two-semester course, all the material in the book can be covered, with the exception of Chapter 7 and the starred sections, which contain technical material and are generally more difficult. In a one-semester course on psychophysical theory, a possible sequence might include the first four sections in Chapter 2, Chapters 4–6, 8–10, 13, and whatever else is deemed important by the instructor in the remaining chapters (again, omitting the starred sections and also the proofs of a number of results).

I have used drafts of the book in several courses, and the students' reactions have been most helpful. I am especially grateful to Charlie Chubb, Ching-Fan Sheu, Martin Gizzi, and John Van Praag for their remarks.

Jean-Paul Doignon, Geoffrey Iverson, and Misha Pavel, my longtime friends and co-workers, also had a positive influence on my writing. Geoffrey's careful reading of drafts of many chapters and his detailed comments have been particularly valuable.

The viewpoint on psychophysics given here owes much to the work of several researchers in the field. Among others, the names of David Krantz, Michael Levine, and especially Duncan Luce, whose contribution was seminal, should be mentioned. It is not that this viewpoint is startlingly new. To the contrary. The novelty of the presentation only resides in an attempt to discuss the concepts of classical psychophysics in the framework of measurement theory, and more generally, in the language of contemporary mathematics. Much more will be said on this matter in the initial chapter, entitled "Preliminaries."

I am indebted to my colleagues at New York University for the intellectually stimulating atmosphere that characterizes our program. I am especially grateful to Murray Glanzer, Lloyd Kaufman, Michael Landy, Tony Movshon, and George Sperling for the encouragement they gave me regarding this project.

At some time or other, Mary Peters, Amy Kritz, Kathleen Williams, Odella Schattin, and Saritha Clements typed drafts of chapters of this book. I am happy to thank them here for their expert, conscientious work, and for their friendly acceptance of my idiosyncrasies. I am also grateful to my daughter Catherine Landergan-Falmagne, who kindly offered to do the artwork. The final appearance of this book owes much to Joan Knizeski-Bossert, from Oxford, whose painstaking vigilance, coupled with patience and understanding, was very helpful in the final stage.

The work reported here was partly supported by grants from the National Science Foundation to New York University. Part of the writing was done during my tenure as a Guggenheim fellow and as a von Humboldt fellow. The support of these institutions is gratefully acknowledged.

I am also thankful to my wife, Cecilia, for her unwavering, good-humored support of what may perhaps have seemed, at times, a rather whimsical activity.

This book is dedicated to Lloyd Kaufman, whose friendship and guidance over the years have been invaluable.

New York City   J.-C. F.
January 1985

Contents

Table of Symbols

Symbol	Meaning	Introduced in
$\varnothing$	Empty set	Preliminaries
$\subset$	Reflexive set inclusion	Preliminaries
$\in, \cup, \cap$	Standard set theoretical symbols	Preliminaries
$\{x \mid \rho(x)\}$	Set of all x satisfying property ρ	Preliminaries
$\precsim$	Often, a weak order	1.14
$\mathscr{F}(R)$	Field of a relation R	1.3
$\mathscr{D}(R), \mathscr{R}(R)$	Domain and range of a relation R	1.3
$\bar{R}$	Negation of R	1.8
$f \circ g$	Composition of g by f	1.11
f^{-1}	Inverse of a $1-1$ function f	1.11
$f^{-1}(A)$	Inverse image of A by f	1.11
$\mathbb{N}$	Set of positive integers	Preliminaries
$\mathbb{Z}$	Set of integers	Preliminaries
$\mathbb{Q}$	Set of rational numbers	Preliminaries
$\mathbb{R}$	Set of real numbers	Preliminaries
(a,b)	Open, real interval; also, an ordered pair	
$[a,b]$	Closed real interval	
$[a,b), (a,b]$	Real, half open intervals	
$\mathbb{P}$	A probability measure	
C	Set of comparable stimuli	4.3
Φ	Often, the distribution function of a standard, normal random variable	
$\mathbf{X}, \mathbf{Y}, \mathbf{Z}, \mathbf{U}, \ldots$ etc.	Random variables	
$\exp x$	Another notation for e^x	
p_a	Psychometric function with standard a	6.2
$\mathscr{F}$	A psychometric family	6.2, 6.4
Δ	Weber function	8.1
ξ	Sensitivity function	8.1
Θ	A collection of payoff matrices	Ch. 10
$p_s(\theta), p_n(\theta)$	Hit and false alarm probabilities with a payoff matrix θ	Ch. 10
ρ	An ROC curve or function	10.1
$\gamma_{o}, \gamma_{sn}, \gamma_{ns}, \gamma_{v}$	Values of the gains in a payoff matrix	10.6
$\mathscr{U}$	Often, a collection of random variables	
$d'(s,n)$	Standard index of detectability	10.10

Elements of Psychophysical Theory

Preliminaries

CLASSICAL VERSUS MODERN PSYCHOPHYSICS

Traditionally, research in psychophysics has attempted to answer the following questions:

Q1. What are the basic "sensation" scales underlying the subject's responses in psychophysical experiments?
Q2. How are these scales related to the physical scales?

These questions prompted a program of research that originated with G. T. Fechner and was remarkably successful in generating a considerable array of useful data as well as a theoretical framework for these data. Over the years, however, Fechner's methods and concepts have been criticized. Today, many consider classical (or Fechnerian) psychophysics outmoded, and of historical interest only. In standard textbooks, it is dispatched rather than expounded, the typical presentation reading like a summary of a treatise that could have been written at the end of the nineteenth century. Little effort is made to analyze the filiation between classical and modern concepts, and the progress realized.

This situation deserves to be corrected. In fact, the influence of Fechner's program on contemporary psychophysics is overwhelming, even though the favored terminology may have evolved somewhat. Rather than Q1 or Q2, a modern psychophysicist would ask:

Q3. How is physical intensity coded by a particular sensory system?

This reformulation of the fundamental questions reflects the tendency of contemporary psychophysics to seek explanations of the data in terms of models or mechanisms. This involves a generalization of the classical viewpoint, embodied in Q1 and Q2, that a stimulus intensity induces an event in the organism, which may be represented by a single number. A less restrictive position is consistent with Q3. The effect of a stimulus intensity on the organism may have a representation as an intricate mathematical object, such as a random variable, or a stochastic process of neural events.

Let us be more concrete. In a discrimination experiment, let $P_{a,b}$ be the probability that a stimulus of intensity a is judged as exceeding a stimulus of intensity b in some sensory attribute. The fundamental equation of classical

3

psychophysics is

$$P_{a,b} = F[u(a) - u(b)] \qquad (1)$$

in which u and F are real valued, strictly increasing, continuous (but otherwise unspecified) functions. Thus, the probability of choosing a over b increases with the difference between these stimuli on the sensory scale u. This scale is taken to be a measure of the magnitude of sensations evoked by the stimuli. (The foundation of this position will be discussed in Chapter 13.) Equation 1 must have a solution, that is, the functions u and F must exist, for Fechner's procedures to be valid. This equation is never discussed, does not even appear, in typical contemporary texts (for an exception, see Kaufman, 1974).[1] However, almost all models for discrimination data considered seriously by working psychophysicists involve generalizations or special cases of this equation (or equivalent ones).[2] For instance, Equation 1 may appear as a consequence of a complicated model. In such a case, the function F may take the form of some distribution function, and $u(a)$, $u(b)$ may be parameters of some stochastic process.

Our presentation will clarify the relations between past and current concepts and methods.[3] An apt title for a large part of this book (Chapters 1–9) would have been "Classical Psychophysics from a Modern Viewpoint.'

ON THE UNIQUENESS OF MODELS
AND REPRESENTATIONS

Questions Q1 and Q2 implicitly presuppose that the sensation scales somehow exist independently of both the experimental paradigm and the mathematical model used to analyze the data, and that they have to be "uncovered." Similarly, but more generally, Q3 may suggest that the stimuli, or more accurately, the effects they produce in the organism, have a mathematical representation the form of which does not depend on paradigm or model. This requires some elaboration. Consider the following typical example of psychophysical lingo, describing a model for the discrimination probabilities $P_{a,b}$ appearing in Equation 1:

> We assume that the presentation of a stimulus of intensity a induces, in some neural location, some excitation of intensity U_a, a random variable. If a pair of stimuli (a,b) is presented in a discrimination paradigm, the subject will choose a over b as the more intense stimulus whenever the excitation induced by stimulus a exceeds that

---

1. In all fairness, it must be admitted that this equation was only implicit in the "Elements of Psychophysics" (Fechner, 1860/1966).

2. Even Stevens's magnitude estimation or cross-modality matching methods (and data) may be formalized by a theory closely related to the Fechnerian Equation 1. (See the Krantz-Shepard relation theory in Chapter 13.)

3. The opposition between Stevens's and Fechner's school of psychophysics has been grossly exaggerated, at the cost of much confusion. It can be argued convincingly that, apart from semantical issues, the two positions are quite consistent.

induced by stimulus b; that is, whenever $\mathbf{U}_a > \mathbf{U}_b$. This means that the discrimination probabilities $P_{a,b}$ satisfy the equation

$$P_{a,b} = \mathbb{P}\{\mathbf{U}_a > \mathbf{U}_b\}, \tag{2}$$

where $\mathbb{P}$ is the probability measure.

This illustrates a convenient and suggestive descriptive style, which we shall use on occasion. It may be misleading, however, if employed carelessly. The quoted text may suggest, for example, that the random variables $\mathbf{U}_a$ and $\mathbf{U}_b$ appearing in (2) are a natural, invariant mathematical representation of the events taking place in the organism as a result of the stimulation. Such a presumption, even though it may very well be logically unassailable (there may be no practical way to disprove it) is nevertheless controversial. It is indeed at odds with the considerable arbitrariness presiding at various important stages of a research enterprise. The most critical choice to be made concerns the model used to explain the data. A particular model, say M, found to provide an acceptable fit to some data, is rarely unique in this regard. There usually are many models fitting the data equally well, and thus equivalent to M in this respect. However, equivalent models may lead to very different representations.

The model of Equation 2 (which, incidentally, generalizes that of Equation 1) will provide an example. Let us suppose that a further stage in the sensory coding of the stimuli is taking place, and that the stimuli are represented by the random variable $g(\mathbf{U}_a)$, $g(\mathbf{U}_b)$, etc., in which g is some real valued, strictly increasing function defined on the real numbers. Thus, the subject's decisions are based on a comparison of the random variables $g(\mathbf{U}_a)$ and $g(\mathbf{U}_b)$, and (1) is replaced by

$$P_{a,b} = \mathbb{P}\{g(\mathbf{U}_a) > g(\mathbf{U}_b)\}. \tag{3}$$

But obviously, (2) and (3) are equivalent. Nothing in the discrimination data considered would justify choosing $\mathbf{U}_a$ over $g(\mathbf{U}_a)$ as being a more genuine representation of the neural effects of stimulus a. Nevertheless, the form of the distributions of the random variables $\mathbf{U}_a$ and $g(\mathbf{U}_a)$ may differ drastically.[4] A researcher taking such representations too literally may be led astray and venture into unwarranted speculations. One might argue that the choice of a representation may be influenced by taking into account additional data, collected with a different paradigm, or even of a different nature (e.g., physiological). Actually, some reflection indicates that, even in light of such data, the situation would not be altered significantly. The arbitrariness of the choice of a representation may be reduced, but does not disappear.

Moreover, models that are not formally equivalent may have predictions that are not distinguishable experimentally. This lack of "uniqueness" of the models is by no means peculiar to psychophysics, but is especially dramatic in this field. The fact is that the data basis is scarce, as compared with the ambitious explanations often entertained by researchers.

---

4. Some important properties will remain. For example, if the random variables $\mathbf{U}_a$ are independent, then the random variables $g(\mathbf{U}_a)$ are also independent.

Such considerations will lead us to adopt, in our presentation of psychophysical theory, a rather sober attitude toward models and scales. But what, one might ask, will then be at the center of the discussion?

LAWS VERSUS MODELS

Two central questions confront the psychophysical researcher:

1. What mechanisms, or models, may serve to explain the observed sensory responses?
2. What regularities, or laws, are suggested by the data?

The relative importance attached to these questions provides an interesting way of classifying workers in the field. One might argue that the opposition that I am hinting at here is artificial, and claim, virtuously, that everyone wants to know how the brain and the sensory systems work, and proceeds to find out by studying the regularities in the data.[5] Nevertheless, I believe that the classification is useful, and that there really are two schools of thought, or at least two research styles.

Classical psychophysics was certainly focused on the second question. Probably influenced by the successful history of physics, the early psychophysicists were searching for regularities or laws, rather than for models or mechanisms, hoping to build up a solid experimental foundation for ulterior, more ambitious, theoretical constructions. Stevens and his followers are direct descendants of Fechner's, while many other contemporary psychophysicists definitely belong in the first school, and see their research as an attempt at discovering mechanisms.

Some would certainly say that too much emphasis on the second question leads to rather dull enterprises, which at best prepare the way for more creative accomplishments. This may very well be the dominant opinion in psychophysics today. Despite this pessimistic appraisal, this book is organized around empirical laws, regularities, or invariants (these may be taken as synonyms). Models will play a role, however, and many will be discussed in detail; but they will appear as illustrations or special cases of more general structures. The main reason for this choice is that laws tend to have a better life expectancy than models. A law may be useful scientific device even when it is known to be falsified systematically in some conditions. Weber's law is a case in point. It is known to hold well at medium intensities, but fails dramatically at the lower end of the stimulus scale (and for some sensory continua, also at the upper end).[6] Nevertheless, Weber's law

5. One might also object that the distinction between models and laws is not clear, and could not easily be formalized, since it is a matter of degree. Both a model and a law define constraints on the data. In the statement of a law, economy of though presides, and a minimum of hypothetical concepts is used. Such preoccupation with economy is less prominent in the statement of a model, the domain of application of which can often be stretched to include the prediction of empirical relations beyond its intended scope, through the evocative power of its concepts.

6. A comparable example in physics is Boyle's law, which fails at low temperature. A more comprehensive description of the data is offered by van der Waal's law.

remains an important criterion for models. A discrimination model is judged acceptable only if, to a good approximation, it is consistent with Weber's law at medium intensities.

The search for regularities tends to be neglected in contemporary psychophysics. The organization of this book is a step toward a change of focus in psychophysical research.[7]

ON THE CONTENT OF THIS BOOK

The Contents of this book may puzzle some readers, who will wonder about the role, in psychophysics, of the esoteric topics of Part I, such as "functional equations" or "extensive measurement." This material is included since we wanted our discussion of psychophysical theory to be accessible to any student with a bit of mathematical training (say, a couple of courses in calculus, maybe one college-level course in algebra), but equipped with a great deal of perseverance. Many fundamental results in psychophysical theory can be obtained through relatively straightforward applications of functional equations or extensive measurement techniques. Unfortunately, these techniques are only presented in specialized texts, and then in a manner which is often not exactly suitable for our purpose. Omitting them in this book would have rendered the task of the thorough student of psychophysical theory much more difficult. The interdependence of some of the most important mathematical results discussed here is illustrated in the following figure, which displays the "mathematical skeleton" of the book.

It is my hope that the efforts made to present the material of Part I in a style congenial to a wide audience will be perceptible and appreciated.

The reader seeking only a survey of psychophysical theory can start on Chapter 4, with the understanding that the proofs of a number of important results may have to be skipped.

Finally, it must be said that not all the topics that could be evoked by the title of this book will be dicussed. Among the regrettable omissions are color theory and multidimensional scaling. A chapter on the historically important question of the sensory threshold had been planned, but was dropped in the final draft and replaced by a few paragraphs in Chapter 10. Green and Luce's counting and timing models are only mentioned in passing (Green and Luce, 1974; Luce and Green, 1972, 1974). Levine's projective geometry representations of magnitude estimation and related data are not discussed (Levine, 1974). Sequential dependencies in psychophysical data, even though they certainly are theoretically significant, and empirically pervasive, are only alluded to.

---

7. This view of the role of models or theories in the scientific enterprise did not originate with the writer. It has been propounded by Ernst Mach, and critized by others, such as Max Planck. In the celebrated words of Mach (1871, English translation published as *History and Root of the Principle of the Conservation of Energy*, 1911): "The aim of natural science is to obtain connections among phenomena. Theories, however, are like withered leaves, which drop off after having enabled the organism of science to breathe for a time." (An account of the debate can be found in Frank, 1941.)

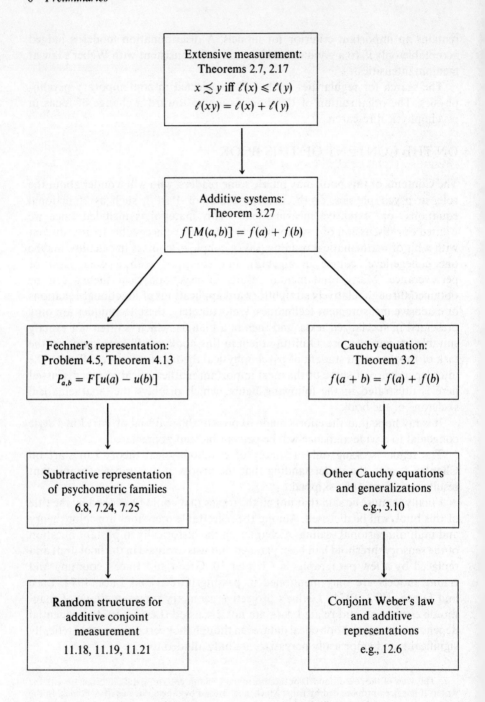

Extensive measurement:
Theorems 2.7, 2.17
$x \precsim y$ iff $\ell(x) \leqslant \ell(y)$
$\ell(xy) = \ell(x) + \ell(y)$

Additive systems:
Theorem 3.27
$f[M(a,b)] = f(a) + f(b)$

Fechner's representation:
Problem 4.5, Theorem 4.13
$P_{a,b} = F[u(a) - u(b)]$

Cauchy equation:
Theorem 3.2
$f(a + b) = f(a) + f(b)$

Subtractive representation
of psychometric families
6.8, 7.24, 7.25

Other Cauchy equations
and generalizations
e.g., 3.10

Random structures for
additive conjoint
measurement
11.18, 11.19, 11.21

Conjoint Weber's law
and additive
representations
e.g., 12.6

Mathematical backbone of the book. Only the main lines are indicated. An arrow linking two boxes indicates that the upper results can be used to infer the lower ones.

The most flagrant gap concerns an important current of contemporary visual and auditory psychophysics in which it is hypothesized that a sensory system is essentially a Fourier analyzer (Gulick, 1971; Kaufman, 1974). This position leads the researcher to construct stimuli that are capable of an enlightening description in terms of their Fourier components. The finding that the sensory system is differentially sensitive to distinct Fourier components suggests the existence of separate sensory channels associated with these components (Campbell and Robson, 1968). To include a comprehensive description of the theoretical developments involved in this line of research would have added substantially to the length of the book.

Any one of these, and other, omissions is unfortunate. As a whole, they have no better justification than that this book had been on the writing table for nearly ten years, and that it was ample time to go public.

NOTATION AND CONVENTIONS

Standard mathematical notation is used throughout. The symbols $\varnothing$, $\in$, $\subset$, $\cup$, and $\cap$ have their usual meaning in set theory. (Notice that $\subset$ is the reflexive inclusion.) The formula $A = \{a|\Phi(a)\}$ stands for the set of all those objects a satisfying property Φ. The logical equivalence "if and only if" will be abbreviated as "iff." We can thus write, for sets A, B, C, and D,

$$\text{if } A = \{a|\Phi(a)\} \qquad \text{then } a \in A \text{ iff } \Phi(a), \tag{4}$$

$$A \subset \varnothing \qquad \text{iff there is no } a \text{ satisfying } a \in A, \tag{5}$$

$$A \subset (B \cup C) \cap D \qquad \text{iff } A \subset (B \cap D) \cup (C \cap D). \tag{6}$$

Each of these statements is, of course, a true sentence in set theory. The reader for whom one of these would evoke the slightest feeling of strangeness should consult a standard text, such as Suppes (1957). The symbol $\mathbb{P}$ denotes a probability measure. The symbols $\mathbb{N}$, $\mathbb{Z}$, $\mathbb{Q}$, and $\mathbb{R}$ stands for particular sets, namely:

$\mathbb{N}$ is the set of natural numbers, $\mathbb{N} = \{1,2,\ldots\}$.
$\mathbb{Z}$ ($\mathbb{Z}^+$) is the set of (positive) integers.
$\mathbb{Q}$ ($\mathbb{Q}^+$) is the set of (positive) rational numbers.
$\mathbb{R}$ ($\mathbb{R}^+$) is the set of (positive) real numbers.

The symbol ■ denotes "end of proof." Starred sections contain more difficult material and may be omitted at first reading. Especially long or difficult proofs are usually put in an appendix to a chapter. Such appendixes are always starred.

Each chapter is subdivided into sections, and each section into titled subsections, which we call paragraphs. For ease of reference, only the paragraphs are numbered. A paragraph is often a definition, a theorem, or a list of remarks.

I
BACKGROUND

1

Ordinal Measurement

Consider the following variations of a classical psychophysical experiment. A human subject is presented with two stimuli: *a,b*.

Variation 1. *a* and *b* are material objects. The subject is given the opportunity to manipulate them. After a moment he or she is asked

$$\text{"Is } a \text{ heavier than } b?\text{"} \tag{1}$$

Variation 2. *a,b* are pure tones of the same frequency, differing in their amplitude, presented monaurally and successively. After listening to the pair (*a,b*) the subject answers the question:

$$\text{"Is } a \text{ louder than } b?\text{"} \tag{2}$$

Variation 3. The subject observes a screen on which two patches of light *a,b* are projected and is asked:

$$\text{"Does } a \text{ contain more red than } b?\text{"} \tag{3}$$

These three variations illustrate the so-called *yes-no-paradigm*, the importance of which is fundamental in psychophysical research—both in view of the considerable amount of data collected, and of the theoretical developments that it inspired. This chapter discusses this paradigm from the viewpoint of theories involving only ordinal constraints on the data. For the subject, the adjective "heavy" (for example) unambiguously refers to a category of sensory impressions. He or she may hesitate before answering (1) for some objects *a,b*. But the subject's hesitation will be due to the unreliability of his or her nervous system, not to the ambiguity of the question. For the mathematically minded student of the data, "heavier than" or "not heavier than" will naturally evoke the order relations > or ⩽ of the real numbers. Conceivably, the objects *a,b,...,* can be assigned numbers $h(a)$, $h(b)$, ..., the assignment depending on how heavy the objects appear to be. Specifically, we have

$$h(a) \leqslant h(b) \qquad \text{iff} \qquad a \text{ does not appear heavier than } b.$$

This chapter deals with a theoretical investigation of the proposition that the data in the yes-no paradigm satisfies some or all of the properties of >, ⩽. We begin by assuming that the subject's responses are reliable. In other words, we assume that repeated presentations of the same pair of stimuli would elicit the same response. This assumption is not always realistic and will be abandoned later on. Set theory provides a very useful coding of the data typically obtained in this paradigm. Suppose that in Variation 1, for example, the experiment involves a set $A = \{a_1, a_2, a_3, a_4, a_5\}$ of stimuli, and that the data take the form of Table (4). We assume that all ordered pairs $(a,b) \in A \times A$ have been considered.

	a_1	a_2	a_3	a_4	a_5
a_1	no	no	no	no	no
a_2	no	no	no	no	no
a_3	yes	yes	no	no	no
a_4	yes	yes	yes	no	no
a_5	yes	yes	yes	no	no

(4)

Thus, the subject's answer to the question

"Is a_3 heavier than a_1?"

is "yes." This data can be summarized by simply listing the ordered pairs $(a,b) \in A \times A$ such that a is judged heavier than b. In other words, the data can be represented by a subset of $A \times A$, that is,

$$\{(a_3,a_1), (a_3,a_2), (a_4,a_1), (a_4,a_2), (a_4,a_3), (a_5,a_1), (a_5,a_2), (a_5,a_3)\}. \tag{5}$$

The corresponding set theoretical notion is that of a "binary relation."

BINARY RELATIONS

1.1. Definition. A set R is called a *binary relation*, or more simply, a *relation* iff there are two sets A,B such that $R \subset A \times B$.[1] In this case, we will occasionally say that R is a relation *from A to B*. If $R \subset A \times A$, we will also say that R is a relation *in A*. A relation is thus a set of ordered pairs. To lighten the writing we will often use the abbreviation aRb to mean that $(a,b) \in R$. Notice in passing an oddity of this definition: the empty set $\varnothing$ is a relation in itself. Indeed, $\varnothing \subset \varnothing \times \varnothing = \varnothing$, since $\varnothing$ is a subset of any set.

1.2. Examples.   Here are some familiar cases of relations:

(a) $\leqslant$, the inequality of the real numbers; thus, as a relation in $\mathbb{R}$.
(b) $>$, the strict inequality, as a relation in $\mathbb{R}$.
(c) $=$, the identity, as a relation in $\mathbb{R}$.
(d) $\subset$, the set inclusion, as a relation in a family of sets; to be specific, say, the set of all subsets of $\mathbb{N}$.

Thus, each of $\leqslant$, $>$, $=$ is a subset of $\mathbb{R}^2$. Taking a geometrical viewpoint, $=$ can be regarded as the first bisector of the Cartesian plane, that is, the set of all those points $(a,b) \in \mathbb{R}^2$ such that $a = b$. (Which subsets of the plane correspond to

---

1. A similar definition can be given of a *ternary relation* (or, in general, of an *n*-ary relation) R by requiring $R \subset A \times B \times C$ for some sets A,B,C (or $R \subset A_1 \times A_2 \times \cdots \times A_n$, for some sets $A_i, 1 \leqslant i \leqslant n$). These notions will not be used, however. Dropping the adjective "binary" in "binary relation" will thus not create ambiguities.

$\leqslant$, $>$?) Relations can also be created artifically. For example:

(e) $S = \{(1,1),(1,2),(2,1),(2,2),(2,3)\}$ is a relation since $S \subset \{1,2\} \times \{1,2,3\}$; notice that S is a relation in $\{1,2,3\}$ since $S \subset \{1,2,3\}^2$.

(f) The data in Table (4) can be recoded in the form of a relation $\succ$ in $A = \{a_1,a_2,a_3,a_4,a_5\}$ defined by: $a \succ b$ iff the subject's answer to the question "is a heavier than b?" is "yes."

The relation $\succ$ can then be conveniently represented by Table (6) or, equivalently, by the listing provided by (5).

	a_1	a_2	a_3	a_4	a_5	
a_1	—	—	—	—	—	
a_2	—	—	—	—	—	
a_3	$\succ$	$\succ$	—	—	—	(6)
a_4	$\succ$	$\succ$	$\succ$	—	—	
a_5	$\succ$	$\succ$	$\succ$	—	—	

(g) A more refined coding of the same data can be made. The subject was asked the following two questions.

"Is a_1 heavier than a_2?"

"Is a_2 heavier than a_1?"

As indicated by Table (4) the answer was "no" to both questions. Thus, we may deduce that a_1 appears to be as heavy as a_2. We formalize "as heavy as" by a relation $\sim$, defined by

$$a \sim b \qquad \text{iff} \qquad a,b \in A, \text{ not } a \succ b \text{ and not } b \succ a.$$

To complete the picture, we also formalize "lighter than" by a relation $\prec$,

$$a \prec b \qquad \text{iff} \qquad a,b \in A, \text{ not } a \sim b \text{ and not } a \succ b.$$

The data are thus recoded as in Table (7).

	a_1	a_2	a_3	a_4	a_5	
a_1	$\sim$	$\sim$	$\prec$	$\prec$	$\prec$	
a_2	$\sim$	$\sim$	$\prec$	$\prec$	$\prec$	
a_3	$\succ$	$\succ$	$\sim$	$\prec$	$\prec$	(7)
a_4	$\succ$	$\succ$	$\succ$	$\sim$	$\sim$	
a_5	$\succ$	$\succ$	$\succ$	$\sim$	$\sim$	

Notice that $A \times A$ is the union of the three relations $\succ$, $\sim$, $\prec$. Finally, we define a relation $\precsim$ in A as the union of $\prec$ and $\sim$ in (7). Clearly,

$$a \precsim b \qquad \text{iff} \qquad a \text{ does not appear heavier than } b.$$

That is, $\precsim$ symbolizes the "no" responses in Variation 1.

Other examples of relations can be found in the exercises. The next definition introduces a number of properties of relations which together provide a convenient classification scheme.

1.3. Definition.   A relation R is called:

(a) *Reflexive on A* iff aRa for all $a \in A$.
(b) *Irreflexive on A* iff aRa for no $a \in A$.
(c) *Symmetric on A* iff aRb implies bRa, for all $a,b \in A$.
(d) *Asymmetric on A* iff aRb implies not bRa, for all $a,b \in A$.
(e) *Antisymmetric on A* iff $a = b$ whenever both aRb and bRa, for all $a,b \in A$.
(f) *Transitive on A* iff aRc whenever both aRb, bRc, for all $a, b, c \in A$.
(g) *Connected on A* iff aRb or bRa, for all $a,b \in A$.
(h) *Weakly connected on A* iff aRb or bRa, whenever $a \neq b$, for all $a,b \in A$.

As usual in mathematics, the "or" in (g) and (h) is the logical disjunction; that is, both aRb and bRa can arise. Notice that a relation R in set A can be reflexive on $B \subset A$ without being reflexive on A. For example, S, in Example 1.2(e), is reflexive on $\{1,2\}$ but is not reflexive on $\{1,2,3\}$. Similar remarks apply to the other parts of Definition 1.3. Occasionally, we say that some relation R is reflexive, irreflexive, etc., without specifying a particular set. This should be taken to mean that R is reflexive, irreflexive, etc., on the set

$$\mathscr{F}(R) = \{a \,|\, aRb \text{ or } bRa, \text{ for some } b\},$$

called the *field* of R. Since aRb implies $a,b \in \mathscr{F}(R)$ by definition, we have

$$R \subset \mathscr{F}(R)^2. \tag{8}$$

Thus, any relation is a relation in its field. In terms of this convention, S is not reflexive, and $\leq$ is reflexive $(\mathscr{F}(S) = \{1,2,3\}, \ \mathscr{F}(\leq) = \mathbb{R})$. The reader can evaluate his or her mastery of these notions by checking the results in Table (9) in which the above definitions have been applied to the examples in 1.2.

	$\leq$	$>$	$=$	$\subset$	S	$\succ$	$\sim$	$\lesssim$
Reflexive	yes	no	yes	yes	no	no	yes	yes
Irreflexive	no	yes	no	no	no	yes	no	no
Symmetric	no	no	yes	no	no	no	yes	no
Asymmetric	no	yes	no	no	no	yes	no	no
Antisymmetric	yes	yes	yes	yes	no	yes	no	no
Transitive	yes	yes	yes	yes	no	yes	yes	yes
Connected	yes	no	no	no	no	no	no	yes
Weakly connected	yes	yes	no	no	no	no	no	yes

(9)

Several remarks must be made about this table. First, S has none of the properties (a) to (h) (on its field, $\mathscr{F}(S) = \{1,2,3\}$). The inequality $>$ is antisymmetric, but "vacuously": There are no $a,b \in \mathbb{R}$ satisfying $a > b, b > a!$ (The reader puzzled by this logical point should spend some time on Exercise 2.) The same remark applies to $\succ$. In fact, this relation has all the properties of $>$, except weak connectedness.

It is useful to notice that the field of a relation R is the union of the two sets

$$\mathscr{D}(R) = \{a \mid aRb \text{ for some } b\},$$

$$\mathscr{R}(R) = \{a \mid bRa \text{ for some } b\},$$

which will be called, respectively, the *domain* and the *range* of R. By definition,

$$R \subset \mathscr{D}(R) \times \mathscr{R}(R),$$

and $\mathscr{D}(R)$, $\mathscr{R}(R)$ are the smallest sets with this property. (If $R \subset A \times B$, then $\mathscr{D}(R) \subset A$ and $\mathscr{R}(R) \subset B$.) Clearly, the domain and the range of a relation need not be disjoint and may in fact be identical, as in Examples 1.2(a) to (d). In Example 1.2(e), we have

$$\mathscr{F}(S) = \mathscr{R}(S) = \{1,2,3\}, \qquad \mathscr{D}(S) = \{1,2\}.$$

Example 1.3(f) gives

$$\mathscr{F}(\succ) = \{a_1, a_2, a_3, a_4, a_5\},$$

$$\mathscr{D}(\succ) = \{a_3, a_4, a_5\}, \qquad \mathscr{R}(\succ) = \{a_1, a_2, a_3\}.$$

Various implications linking properties (a) to (h) can be derived. Some of them are immediate: A connected relation is also reflexive and weakly connected; an asymmetric relation is irreflexive. The result below is perhaps slightly less obvious.

1.4. Theorem. *An irreflexive and transitive relation is asymmetric.*

Proof. Let R be a transitive, irreflexive relation and suppose that aRb, bRa for some a,b. (We assume thus that R is not asymmetric.) By transitivity, we derive aRa, contradicting the hypothesis that R is irreflexive. ∎

This simple argument provides our first example of a proof of a theorem. Many proofs will, however, tend to be longer, some considerably longer. A serious study will then be required. When a needed argument is not more difficult than that of the above proof, it will often be left to the reader. Another, somewhat more difficult example, is given below.

1.5. Theorem. *Let R be a connected, transitive relation. Define a relation E by*

$$aEb \qquad iff \qquad both \ aRb \ and \ bRa.$$

Then E is a reflexive, transitive, and symmetric relation. Moreover, $\mathscr{F}(R) = \mathscr{F}(E)$.

Proof.   Remember that since R is connected, it is also reflexive. First, we show that $\mathscr{F}(R) = \mathscr{F}(E)$. Clearly, $\mathscr{F}(E) \subset \mathscr{F}(R)$. Indeed, $a \in \mathscr{F}(E)$ implies

$$aEb \quad \text{or} \quad bEa$$

for some b (by definition of the field of E), which in turn implies

$$aRb \quad \text{and} \quad bRa.$$

This gives $a \in \mathscr{F}(R)$. Conversely, if we assume that $a \in \mathscr{F}(R)$, we obtain aRa since R is reflexive. Thus aEa, and we have $a \in \mathscr{F}(E)$. Thus $\mathscr{F}(R) \subset \mathscr{F}(E)$, and we conclude that $\mathscr{F}(R) = \mathscr{F}(E)$, as asserted. The reflexitivity of E follows from that of R: For any $a \in \mathscr{F}(E) = \mathscr{F}(R)$, we have aRa, which implies aEa by definition of E. Similarly, the transitivity of E is a straightforward consequence of the transitivity of R. Finally, the symmetry of E is derived from sentential calculus: If aEb, then aRb and bRa by definition—the "and" being the logical conjunction—thus bRa and aRb, that is, bEa. ■

This proof was given in considerable detail. In the future, a more compact style will be adopted progressively. Otherwise, the size of this book would quickly become unmanageable and, more important, key substantive issues would become lost in a mass of minor technical details.

EQUIVALENCE RELATIONS, PARTITIONS, FUNCTIONS

The above theorem implicitly introduces an important concept. A couple of examples of relations that are simultaneously reflexive, transitive, and symmetric have been encountered before, that is, (cf. Table (9)) the equality of the real numbers and the relation $\sim$ symbolizing "as heavy as" in Example 1.2(g). In this last case, we had

$$\sim = \{(a_1,a_1),(a_2,a_2),(a_1,a_2),(a_2,a_1),(a_3,a_3),(a_4,a_4),(a_5,a_5),(a_4,a_5),(a_5,a_4)\}.$$

Examination of this expression suggests a natural classification of the elements of the set $A = \{a_1,a_2,a_3,a_4,a_5\}$ into three subsets

$$A_1 = \{a_1,a_2\}, \qquad A_2 = \{a_3\}, \qquad A_3 = \{a_4,a_5\}$$

having the following properties: for any $i,j \in \{1,2,3\}$

1. $A_i \neq \varnothing$;
2. if $i \neq j$, then $A_i \cap A_j = \varnothing$;
3. $A_1 \cup A_2 \cup A_3 = A$.

Notice the correspondence between $\sim$ and the sets A_i: If $a,b \in A_i$, then $a \sim b$ and $b \sim a$; if $i \neq j$, $a \in A_i$, and $b \in A_j$, then not $a \sim b$ and not $b \sim a$. Some reflection indicates that the situation in the case of $=$, the equality of the real numbers, is similar. Here, each $x \in \mathbb{R}$ is in the set $\{x\}$. Thus, we have as many classes as we have elements in $\mathbb{R}$. These remarks prepare us for the next definition and theorem.

1.6. Definition. A relation E in a set A that is reflexive, transitive, and symmetric (on A) will be called an *equivalence relation* (on A).

Let **A** be a family of subsets of A, satisfying the following conditions:

1. $\alpha \neq \varnothing$ for any $\alpha \in \mathbf{A}$.
2. $\alpha \cap \beta \neq \varnothing$ for any $\alpha, \beta \in \mathbf{A}$ such that $\alpha \neq \beta$.
3. $\bigcup_{\alpha \in \mathbf{A}} \alpha = A$.

In words: each $\alpha \in \mathbf{A}$ is not empty; any two distinct members of **A** are disjoint; the union of all the sets in **A** is equal to A. Then, **A** is called a *partition of* A; and any $\alpha \in \mathbf{A}$ is called a *class* of that partition.

The theorem below indicates that our example involving $\sim$ and the three sets $\{a_1, a_2\}$, $\{a_3\}$, and $\{a_4, a_5\}$ illustrates a general situation.

1.7. Theorem. *Let E be an equivalence relation on a set A. For any $a \in A$, define*

$$\mathbf{a}_E = \{b \,|\, aEb\}, \qquad and \qquad \mathbf{A}_E = \{\mathbf{a}_E \,|\, a \in A\}.$$

*Then $\mathbf{A}_E$ is a partition of A. Conversely, let **A** be a partition of a set A. Define a relation $E_\mathbf{A}$ in A by*

$$aE_\mathbf{A}b \qquad iff \qquad a, b \in \alpha \text{ for some } \alpha \in \mathbf{A}.$$

Then $E_\mathbf{A}$ is an equivalence relation on A.

In the sequel, $\mathbf{A}_E$ will be called the *partition* (of A) *induced by E*, and $E_\mathbf{A}$ will be called *the equivalence relation* (on A) *induced by **A***. When no ambiguity can arise (i.e., when only one equivalence relation or one partition is under discussion), we will simply write **a**, **A**, E, respectively, for $\mathbf{a}_E, \mathbf{A}_E, E_\mathbf{A}$. We do so in the proof below. We only prove the first part of the theorem and leave the second to the reader (see Exercise 5 at the end of the chapter).

Proof. Let E be an equivalence relation on a set A. We show that $\mathbf{A} = \{\mathbf{a} \,|\, a \in A\}$ (with $\mathbf{a} = \{b \,|\, aEb\}$) is a family of subsets of A satisfying conditions 1 to 3 of a partition of A. Clearly, any $\mathbf{a} \in \mathbf{A}$ is not empty. (Indeed, $a \in \mathbf{a}$, since E is reflexive.) Take $\mathbf{a}, \mathbf{b} \in \mathbf{A}$ and suppose that $c \in \mathbf{a} \cap \mathbf{b}$. By definition, we have aEc, bEc. Using the symmetry and transitivity of E, we obtain cEb, aEb, and bEa. For any $d \in A$ we have, successively,

$d \in \mathbf{a}$	iff	aEd	(definition of **a**)
	iff	dEa	(symmetry of E)
	iff	dEb	(aEb and transitivity of E)
	iff	bEd	(symmetry of E)
	iff	$d \in \mathbf{b}$	(definition of **b**)

Thus, we have $\mathbf{a} = \mathbf{b}$. Summarizing, we obtain: If $\mathbf{a}, \mathbf{b}$ are not disjoint they are identical; or equivalently, if $\mathbf{a}, \mathbf{b}$ are distinct sets, they are disjoint. We also have

$$A = \bigcup_{a \in \mathbf{A}} \mathbf{a}.$$

Indeed, $a \in \mathbf{a}$ for any $a \in A$, yielding $A \subset \bigcup_{\mathbf{a} \in \mathbf{A}} \mathbf{a}$, and if $c \in \bigcup_{\mathbf{a} \in \mathbf{A}} \mathbf{a}$, then $c \in \mathbf{b}$ for some $\mathbf{b} \in \mathbf{A}$. This gives bEc, $c \in A = \mathscr{F}(E)$ (E is reflexive on A). Finally, $\mathbf{a} \subset A$ for any $\mathbf{a} \in \mathbf{A}$ is obtained from a practically identical argument. $\mathbf{A}$ is thus a family of subsets of A. We conclude that $\mathbf{A}$ is a partition of A. ∎

We introduce next the important notion of the "negation" of a relation. Consider the relation F in the set of human beings, defined by

$$aFb \quad \text{if} \quad a \text{ is the father of } b.$$

It seems reasonable to define the "negation" of F as the set of all pairs (a,b) of human beings, such that a is not the father of b. This idea is formalized in the definition below.

1.8. Definition. Let R be a relation; then the set

$$\bar{R} = \mathscr{F}(R)^2 - R$$

is called the *negation* of R, or *not R*. In words: $\bar{R}$ contains all those (a,b) elements of $\mathscr{F}(R)^2$ such that not aRb. By definition,

$$\bar{R} \subset \mathscr{F}(R)^2, \tag{10}$$

thus $\bar{R}$ is a relation. Notice the following properties: $\bar{R} \cap R = \varnothing$, $\mathscr{F}(R)^2 = R \cup \bar{R}$. For instance, in Example 1.2(e),

$$\bar{S} = \{1,2,3\}^2 - S$$
$$= \{(3,3),(3,2),(1,3),(3,1)\}.$$

The negation of $\leqslant$ in Example 1.2(a) is $>$. The notation $\bar{\leqslant}$ is thus not used here. Similarly, we will use $>$ rather than $\bar{\precsim}$, to denote the negation of $\precsim$, for any arbitrary relation $\precsim$. Notice that we also have $\mathscr{F}(\bar{S}) = \mathscr{F}(S)$, $\mathscr{F}(\leqslant) = \mathscr{F}(>)$. In these two examples, a relation and its negation have the same field. This is not always true. Indeed:

1.9. Theorem. *If R is a relation, then*

$$\mathscr{F}(\bar{R}) \subset \mathscr{F}(R) \tag{11}$$

and

$$\bar{\bar{R}} \subset R. \tag{12}$$

The converse inclusions do not hold in general. ($\bar{\bar{R}}$ means the negation of $\bar{R}$.)

Proof. If $a \in \mathscr{F}(\bar{R})$, then $a\bar{R}b$ or $b\bar{R}a$ for some b, by definition. Using (10), we obtain $a \in \mathscr{F}(R)$, establishing (11). Successively,

$$\bar{\bar{R}} = \mathscr{F}(\bar{R})^2 - \bar{R} \quad \text{(by definition)}$$
$$\subset \mathscr{F}(R)^2 - \bar{R} \quad \text{(by (11))}$$
$$= R.$$

To see that the converse inclusions in (11) and (12) are not generally true, define a relation R in $A = \{a,b,c\}$ by the table

	a	b	c
a	—	R	—
b	R	R	R
c	—	R	—

Then, successively, $\mathscr{F}(R) = A$, $\bar{R} = \{(a,a),(a,c),(c,a),(c,c)\}$, $\mathscr{F}(\bar{R}) = \{a,c\}$, $\bar{\bar{R}} = \varnothing$. ∎

Thus, $\bar{\bar{R}}$ is not, in general, identical to R. In some instances, it will be convenient to restrict considerations to the cases where $\bar{\bar{R}} = R$ holds. The situation is analyzed in the next theorem.

1.10. Theorem. *Let R be a relation. Then the following three conditions are equivalent:*

(i) *If $a \in \mathscr{F}(R)$, then there exists some $b \in \mathscr{F}(R)$ such that not aRb, or not bRa.*
(ii) $\mathscr{F}(\bar{R}) = \mathscr{F}(R)$.
(iii) $\bar{\bar{R}} = R$.

Proof. It is easy to see that since

$$\bar{R} \cup \bar{\bar{R}} = \mathscr{F}(\bar{R})^2, \qquad \bar{R} \cup R = \mathscr{F}(R)^2$$

and

$$\bar{R} \cap \bar{\bar{R}} = \bar{R} \cap R = \varnothing,$$

Conditions (ii) and (iii) are equivalent. We show that (i) implies (ii). Let $a \in \mathscr{F}(R)$; then not aRb, or not bRa for some $b \in \mathscr{F}(R)$. This means that either (a,b) or (b,a) is in the set

$$\mathscr{F}(R)^2 - R = \bar{R} \subset \mathscr{F}(\bar{R})^2.$$

That is, $a \in \mathscr{F}(\bar{R})$. We have thus $\mathscr{F}(R) \subset \mathscr{F}(\bar{R})$. Since $\mathscr{F}(\bar{R}) \subset \mathscr{F}(R)$ by Theorem 1.9, we conclude that $\mathscr{F}(\bar{R}) = \mathscr{F}(R)$. Finally, (ii) implies (i), for if $a \in \mathscr{F}(R) = \mathscr{F}(\bar{R})$, then $a\bar{R}b$ or $b\bar{R}a$ for some $b \in \mathscr{F}(\bar{R})$ by definition of the field of $\bar{R}$. That is, not aRb, or not bRa for some $b \in \mathscr{F}(R) = \mathscr{F}(\bar{R})$. ∎

The next definition is a reminder of some standard terminology regarding the notion of *function* (considered to be a special kind of relation).

1.11. Definition. A relation f is a *function* iff $b = c$ whenever both afb, afc for all a, b, c. When a relation f is a function, we usually write $f(a) = b$ or, sometimes, $f_a = b$ to mean $(a,b) \in f$; we call b the *image* of a. The notion of image can be extended to sets. For any set C, the *image of C by the function f* is the set

$$f(C) = \{b \mid f(a) = b \text{ for some } a \in C\}.$$

The *inverse image of C by f* is the set

$$f^{-1}(C) = \{a \mid f(a) \in C\}.$$

Occasionally, the expression $a \mapsto f(a)$ will be used to denote the function f, and simultaneously specify a typical element in its domain. Let A,B be sets. A function f is said to be

(a) *(Defined) on A* iff $A = \mathcal{D}(f)$.
(b) *Mapping A onto* (respectively *into*) B iff $\mathcal{D}(f) = A$ and $\mathcal{R}(f) = B$ (respectively $\mathcal{R}(f) \subset B$); when $\mathcal{R}(f) \subset \mathbb{R}$, we will occasionally say that f is *real valued*.
(c) An *identity* iff $f(a) = a$ for all $a \in \mathcal{D}(f)$.
(d) A *one-to-one* (1–1) function iff the set

$$f^{-1} = \{(a,b) \mid f(b) = a\}$$

is a function. In such case, f^{-1} is called the *inverse* of f.

If f, g are functions then the set

$$f \circ g = \{(a,b) \mid g(a) = c, f(c) = b, \text{ for some } c\}$$

is called *the composition of g by f*. It is easy to show that f is a function. The following three expressions are equivalent:

$$(a,b) \in f \circ g, \qquad (f \circ g)(a) = b, \qquad f[g(a)] = b.$$

Let f,h, be two functions, respectively defined on A,B with $A \subset B$ and satisfying the condition

$$f(a) = h(a) \text{ for all } a \in A.$$

Then $h|_A = f$ is called the *restriction* of the function h *to* the set A, and h is called an *extension* of the function f to the set B. More generally, a relation R is a *restriction* of a relation S, or S an *extension* of R iff $R \subset S$.

The last definition of this section introduces the important relation of *equipollence* between sets. Intuitively, two sets are *equipollent* iff they have the same number of elements. For large sets, this intuitive "definition" may lead to erroneous conclusions. The definition below removes any ambiguity.

1.12. Definition. Let $\mathbb{N}(n)$ denote the set containing the first n natural numbers, that is, $\mathbb{N}(n) = \{j \in \mathbb{N} \mid 1 \leqslant j \leqslant n\}$. Two sets A,B are called *equipollent* iff there exists a 1–1 function mapping A onto B. A set is called:

(a) *Finite* iff it is equipollent to $\mathbb{N}(n)$ for some $n \in \mathbb{N}$.
(b) *Infinite* iff it is not finite.
(c) *Countable* iff it is equipollent to $\mathbb{N}$.
(d) *At most countable* iff it is either finite or countable.
(e) *Uncountable* iff it is neither finite nor countable.

Obviously, $\mathbb{N}$ is countable and $\mathbb{N}(n)$ is finite, for any $n \in \mathbb{N}$. (Use the identity on $\mathbb{N}, \mathbb{N}(n)$.) Some other well-known consequences of this definition are: a countable set is not finite, $\mathbb{Z}, \mathbb{Q}$ are countable; $\mathbb{R}$ is uncountable, and equipollent to $\mathbb{R}^n$, for any $n \in \mathbb{N}$ (cf. Rudin, 1964 or Suppes, 1960).

Defining for sets A,B

$$A \approx B \quad \text{iff} \quad A,B \text{ are equipollent,}$$

it is easy to show that $\approx$ is an equivalence relation (Exercise 9). When $A \approx B$, we say that the sets A,B *have the same cardinal number*. The *cardinal number* of a set means, intuitively, the number of elements that it contains. For any set A, we will denote its cardinal number by $|A|$. If A is finite, the meaning of this notation is clear: $|\{a,b,c\}| = 3$; if $A \approx \mathbb{N}(n)$, then $|A| = n$. It can also be made precise in the case of infinite sets, but such developments will neither be included nor needed here (cf., for example, Suppes, 1960).

ALGEBRAIC THEORY—WEAK ORDERS

Let us go back to the yes-no paradigm, and the hypothetical data of Table (4). We adopt the following notation. As in Example 1.2(g), we write: $a \precsim b$ iff the subject's answer to the question

"Is a heavier than b?"

is "No." We obtain Table (13).

	a_1	a_2	a_3	a_4	a_5
a_1	$\precsim$	$\precsim$	$\precsim$	$\succsim$	$\succsim$
a_2	$\succsim$	$\succsim$	$\succsim$	$\succsim$	$\succsim$
a_3	—	—	$\precsim$	$\succsim$	$\succsim$
a_4	—	—	—	$\succsim$	$\succsim$
a_5	—	—	—	$\precsim$	$\succsim$

$$(13)$$

Notice that these data are realistic, in the sense that it would be easy empirically to find five objects generating Table (13). Does $\precsim$ behave like $\leqslant$, the inequality of the real numbers? One interpretation of this somewhat ambiguous question leads to the investigation of whether $\precsim$ and $\leqslant$ satisfy the same properties. The answer is no. Examination of Table (9) shows that $\precsim$ and $\leqslant$ have many properties in common, but $\leqslant$ is antisymmetric while $\precsim$ is not. Some reflection leads to a more fruitful interpretation. Can we *represent* $\precsim$ by $\leqslant$ in the following sense: Can we assign to the stimuli $a_1,\ldots,a_5$, numbers $h(a_1),\ldots,h(a_5)$ in such a way that

$$h(a_i) \leqslant h(a_j) \quad \text{iff} \quad a_i \precsim a_j?$$

This suggests the following generalization:

1.13. Problem. Let $\precsim$ be a relation in a set A. Under which conditions on the pair $(A,\precsim)$ does there exists a function h mapping A into $\mathbb{R}$ satisfying

$$h(a) \leqslant h(b) \quad \text{iff} \quad a \precsim b, \quad (14)$$

for all $a,b \in A$?

Connectedness is a necessary property. Suppose indeed that some function h satisfying (14) exists. Standard properties of the natural ordering of real numbers imply that, for $a,b \in A$

$$\text{either} \quad h(a) \leqslant h(b) \quad \text{or} \quad h(b) \leqslant h(a).$$

Using (14), we derive

$$a \precsim b \quad \text{or} \quad b \precsim a.$$

The necessity of transitivity is derived by a similar argument. On the other hand, antisymmetry is not necessary. To show this, we use Table (13) (where antisymmetry fails; since, for example $a_1 \precsim a_2, a_2 \precsim a_1, a_1 \neq a_2$) and define

$$2 = h(a_5) = h(a_4) > 1 = h(a_3) > 0 = h(a_2) = h(a_1).$$

It is easy to check that (14) holds. Taken alone, connectedness and transitivity are not sufficient to ensure the existence of a function h satisfying (14). We analyze an example proving this fact in 1.36. A sufficient set of conditions is given in Theorem 1.17. We first cover some preliminary material.

1.14. Definition.   Let R be a relation in a set A. If R is transitive and connected on A, then (A,R) is called a *weak order*. A weak order (A,R) is a *simple order* iff R is antisymmetric on A. To mean that (A,R) is a weak order we occasionally say that R is a *weak order on A*. A similar convention applies to a simple order.

Examples of these notions have been encountered earlier: Table (13) provides an example of a weak order; $(\mathbb{R}, \leqslant)$ is a simple order. Various other examples are contained in the exercises. From Theorem 1.5 and Definition 1.6, it follows that if (A,R) is a weak order, then the relation E defined by

$$aEb \quad \text{iff} \quad \text{both } aRb, bRa$$

is an equivalence relation on A. We call E the *equivalence relation induced by R* (on A). By Theorem 1.7, we know that E itself induces a partition $\mathbf{A}$ of A. By extension, $\mathbf{A}$ will be called *the partition of A induced by R* (via E). For example, the relation $\sim$ of Table (7) is the equivalence relation on $\{a_1,a_2,a_3,a_4,a_5\}$ induced by $\precsim$; $\{\{a_1,a_2\},\{a_3\},\{a_4,a_5\}\}$ is the partition induced by $\precsim$. It will be both natural and convenient to further extend the above convention to subsets B of A. In particular, if $\mathbf{A}$ is a partition of A induced by some weak order R (or by some equivalence relation E), we will refer to

$$\mathbf{B} = \{\mathbf{b} \,|\, \mathbf{b} = \mathbf{a} \cap B \text{ for some } \mathbf{a} \in \mathbf{A}\}$$

as the partition of B induced by R (or E) even though R (or E) is not a relation in B.

1.15. Theorem.   *Let (A,R) be a weak order; let $\mathbf{A}$ be the partition of A induced by R; define a relation $\mathbf{R}$ in $\mathbf{A}$ by*

$$\mathbf{aRb} \quad \text{iff} \quad aRb \tag{15}$$

for some $a \in \mathbf{a}$ and $b \in \mathbf{b}$. Then $(\mathbf{A},\mathbf{R})$ is a simple order.

Proof. Clearly by (15), the transitivity and connectedness of R (on A) imply the transitivity and connectedness of $\mathbf{R}$ (on $\mathbf{A}$). Let E be the equivalence relation on A induced by R, in the sense of Theorem 1.5; thus $\mathbf{a} = \{b \,|\, aEb\}$. Suppose that

$$\mathbf{aRb} \qquad \text{and} \qquad \mathbf{bRa}.$$

Then, successively

$$aRb \qquad \text{and} \qquad bRa; \qquad\qquad \text{(by (15))}$$

$$aEb. \qquad\qquad \text{(by def. of } E)$$

Thus $b \in \mathbf{a} \cap \mathbf{b}$, which implies $\mathbf{a} = \mathbf{b}$, since two classes of a partition are either disjoint, or indistinguishable. ■

1.16. Theorem. *Let $(A, \leqslant)$ be a simple order; let $>$ be the negation of $\leqslant$. Then for any $a,b \in A$, exactly one of the following holds*

$$a > b, \qquad a = b, \qquad b > a.$$

This condition is usually referred to as the *trichotomy property.*

Proof. By connectedness, for any $a,b \in A$, we have

$$a \leqslant b \qquad \text{or} \qquad b \leqslant a.$$

If both hold, then $a = b$ by antisymmetry. If not $b \leqslant a$, then $a > b$; if not $a \leqslant b$, then $b > a$. ■

1.17. Theorem. *Let $(A, \precsim)$ be a weak order. If the partition of A induced by $\precsim$ is at most countable, then there exists a function h mapping A into the reals, such that*

$$h(a) \leqslant h(b) \qquad \text{iff} \qquad a \precsim b \qquad\qquad (16)$$

for all $a,b \in A$. Moreover, whether or not the assumption of finiteness or countability holds, if h_1, h_2 are two real-valued functions satisfying (16), then $h_2 = f \circ h_1$ for some strictly increasing function f mapping $\mathcal{R}(h_1)$ onto $\mathcal{R}(h_2)$.

(We recall that a function f mapping a subset of the reals into the reals is called strictly increasing iff $s > t$ implies $f(s) > f(t)$ for all $s,t \in \mathscr{D}(f)$.) This theorem, which is due to Cantor (1895; see also Birkhoff, 1967; Krantz, Luce, Suppes, & Tversky, 1971) is the key result of this section. Actually, the condition that the partition induced by $\precsim$ is at most countable is not necessary: for example, take $(\mathbb{R}, \leqslant)$ the natural order of the reals, and define h in (16) as the identity on $\mathbb{R}$. A complete answer to Problem 1.13, which involves a necessary and sufficient set of conditions, is somewhat technical. It is relegated to the Complements section of this chapter. The last proposition in Theorem 1.17 deserves some attention. It contains an answer to what is usually referred to as a *uniqueness problem*: how unique is the function h satisfying (16) for a given weak order $(A, \precsim)$? A typical answer involves a characterization—that is, a complete description—of the class of all functions h satisfying (16). Notice that such a characterization is provided (implicitly) by the theorem: the class of functions h can be generated from one function h_0 satisfying (16), by the equation $h = f \circ h_0$, where f ranges over the set of all strictly increasing functions mapping $\mathscr{R}(h_0)$ into $\mathbb{R}$. Many other examples of such *uniqueness problems* will be encountered in this book. A frequent terminology used in this connection involves the notion of the *scale type* of h (cf. Suppes & Zinnes, 1963). In this terminology, h would be referred to as an *ordinal scale*, reflecting the fact that the weak order $(A, \precsim)$ of the theorem only defines h up to an arbitrary strictly increasing transformation. This terminology is discussed in Chapter 13.

Proof. We first assume that A is countable. Its elements can thus be listed as $a_1, a_2, \ldots, a_i, \ldots$. Define, for any $i, j \in \mathbb{N}$

$$s_{ij} = \begin{cases} 1 & \text{if} & a_i \precsim a_j, \\ 0 & \text{otherwise;} \end{cases}$$

and define a function h on A by

$$h(a_j) = \sum_{i=1}^{\infty} 2^{-i} s_{ij} \tag{17}$$

(Notice that (17) converges, since $\sum_{i=1}^{n} 2^{-i}$ converges. The idea of this construction is due to David Radford; cf. Roberts, 1979, p. 110.) Suppose that $a_n \precsim a_m$. Then, for any $a_i \in A$, $a_i \precsim a_n$ implies $a_i \precsim a_m$, and thus $h(a_n) \leqslant h(a_m)$ by definition of h.

Conversely, if not $(a_n \precsim a_m)$, then $a_m \precsim a_n$ by connectedness, and $h(a_m) \leqslant h(a_n)$ follows. By the construction of h, however, we cannot have $h(a_m) = h(a_n)$ since $a_n \precsim a_n$ but not $a_n \precsim a_m$.

If A is uncountable, we consider the partition **A** and the simple order $\leqslant$ induced by $\precsim$ on **A** in the sense of Theorem 1.15. By the above argument, there exists a mapping h^* of **A** into the reals, such that for any $\mathbf{a}, \mathbf{b} \in \mathbf{A}$,

$$\mathbf{a} \leqslant \mathbf{b} \quad \text{iff} \quad h^*(\mathbf{a}) \leqslant h^*(\mathbf{b}).$$

Defining h on A by $h(a) = h^*(\mathbf{a})$, it is easy to check that (16) is satisfied. We leave the finite case to the reader.

Suppose that h_1, h_2 are two functions satisfying (16). Define f on $\mathscr{R}(h_1)$ by

$$f[h_1(a)] = h_2(a).$$

(It follows from (16) that f is well defined.) Take any $s, t \in \mathscr{D}(f)$, with, say, $s = h_1(a)$, $t = h_1(b)$, then, successively,

$$h_1(a) = s > t = h_1(b) \quad \text{iff} \quad \text{not } a \precsim b$$
$$\text{iff} \quad h_2(a) > h_2(b)$$
$$\text{iff} \quad f[h_1(a)] > f[h_1(b)]$$
$$\text{iff} \quad f(s) > f(t).$$

The function f is thus strictly increasing. ∎

We consider next the possibility that the binary relation $\precsim$ is not connected. The basic idea here is that, if the experimenter has strong reasons to believe that a weak order can be constructed by comparing the objects from the viewpoint of the characteristic, he or she may decide to save time and skip some of the comparisons: in some cases, only a small fraction of the number of all possible comparisons is required to generate the weak order. The following table, defining a relation $\precsim$ that is neither connected nor transitive, illustrates this remark. We have neither $a_1 \precsim a_4$, nor $a_4 \precsim a_1$. However, we can infer that $a_1 \precsim a_4$ would result from a comparison of a_1 and a_4 since

$$a_1 \precsim a_2 \qquad \text{and} \qquad a_2 \precsim a_4.$$

	a_1	a_2	a_3	a_4	a_5
a_1	$\precsim$	$\precsim$	$\precsim$	—	—
a_2	$\succsim$	$\precsim$	$\succsim$	$\succsim$	—
a_3	—	—	$\precsim$	$\succsim$	—
a_4	—	—	—	$\precsim$	$\precsim$
a_5	—	—	—	$\succsim$	$\succsim$

This suggests adding (a_1, a_4) to $\precsim$, forming a new relation

$$\precsim \cup \{(a_1, a_4)\}.$$

By a similar argument, we can also add the pair (a_3, a_5), since $a_3 \precsim a_4$, $a_4 \precsim a_5$; then, successively, we can add (a_2, a_5), (a_1, a_5), finally forming the relation

$$\precsim' = \precsim \cup \{(a_1, a_4), (a_3, a_5), (a_2, a_5), (a_1, a_5)\}.$$

Notice that $\precsim'$ is connected and transitive, that is, $\precsim'$ is a weak order. Using Theorem 1.17, we can thus assert the existence of a real-valued function h satisfying

$$a_i \precsim' a_j \qquad \text{iff} \qquad h(a_i) \leqslant h(a_j).$$

Thus, in particular, whenever a_i has been compared to a_j,

$$a_i \precsim a_j \qquad \text{iff} \qquad h(a_i) \leqslant h(a_j).$$

The next couple of definitions and theorems generalize this idea.

1.18. Definition. Let A be a set; let $\precsim$ be a relation in A. Then $(A, \precsim)$ is a *local weak order*, or more simply, a *low order* iff for all $m \in \mathbb{N}$ and $a, b, c, b_1, b_2, \ldots, b_m \in A$,

1. If $(a \precsim b$ and $a \precsim c)$ or $(b \precsim a$ and $c \precsim a)$, then $(b \precsim c$ or $c \precsim b)$.
2. There exist $n \in \mathbb{N}$ and $a_1, a_2, \ldots, a_n \in A$ such that $a_1 = a, a_n = b$, and for $1 \leqslant i \leqslant n - 1$, either $a_i \precsim a_{i+1}$ or $a_{i+1} \precsim a_i$.
3. If $b_j \precsim b_{j+1}$ for $1 \leqslant j \leqslant m - 1$, and $b_m \precsim b_1$, then $b_{j+1} \precsim b_j$ for $1 \leqslant j \leqslant m - 1$.

When $(A,\precsim)$ is a low order, we will occasionally say equivalently that $\precsim$ is a *low order (on A)*. It will also be convenient to say, when $a\precsim b$ or $b\precsim a$, that *a is comparable to b*. Axiom 1 essentially defines the field of $\precsim$ as the set of all pairs (a,b) such that a is "not too far" from b in the latent weak ordering.[2] Intuitively, Axiom 2 means that if a and b are two "distant" objects and are not comparable, they can nevertheless be compared via a sequence of "local" comparisons. Axiom 3 is a weakened version of transitivity. Writing

$$a \prec b \qquad \text{for} \qquad (a\precsim b \text{ and not } b\precsim a),$$

this axiom states that there exists no "cycle"

$$b_1 \precsim \cdots \prec b_j \precsim \cdots \precsim b_m \precsim b_1.$$

It follows easily from Axioms 2 and 3 that $\precsim$ is reflexive. The relation defined in the preceding table provides an example of a low order. The following result is immediate.

1.19. Theorem.   *Any weak order is a low order.*

We have seen that a low order could sometimes be extended to a weak order. As shown in Theorem 1.22, this example illustrates a general situation. A preliminary definition is needed.

1.20. Definition.   Let R be a relation. Then R^t is the *transitive closure* of R iff R^t is a relation defined by $aR^t b$ iff $a,b \in \mathscr{F}(R)$, and there exist $n \in \mathbb{N}$ and $a_1 = a, a_2, \ldots, a_n = b$ such that $a_i R a_{i+1}$ for $1 \leqslant i \leqslant n-1$.

Thus, R^t is a transitive relation containing R. (Actually, R^t is the smallest relation satisfying these conditions; that is, if T is a transitive relation with $R \subset T$, then $R^t \subset T$.) Clearly, $R = R^t$ iff R is transitive.

1.21. Examples.   (a) Let $S = \{(1,2), (2,1), (2,2), (2,3), (3,3)\}$; then

$$S^t = S \cup \{(1,1), (1,3)\}.$$

Notice that S^t is a weak order, but that S is not a low order since $(1,1) \notin S$.

(b) Define a relation R in $\mathbb{R}$ by

$$aRb \qquad \text{iff} \qquad a \leqslant b \qquad \text{and} \qquad b - a < 1.$$

Then, R is a low order on $\mathbb{R}$ and $R^t = \leqslant$, the inequality of the real numbers.

(c) Let M,F be two relations in the set H of human beings (alive or dead), defined by

$$aMb \qquad \text{iff} \qquad a \text{ is the mother of } b,$$

$$aFb \qquad \text{iff} \qquad a \text{ is the father of } b.$$

Define a relation T in H by

$$T = (M \cup F)^t.$$

---

2. Axiom 1 is referred to as *conditional connectedness* by Luce & Roberts (1968).

Then, aTb means that a is a parent, a grandparent, or an ancestor of b. This example correctly suggests that, if P,Q are two relations, then

$$(P^t \cup Q^t) \subset (P \cup Q)^t$$

The equality does not hold in general, since

$$M^t \cup F^t \neq (M \cup F)^t.$$

1.22. Theorem.   *The transitive closure of a low order is a weak order.*

Example 1.21(a) shows that the converse proposition—if S^t is a weak order, then S is a low order—does not hold.

Proof.   Let $\precsim$ be a low order. We only have to prove that $\precsim^t$ is connected. Take any $a,b \in \mathscr{F}(\precsim) = \mathscr{F}(\precsim^t)$. By Axiom 2 in 1.18, there exists a finite sequence $a_1 = a, a_2, \ldots, a_n = b$, such that a_i is comparable to a_{i+1} for $1 \leqslant i \leqslant n - 1$. We have exactly four cases:

1. $a_1 \precsim a_2 \precsim \cdots \precsim a_n$.
2. $a_n \precsim a_{n-1} \precsim \cdots \precsim a_1$.
3. $a_{i-1} \precsim a_i, a_{i+1} \precsim a_i$, for some index i.
4. $a_i \precsim a_{i-1}, a_i \precsim a_{i+1}$, for some index i.

Cases 1 and 2 give, respectively, $a_1 \precsim^t a_n, a_n \precsim^t a_1$. In either Case 3 or 4 we use Axiom 1 to assert that a_{i-1} is comparable to a_{i+1}. This means that the term a_i can be eliminated from the sequence $\{a_i\}$, yielding (after appropriate renaming of the terms) a sequence

$$a = a_1', a_2', \ldots, a_{n-1}' = b,$$

with a_i' comparable to a_{i+1}' for $1 \leqslant i \leqslant n - 2$. This elimination process can be pursued until Case 1 or Case 2 is obtained. We conclude that either $a \precsim^t b$ or $b \precsim^t a$. That is, $\precsim^t$ is connected. ∎

Theorem 1.23, generalizing the existence result in Theorem 1.17, follows immediately from Theorems 1.22 and 1.17.

1.23. Theorem.   *Let $(A, \precsim)$ be a low order. If the partition of A induced by $\precsim^t$ is at most countable, then there exists a function h mapping A into the reals, such that*

$$a \precsim b \qquad \text{iff} \qquad h(a) \leqslant h(b)$$

whenever a is comparable to b.

The uniqueness of the function h is identical to that stated in Theorem 1.17.

1.24. Remarks.   The conditions defining a weak order constitute a genuine empirical theory for the type of data collected in the yes-no paradigm. In principle, we can check whether connectedness and transitivity are satisfied in some data collected using Variation 1, for example. If these conditions are satisfied, we know by Theorem 1.17 that the function h can be obtained (since in any realistic experiment the number of stimuli will be finite). Indeed, h can be constructed by the very procedure used in the proof of Theorem 1.17.

This function is then a candidate scale for measuring "heaviness." If the number of stimuli is large, then the testing of the conditions and the construction of the function may require a computer. There are various reasons why this theory might fail to provide a satisfying explanation of a given set of data. Some types of failure appear fundamental and lead to a clear rejection of the theory. Consider, for example, a situation in which a subject is required to compare the stimuli in a mixed collection C: some of these stimuli are pure tones, others are visual flashes.[3] In the notation of Theorem 1.17 we write (for any $c,d \in C$) $c \precsim d$ iff the subject answers "No" to the question: "Does c appear subjectively more intense than d?" Let x be a visual flash, and let a,b be two tones. Suppose that the physical intensity of a markedly exceeds that of b—say there is a 15-dB difference between a and b. The following data is quite conceivable.

$$a \precsim x, \qquad x \precsim b, \qquad \text{not } a \precsim b \qquad (18)$$

contradicting transitivity. Such data would result if the subject experiences difficulty in comparing the subjective intensity of stimuli across different sensory modalities.

Other types of failure appear relatively trivial and require only minor adaptations of the theory. In particular, the present theory is deterministic. If a violation of transitivity, such as (18), is observed, this theory should, in principle, be rejected. In an experimental context different from the one described above, this may seem needlessly harsh. One might argue that this single failure may be due to the subject being tired or absent minded. This viewpoint is quite reasonable and suggests the construction of a more flexible theory embodying the same basic ideas, for example, in a probabilistic framework. How such theory may be developed is outlined in Exercises 26 to 29.

BIORDERS

Consider Variation 2 of the yes-no paradigm. The stimuli a,b are presented sequentially to the subject; first a, then b. Given the nature of the stimuli (tones), this asymmetry is practically unavoidable. It is likely, moreover, that it would have some effect on the data. For instance, the subject's task may be conceptualized as involving a comparison of the *trace* of a in (acoustic) memory, with the current perception of b. It is conceivable that the trace of a stimulus is weaker than the current perception of the same stimulus. Other interpretations are possible. In general, this suggests a theory in which the number assigned to a stimulus a depends on whether a is the first or the second term in a pair offered for comparison. These ideas are expressed more precisely in the problem below, which generalizes Problem 1.13.

---

3. A similar counterexample was proposed by Savage (cf. Luce & Suppes, 1965, pp. 334–335), in the context of a probabilistic theory of utility.

1.25. Problem. Let A,X be sets; let R be a relation from A to X. Under which conditions on the triple (A,X,R) does there exist a pair h,g of functions, mapping A,X, respectively, into the reals, such that

$$h(a) \leqslant g(x) \qquad \text{iff} \qquad aRx \qquad (19)$$

whenever $a \in A, X \in X$?

In Variation 2, we have $A = X$, but the case $A \neq X$ is also of interest (see, in particular, Example 1.27(b)). We will develop the theory in the general case. Suppose that

$$aRx, \text{ not } bRx, bRy.$$

Suppose also that h,g exist satisfying (19). We derive

$$h(a) \leqslant g(x), \qquad g(x) < h(b), \qquad h(b) \leqslant g(y)$$

yielding

$$h(a) < g(y)$$

which implies

$$aRy.$$

We conclude that for h,g to exist satisfying (19), it is necessary that

$$\text{if } aRx, \text{ not } bRx, bRy, \text{ then } aRy, \qquad (20)$$

whenever $a,b \in A, x,y \in X$. Extending an earlier convention, we will occasionally (in particular, when the sets A,X are small) represent the relation R by a rectangular table, an example of which is given in Table (21).

	x_1	x_2	x_3	x_4
a_1	—	—	R	R
a_2	R	R	R	R
a_3	—	—	R	—
a_4	—	—	R	R
a_5	R	—	R	R

(21)

$$A = \{a_1,a_2,a_3,a_4,a_5\}, \; X = \{x_1,x_2,x_3,x_4\}.$$

Formula (20) means that such a table cannot contain a subtable of the form in Table (22).

	x	y
a	R	—
b	—	R

(22)

The reader can check that this property is satisfied in Table (21). In such a case, the lines and columns of the table can be interchanged in such a way that the letters R are all contained in a triangular region. This is illustrated in Table (23), which is equivalent to Table (21).

	x_3	x_4	x_1	x_2	
a_2	R	R	R	R	
a_5	R	R	R	—	
a_1	R	R	—	—	(23)
a_4	R	R	—	—	
a_3	R	—	—	—	

Relations satisfying (20) have been studied by Riguet (1951; cf. Ore, 1962), under the name *Ferrers relations*. Triangular tables of the type exemplified by (23) have been used extensively in attitude scaling (Guttman, 1944; Stouffer, Guttman, Schuman, Lazarsfeld, Starr, & Clausen, 1950). In this context, Table (23) is an example of a so-called *Guttman scale*; $a_1, a_2, \ldots$, would usually represent different subjects; $x_1, x_2, \ldots$, would represent different questions of a questionnaire; $a_i R x_j$ would mean that subject a_i answered "no" to question x_j. Problem 1.25 has been analyzed by Ducamp and Falmagne (1969). Other references are given in the last paragraph of this section.

1.26. Definition.   Let A, X be sets; let R be a relation from A to X. Then, the triple (A, X, R) is called a (*weak*) *biorder*, or equivalently, R is called a (*weak*) *biorder from A to X* iff whenever $a, b \in A$, $x, y \in X$.

$$a R x, \; b \bar{R} x, \; b \bar{R} y \qquad \text{imply} \qquad a R y.$$

A close examination of this concept shows that this terminology—in particular, the adjective "weak"—is consistent with our definition of a weak order in 1.14. However, since only one type of biorder will be analyzed in this chapter, we will drop the adjective "weak" in further references to this concept (see Exercises 23 and 24, however).

An example of a biorder was given in Table (23). A couple of additional examples follow.

1.27. Examples.   (a) Let $\ll$ be a relation on $\mathbb{R}$, defined by $s \ll t$ iff $s < t$, $s \in \mathbb{Q}, t \in \mathbb{R} - \mathbb{Q}$. The triple $(\mathbb{Q}, \mathbb{R} - \mathbb{Q}, \ll)$ is a biorder. Notice that $\mathbb{Q}$ is countable while $\mathbb{R} - \mathbb{Q}$ is uncountable.

(b) We modify slightly the procedure in Variation 1 of the yes-no paradigm. Consider a set $A = \{a_1, a_2, a_3, a_4, a_5\}$ of stimuli. The stimuli are presented to the subject one at a time. He or she is asked whether each stimulus seems to be (1) very light, (2) light, (3) neutral, (4) heavy, or (5) very heavy.

For each stimulus a_i, the subject chooses one of the five responses. For simplicity, we represent the response by its number. The data are recoded in terms of relation $\lhd$ defined by: $a_i \lhd j$ iff the subject's response is j or smaller. Some hypothetical data are given in Table (24).

	1	2	3	4	5
a_1	◁	◁	◁	◁	◁
a_2	◁	◁	◁	◁	◁
a_3	—	—	◁	◁	◁
a_4	—	—	—	◁	◁
a_5	—	—	—	◁	◁

$$(24)$$

There are obvious resemblances between the yes-no paradigm and this one, and in fact, between data Tables (13) and (24). Both tables indicate that a_4 seems indistinguishable from a_5, and a_1 from a_2; moreover, a_4 and a_5 seem heavier than a_3, itself appearing heavier than either a_1 or a_2. Clearly, however, $\precsim$ and $\lhd$ differ in a critical way: $\precsim$ is a relation in $\{a_1,a_2,a_3,a_4,a_5\}$ while $\lhd$ is a relation from $\{a_1,a_2,a_3,a_4,a_5\}$ to $\mathbb{N}(5)$. Comparing Problem 1.13 and Problem 1.25 clarifies the situation.

(c) At each trial of an experiment, a subject is presented with a circular patch of monochromatic light s, on a background b of the same chroma; s,b are numerical values on an intensity scale. The stimulus is separated from the background by a thin, dark annulus. The subject is asked whether the stimulus appears dimmer than the background. In this case, the experimenter writes sDb. Suppose that the intensity values for both stimulus and background vary in some numerical interval I. Thus, D is a relation in I. Some reflection on this situation leads to the conjecture that (I,I,D) is a biorder. Suppose indeed that the experimenter observes sDb and $s'\bar{D}b$ for some $s, b, s' \in I$. Thus, s appears dimmer than b while s' does not. It is reasonable to conclude that $s < s'$ (if we assume, as is customary, that the brightness scale is strictly increasing with intensity). If we also have $s'Db'$, a similar argument gives $b < b'$, which in view of sDb, leads to the hypothesis sDb'. In other terms, D satisfies the defining formula of a biorder from I to I.

(d) Let $(A,\precsim)$ be a weak order; then $\precsim$ is a biorder from A to A (check this); in particular the inequality of the real numbers, $\leqslant$, is a biorder from $\mathbb{R}$ to $\mathbb{R}$. Notice that the $<$, the strict inequality of the reals, is also a biorder.

Thus, the functions of h,g of Problem 1.25 exist only if R is a biorder from A to X. This condition is sufficient in the finite or countable case (cf. Theorem 1.32), but not in general (see Exercise 16). Notice that, implicitly, Problem 1.25 involves the existence of two weak orders on each of A,X (corresponding to the two functions h,g). As a preliminary step, we will analyze the exact connection between these two orderings and the biorder. We first establish a simple, but useful result.

1.28. Definition. Let R be a relation. Define a relation R^{-1}, called the *converse* of R, by

$$aR^{-1}b \qquad \text{iff} \qquad bRa.$$

Notice that the negation of the converse of a relation R is identical to the converse of the negation of R:

$$(\bar{R})^{-1} = \overline{(R^{-1})},\tag{25}$$

since

$$a(\bar{R})^{-1}b \quad \text{iff} \quad b\bar{R}a \quad \text{iff} \quad \text{not}\,(aRb) \quad \text{iff} \quad \text{not}\,(bR^{-1}a) \quad \text{iff} \quad b\overline{(R^{-1})}a.$$

for all $a,b \in \mathcal{F}(R)$. There is thus no ambiguity in the notation $\bar{R}^{-1}$. The notion of the converse of a relation generalizes that of the inverse of a function (cf. Definition 1.11). Extending an earlier convention, we will write $\succsim$ rather than $\precsim^{-1}$ for the converse of $\precsim$, and $\prec$ for the negation of $\succsim$, for any relation $\precsim$.

1.29. Theorem. (A,X,R) *is a biorder iff* (X,A,R^{-1}) *is.*

Indeed, in view of (25), the two following propositions are equivalent:

$$aRx,\, b\bar{R}x,\, bRy \quad \text{imply} \quad aRy;$$

$$yR^{-1}b,\, x\bar{R}^{-1}b,\, xR^{-1}a \quad \text{imply} \quad yR^{-1}a.$$

1.30. Theorem. *Let R be a relation from A to X; let $\sim$, $\precsim$ be two relations in A satisfying* (cf. Ore, 1962, p. 194)

$$a \sim b \quad \text{iff} \quad (aRx \text{ iff } bRx, \text{ for all } x \in X); \tag{26}$$

$$a \precsim b \quad \text{iff} \quad a \sim b \text{ or } (aRx,\, b\bar{R}x \text{ for some } x \in X) \tag{27}$$

then (A,X,R) is a biorder iff $(A,\precsim)$ is a weak order and $\sim$ is the equivalence relation on A induced by $\precsim$ (in the sense of Definition 1.14).

By Theorem 1.29, a similar result holds for the set X.

Proof. Sufficiency. Suppose that

$$aRx,\, b\bar{R}x,\, bRy,\, a\bar{R}y \tag{28}$$

for some $a,b \in A$, $x,y \in X$. From (27), we derive

$$a \precsim b, \qquad b \precsim a,$$

which implies

$$a \sim b,$$

and (28) together with (26) involves a contradiction. Thus $aRx,\, b\bar{R}x,\, bRy$ imply aRy; that is, (A,X,R) is a biorder.

Necessity. Clearly, $\sim$ is an equivalence relation on A. Define a relation $\prec$ on A by

$$a \prec b \quad \text{iff} \quad aRx,\, b\bar{R}x \text{ for some } x \in X.$$

Thus, $\precsim$ is the union of $\sim$ and $\prec$. Suppose that $a \precsim b$, $b \precsim c$. By definition, we have four cases: (i) $a \sim b$, $b \sim c$; (ii) $a \prec b$, $b \sim c$; (iii) $a \sim b$, $b \prec c$; and (iv) $a \prec b$, $b \prec c$. In case (i), $a \sim c$ and thus $a \precsim c$, follow from the transitivity of $\sim$. In cases (ii), (iii), $a \precsim c$ is obtained immediately from the definitions. Suppose that $a \prec b$, $b \prec c$. This implies

$$aRx,\, b\bar{R}x,\, bRy,\, c\bar{R}y \tag{29}$$

for some $x,y \in X$. Since, by hypothesis, R is a biorder, the first three terms in (29) imply aRy, and thus

$$aRy, \quad c\bar{R}y,$$

which implies $a \precsim c$. We conclude that $\precsim$ is transitive on A. To show that $\precsim$ is also connected, take any $a,b \in A$ and suppose that not $a \sim b$. Then for some $x \in X$

$$aRx, b\bar{R}x \quad \text{or} \quad a\bar{R}x, bRx;$$

thus

$$a \precsim b \quad \text{or} \quad b \precsim a.$$

On the other hand, it is easy to check that

$$a \sim b \quad \text{iff} \quad a \precsim b \quad \text{and} \quad b \precsim a.$$

Thus, $\precsim$ is connected on A, and $\sim$ is the equivalence relation on A induced by $\precsim$. ∎

1.31. Remark. As indicated, a similar theorem holds for the set X. In particular, if (A,X,R) is an biorder, we can define a weak order $\precsim'$ on X by

$$x \precsim' y \quad \text{iff} \quad \begin{cases} \text{either } (a\bar{R}x, aRy \text{ for some } a \in A) \\ \text{or } (aRx \text{ iff } aRy \text{ for all } a \in A) \end{cases}$$

This means that any biorder R from a set A to a set X naturally induces two partitions $\mathbf{A},\mathbf{X}$, respectively of A,X. To illustrate this remark, we go back to the biorder in Table (23) and construct $\precsim'$, $\precsim$ (defined as in Theorem 1.30), together with the partitions induced on $A = \{a_1,a_2,a_3,a_4,a_5\}$ and $X = \{x_1,x_2,x_3,x_4\}$. We obtain

	a_2	a_5	a_1	a_4	a_3
a_2	$\precsim$	$\precsim$	$\precsim$	$\precsim$	$\precsim$
a_5	—	$\precsim$	$\precsim$	$\precsim$	$\precsim$
a_1	—	—	$\precsim$	$\precsim$	$\precsim$
a_4	—	—	$\precsim$	$\precsim$	$\precsim$
a_3	—	—	—	—	$\precsim$

$$\mathbf{A} = \{\{a_2\}, \{a_1,a_4\}, \{a_5\}, \{a_3\}\};$$

	x_2	x_1	x_4	x_3
x_2	$\precsim'$	$\precsim'$	$\precsim'$	$\precsim'$
x_1	—	$\precsim'$	$\precsim'$	$\precsim'$
x_4	—	—	$\precsim'$	$\precsim'$
x_3	—	—	—	$\precsim'$

$$\mathbf{X} = \{\{x_1\}, \{x_2\}, \{x_3\}, \{x_4\}\}.$$

In Example 1.27(a), the biorder $\ll$ from $\mathbb{Q}$ to $\mathbb{R} - \mathbb{Q}$ induces the two weak orders $(\mathbb{Q}, \leqslant_1)$, $(\mathbb{R} - \mathbb{Q}, \leqslant_2)$, with $\leqslant_1$, $\leqslant_2$ denoting the natural ordering of the real numbers restricted to $\mathbb{Q}, \mathbb{R} - \mathbb{Q}$, respectively. In this example, interestingly, one of the two partitions induced by $\ll$ is countable while the other is not. Indeed, these two partitions are

$$\{\{s\} \,|\, s \in \mathbb{Q}\}, \{\{s\} \,|\, s \in \mathbb{R} - \mathbb{Q}\}\}.$$

This condition is not necessary: $\leqslant$, the natural ordering of the real numbers, is a biorder from $\mathbb{R}$ to $\mathbb{R}$, and induces two identical, uncountable partitions of $\mathbb{R}$ (cf. Example 1.27(d)).

In the following Theorem, which is due to Ducamp and Falmagne (1969), we only consider the finite case, which allows a very short proof. A complete solution to Problem 1.25 can be found in Doignon, Ducamp, and Falmagne (1984).

1.32. Theorem.   *Let (A, X, R) be a biorder and suppose that at least one of the two partitions of A, X induced by R (in the sense of Remark 1.31) is finite. Then there exists a pair h, g of functions, mapping respectively A, X into $\mathbb{R}$ such that for all $a \in A, x \in X$*

$$h(a) \leqslant g(x) \qquad iff \qquad aRx. \tag{30}$$

By analogy with Theorem 1.17, it may be conjectured that if h_0, g_0 is another pair of functions satisfying (30), then

$$h_0 = f \circ h, \qquad g_0 = f \circ g$$

for some strictly increasing function f mapping $\mathscr{R}(h) \cup \mathscr{R}(g)$ onto

$$\mathscr{R}(h_0) \cup \mathscr{R}(g_0).$$

This conjecture is false (see Exercise 18).

Proof.   To avoid trivialities, we assume that the sets A, R, X are nonempty. Suppose that the partition of A induced by R is finite. (In view of Theorem 1.29, this involves no loss of generality.) Let $\precsim, \sim$ be as in Theorem 1.30. Thus, $(A, \precsim)$ is a weak order and there exists a function h mapping A into $\mathbb{R}$ and satisfying

$$h(a) \leqslant h(b) \qquad \text{iff} \qquad a \precsim b \tag{31}$$

or explicitly,

$$h(a) \leqslant h(b) \qquad \text{iff} \qquad \begin{cases} \text{either } (aRx \text{ iff } bRx, \text{ for all } x \in X) \\ \text{or } (aRx, b\bar{R}x, \text{ for some } x \in X). \end{cases}$$

The function h is bounded ($h(A)$ is a finite set); that is, $|h| < \xi$ for some positive real number ξ. Take any $x \in X$, and consider the set

$$\{h(a) \,|\, aRx\}.$$

If this set is empty, that is, if $a\bar{R}x$ for all $a \in A$, define $g(x) = -\xi$. Otherwise, define

$$g(x) = \max\{h(b)\,|\,bRx\}$$

Clearly, aRx implies $h(a) \leqslant g(x)$. Conversely, suppose that $h(a) \leqslant g(x)$ and $a\bar{R}x$. We cannot have $h(a) \leqslant -\xi = g(x)$ (by hypothesis, $-\xi < h < \xi$). This implies that $\{h(b)\,|\,bRx\} \neq \varnothing$. Since

$$a\bar{R}x, \, bRx$$

together give $h(b) < h(a)$, we obtain

$$\max\{h(b)\,|\,bRx\} = g(x) < h(a),$$

a contradiction. ∎

1.33. Remarks. Various special cases of this theorem have been worked out. For instance, Luce (1956) proposed the notion of a *semiorder*, involving a pair (A,R) such that for some function g mapping A into $\mathbb{R}$,

$$g(a) + 1 \leqslant g(b) \qquad \text{iff} \qquad aRb. \tag{32}$$

Clearly, (32) is a special case of (30), with $A = X$ and $h = g + 1$. Thus, R is a biorder from A to A, which also satisfies additional constraints. The intuition behind (32) is closely related to a traditional concept of psychophysics, that of "just noticeable difference," or Jnd. Suppose, for example, that A is a set of pure tones differing in intensity, and that aRb means that tone a is not perceived as louder than tone b. Equation 32 symbolizes the notion that a is judged louder than b only if its loudness exceeds that of b by more than one Jnd. The Jnd is represented here by the constant 1. A detailed discussion of (32), including references and a proof of a representation theorem in the style of 1.32, will be found in the Complements section of this chapter. The notion of Jnd is discussed in Chapter 8. A related notion is that of an *interval order* that is, an irreflexive biorder (A,R). Under appropriate side conditions, this yields the representation

$$g(a) + u(a) \leqslant g(b) \qquad \text{iff} \qquad aRb$$

with the function u mapping A into the positive reals (Fishburn, 1970a, 1970b, 1973; Doignon, Ducamp, and Falmagne, 1984). This representation generalizes (32). In a psychophysical context, it can be interpreted as involving the concept of a variable Jnd. The notions defining a (weak) biorder can be relaxed along lines similar to those which, in the preceding section, led from a weak order to a low order. The motivation would be identical: if the experimenter is practically certain that a (weak) biorder can be extracted from the data of a complete experiment, she or he may find it expedient to save some time and omit some redundant comparisons. The appropriate notion to be captured here is that of a *local weak biorder*, or more briefly, a *low biorder*. Such developments will not be included here (Exercise 24). We point out, however, that more than an intellectual exercise is involved. Appropriately defined, the notion of a low biorder is closely related to some "tailored resting" techniques in psychometrics (McCormick, 1978; Cliff, Cudeck, & McCormick, 1979).

1.34. Applications. The conceptual importance of the algebraic theories discussed in this chapter is clear. Somewhat surprisingly, these theories did not lead to systematic empirical testing. An important exception, however, is provided by the biorder which, as indicated earlier, has been widely applied in the social sciences under the name *Guttman scale* (Coombs, 1964; Guttman, 1944; Stouffer, Guttman, Lazarsfeld, Starr, & Clausen, 1950). A serious difficulty encountered in such applications arises in connection with the presence of "errors" in the data. By an "error," we mean a case such as the one shown in the following table, that is, a violation of the defining condition of a biorder.

	x	y
a	R	—
b	—	R

A goodness-of-fit index was proposed, based on of the proportion of such cases. As Faverge (1965) pointed out, this index lacks a theoretical foundation and its values are difficult to interpret. The proper context for an analysis of such "errors" is that of a probabilistic theory. How such theory can be developed, in this and various related situations, is considered in detail in Chapters 4 to 8 of this book (see also Exercises 26 to 29).

1.35. References. The material covered in this chapter by no means exhausts the subject covered by its title. Our choice of topics in a quickly expanding field was determined by a tight criterion of relevance to psychophysics, as far as we could realistically foresee it. Much of the recent theoretical work in this area is due to Fishburn (1970c) and Roberts (1970). These papers are actually survey articles and contain extensive references. Other surveys and sources of references are Roberts (1979) and Krantz et al. (in preparation). Biorders have been investigated by Bouchet (1971), Cogis (1976, 1979, 1980, 1982a, 1982b) and Doignon, Ducamp, and Falmagne (1984). In the concluding section of this chapter, we go back to a number of questions raised earlier, but so far left unanswered.

*COMPLEMENTS

In our discussion of Problem 1.13, we stressed the fact that the conditions defining a weak order $\precsim$ (transitivity, connectedness) on some arbitrary set A, were not sufficient to ensure the existence of a function h mapping A into $\mathbb{R}$ and satisfying

$$a \precsim b \quad \text{iff} \quad h(a) \leqslant h(b). \tag{33}$$

We now prove this fact by a counterexample.

1.36. Example. *The lexicographic counterexample.* Let $\precsim$ be a relation in $\mathbb{R}^2$, defined by

$$(x,y) \precsim (x',y') \quad \text{iff} \quad \text{either } x < x' \quad \text{or} \quad (x = x' \text{ and } y \leqslant y')$$

It is easy to check that $(\mathbb{R}^2, \precsim)$ is a simple order (Exercise 12). The relation $\precsim$ is sometimes referred to as the *lexicographic ordering* of $\mathbb{R}^2$. Suppose that h is a function mapping $\mathbb{R}^2$ into $\mathbb{R}$, such that

$$h(x,y) \leqslant h(x',y') \quad \text{iff} \quad (x,y) \precsim (x',y').$$

We have, in particular,

$$h(x,1) > h(x,0)$$

for all $x \in \mathbb{R}$. From the theory of real numbers, we know that there exist a rational number $\rho(x)$, with

$$h(x,1) > \rho(x) > h(x,0).$$

In fact, ρ is a 1-1 function mapping $\mathbb{R}$ into $\mathbb{Q}$. Clearly, $\mathscr{D}(\rho) = \mathbb{R}$ and $\mathscr{R}(\rho) \subset \mathbb{Q}$, and ρ is 1-1 since $x' > x$ implies $(x',0) \succ (x,1)$ (writing, as before, $\succ$ for not $\precsim$), and thus

$$\rho(x') > h(x',0) > h(x,1) > \rho(x).$$

This argument establishes the existence of a 1-1 function ρ, mapping the uncountable set $\mathbb{R}$ into a set that is at most countable. This contradiction proves that no such function h can exist.

A set of necessary and sufficient conditions is contained in the next theorem.

1.37. Definition. Let $(A, \precsim)$ be a weak order. Then $B \subset A$ is called *order dense* in A iff for any $a,b \in A$ satisfying $a \succ b$, there exist $c \in B$ such that $b \precsim c \precsim a$.

1.38. Examples. (a) The set $\mathbb{Q}$ of all rational numbers is dense in $\mathbb{R}$, for the natural ordering $\leqslant$ of the real numbers. (b) Note that $\mathbb{Q}^2$ is not dense in $\mathbb{R}^2$ for the lexicographic ordering $\precsim$ of $\mathbb{R}^2$ defined in Example 1.30. Indeed, if x is irrational, and $(x,y) \succ (x,y')$, then there is no $(z,w) \in \mathbb{Q}^2$ satisfying

$$(x,y') \precsim (z,w) \precsim (x,y), \tag{34}$$

for (34) implies $x = z$.

1.39. Theorem. (Birkhoff, 1967.) *Let $\precsim$ be a relation in a set A. The two following conditions are equivalent:*

(i) *There exists a function h mapping A into $\mathbb{R}$ and satisfying*

$$h(a) \leqslant h(b) \quad \text{iff} \quad a \precsim b.$$

(ii) *$(A, \precsim)$ is a weak order and A contains an order dense subset B, such that the partition of B induced by $\precsim$ is at most countable.*

The proof of this theorem is sketched in Exercises 19 and 20. A version of this theorem also holds in the case of a low order (cf. Exercise 25). We next discuss the notion of a *semiorder*, introduced in Remarks 1.33.

1.40. Definition.   Let R be a relation in a set A, satisfying the following conditions.

   (i) R is a biorder from A to A.
   (ii) R is irreflexive on A.
   (iii) Whenever aRb and bRc, then aRd or dRc for all $a, b, c, d \in A$.

Then, (A,R) is a *semiorder*, or equivalently, R is a *semiorder* on A. Notice that $<$ is a semiorder on $\mathbb{R}$. More generally, if $(A,\lesssim)$ is a weak order, then $(A,\succ)$ is a semiorder (Exercise 21). The converse, however, is false. The notion of a semiorder is well illustrated by the following result.

1.41. Theorem.   *Let A be a finite set. Then (A,R) is a semiorder iff there exists a function g, mapping A into $\mathbb{R}$ and satisfying*

$$g(a) + 1 < g(b) \qquad \text{iff} \qquad aRb, \tag{35}$$

for all $a,b \in A$.

We observe that this theorem also holds if in (35), $<$ is replaced by $\leqslant$. Indeed, if A is finite and g,R satisfy (35), then, with

$$\delta = \min\{g(b) - g(a)|aRb\} > 1,$$

we have

$$aRb \qquad \text{iff} \qquad g(a) + \delta \leqslant g(b) \qquad (\text{since } \delta > 1)$$
$$\text{iff} \qquad g_0(a) + 1 \leqslant g_0(b),$$

with $g_0 = g/\delta$. It is also easy to check that if

$$aRb \qquad \text{iff} \qquad g(a) + 1 \leqslant g(b)$$

for some real valued function g, then R is a semiorder on its field.

A constructive proof of Theorem 1.41, in the style of the proof of Theorem 1.17, can be found in Scott and Suppes (1958) or Suppes and Zinnes (1963). Another proof is given here, which has the merit of illustrating a general method of proof of theorems of this kind, due to Scott (1964). Some preparatory material is needed.

1.42. Definition.   Let R,S be two relations. We call

$$RS = \{(a,b)\,|\,aRc,\ cSb \text{ for some } c\}$$

the *(relative) product of R by S*. Clearly, RS is a relation since $RS \subset \mathscr{D}(R) \times \mathscr{R}(S)$.

Notice that this notion extends that of the composition of functions. In fact, we have for two functions f,g,

$$f \circ g = gf,$$

with the left member defined by 1.11. It is easy to check that the product of relations is an associative operation; that is,

$$R(ST) = (RS)T,$$

for any relations R,S,T. There is thus no ambiguity in writing

$$R_1 R_2 \cdots R_n$$

for the product of n relations $R_1,R_2,\ldots,R_n$. For any relation R, we write $R^2 = RR, R^3 = RRR$, and, in general, $R^n = RR^{n-1}$. Various useful properties of this operation are listed in Theorem 1.43, the proof of which is left for the exercises.

1.43. Theorem. *Let R, S, T and W be four relations. Then*

(i) $(RS)^{-1} = S^{-1}R^{-1}$.
(ii) *if $R \subset S$ then $WRT \subset WST$.*
(iii) $R(S \cup T) = RS \cup RT$.
(iv) $R(S \cap T) \subset RS \cap RT$.
(v) $R^t = \bigcup_{n=1}^{\infty} R^n$.

As illustrated in (ii), (iii), and (iv), and in order to avoid multiplying the parentheses, we use the convention that the relative product operation "precedes" the other basic operations and relations of set theory, such as $\cup, \cap, -, \subset$. For example, (iv) means, more explicitly,

$$[R(S \cap T)] \subset (RS) \cap (RT).$$

A very compact and convenient notational system is now available. It is easy to see, for example, that a relation R is transitive iff

$$RR \subset R,$$

and asymmetric iff

$$R \cap R^{-1} = \varnothing.$$

A couple of other examples of such rewriting are given in Theorem 1.44.

1.44. Theorem. *Let R be a semiorder (on its field); then*

(i) $R\bar{R}^{-1}R \subset R$.
(ii) $R \cap I = \varnothing$, where $I = \{(a,a) | a \in \mathscr{F}(R)\}$ *is the identity on $\mathscr{F}(R)$; that is, R is irreflexive.*
(iii) $RR\bar{R}^{-1} \subset R$.
(iv) $RR \subset R$, *that is, R is transitive.*
(v) $\bar{R}^{-1}\bar{R}^{-1}R \subset \bar{R}^{-1}$.

Proof. Each of (i) to (iii) is equivalent to the corresponding condition in Definition 1.40, and both (iv) and (v) are consequences of (ii) and (iii). We prove (i) and (iv) and leave the remaining conditions to the reader. Suppose that

$$aR\bar{R}^{-1}Rb;$$

then

$$aRc, \quad c\bar{R}^{-1}d \quad \text{and} \quad dRb$$

for some $c,d \in \mathscr{F}(R)$, which implies

$$aRb,$$

since R is a biorder. This establishes (i). To prove (iv), we assume that

$$aRRb \quad \text{and not} \quad aRb.$$

This implies

$$aRR\bar{R}^{-1}a,$$

yielding

$$aRa,$$

by (iii), contradicting (ii). ∎

The proof of Theorem 1.41 is based on the following result from linear algebra.

1.45. Definition. A vector $v \in \mathbb{R}^n$ is called *rational* iff all the coordinates of v are rational numbers. A subset W of $\mathbb{R}^n$ is called *rational* iff all $v \in W$ are rational; $W \subset \mathbb{R}^n$ is called *symmetric* iff $v \in W$ implies $-v \in W$ for all $v \in \mathbb{R}^n$. For any subset M of $\mathbb{R}^n$, we denote $-M = \{v \mid -v \in M\}$.

1.46. Theorem. *Let V be a finite dimensional, real vector space; let $W \subset V$ be finite, rational, and symmetric; let $\{M,N\}$ be a partition of W, such that $-M = N$. Then, the two following conditions are equivalent.*

(i) *There is a linear functional f satisfying*

$$v \in M \quad \text{iff} \quad f(v) > 0,$$

for all $v \in W$.

(ii) *There is no sequence $v_1, v_2, \ldots, v_n \in M$ such that*

$$v_1 + v_2 \cdots + v_n = 0.$$

This result is an application of the so-called *Theorem of the Alternative* (Kuhn & Tucker, 1956). Its proof is beyond the scope of this book. Theorem 1.46 is a special case of a theorem of Scott (1964). It provides a general algorithm for the proof of theorems such as 1.17, 1.32, or 1.41, which is applicable whenever the set(s) under consideration are finite. Examples of applications can be found in Scott (1964), Tversky (1964), Adams (1965), Krantz et al. (1971), and Ducamp (1978). In the following proof, we use Ducamp's version of Scott's technique.

1.47. Proof of Theorem 1.41. The sufficiency is left to the reader. Let V be the vector space of all real-valued functions on $B = A \cup \{e\}$, where $e \notin A$ is a fixed, arbitrary element (corresponding to the number 1 in $g(a) + 1 < g(b)$). We identify each $a \in B$ with its indicator function $1_{\{a\}} \in V$,

$$1_{\{a\}}(b) = \begin{cases} 1 & \text{if } a = b, \\ 0 & \text{otherwise;} \end{cases}$$

that is, we simply write a for $1_{\{a\}}$. By abuse of notation, B is a linear basis of V. Define

$$M_R = \{b - (a + e) | aRb\},$$

$$M_{\bar{R}} = \{(a + e) - b | a\bar{R}b\},$$

$$M = M_R \cup M_{\bar{R}},$$

$$N = -M,$$

$$W = M \cup N.$$

Clearly, $W \subset V$ is finite, rational, and symmetric. Note that W contains all the vectors of the form

$$b - (a + e), \qquad (a + e) - b, \qquad \text{for } a,b \in A.$$

It is also easy to see that $\{M,N\}$ is a partition of W. If we can show that, under the conditions defining a semiorder, there cannot be a sequence $v_1, v_2, \ldots, v_n \in M$ satisfying $\sum_{i=1}^{n} v_i = 0$, we can then assert, by Theorem 1.46, the existence of a linear functional f such that for all $v \in W$,

$$f(v) > 0 \qquad \text{iff} \qquad v \in M.$$

In particular, aRb implies $[b - (a + e)] \in M_R$, yielding

$$f[b - (a + e)] > 0 \tag{36}$$

or, equivalently,

$$f(a) + f(e) < f(b). \tag{37}$$

Conversely, if either of (36) or (37) holds, then $[b - (a + e)] \in M$, and we cannot have

$$[b - (a + e)] = [(c + e) - d] \in M_{\bar{R}}$$

for some $c,d \in A$, since a, b, c, d, e, are linearly independent. Thus

$$[b - (a + e)] \in M_R,$$

and we obtain aRb. If $f(e) > 0$, we define g on A by $g(a) = f(a)/f(e)$, yielding

$$aRb \qquad \text{iff} \qquad g(a) + 1 < g(b). \tag{38}$$

Notice that we cannot have $f(e) < 0$, since then

$$f(a) + f(e) < f(a)$$

implying aRa, and contradicting the assumption that R is irreflexive. It is possible, however, that $f(e) = 0$. In that case, with

$$\delta = \tfrac{1}{2}[\min\{f(b) - f(a) \,|\, aRb\}] > 0,$$

we have

$$f(a) + \delta < f(b) \qquad \text{iff} \qquad aRb,$$

and defining $g = f/\delta$, we again obtain (38). It remains to prove that Condition (ii) of Theorem 1.46 holds, under the assumption that (A,R) is a semiorder. We proceed by contradiction.

Suppose that $v_1, v_2, \ldots, v_n \in M$, with $\sum_{i=1}^{n} v_i = 0$. Notice that $v_{i_0} \in M_R$ for at least one index $i_0, 1 \leqslant i_0 \leqslant n$ since otherwise each v_i is of the form $v_i = (a_i + e) - b_i$, which with

$$\sum_{i=1}^{n} v_i = \sum_{i=1}^{n} [(a_i + e) - b_i] = 0$$

yields

$$e = (1/n) \sum_{i=1}^{n} (b_i - a_i).$$

This cannot be, since the vectors in B are linearly independent. Assume that

$$v_{i_0} = a_1 - (a_0 + e).$$

Again using linear independence, we can assert the existence of at least one index i_1 such that

$$v_{i_1} = a_2 - a_1 + e_1,$$

for some a_2 and with either $e_1 = e$ or $e_1 = -e$. If $a_2 \neq a_0$, we have, similarly, for some index i_2,

$$v_{i_2} = a_3 - a_2 + e_2,$$

with $e_2 = e$ or $e_2 = -e$. Pursuing this path, the set of indices being finite, we end up with a vector

$$v_{i_k} = a_{k+1} - a_k + e_k,$$

$k \leqslant n - 1$, such that $a_{k+1} = a_0$, and $e_k = e$ or $e_k = -e$. We obtain

$$\sum_{j=0}^{k} v_{i_j} = p \cdot e, \tag{39}$$

where p is an integer. We can assume that $p \leqslant 0$, since, if $k = n - 1$, then

$$\sum_{j=0}^{k} v_{i_j} = \sum_{i=1}^{n} v_i$$

and $p = 0$, and if $k < n - 1$ with $p > 0$, we can extract a new subsequence $\{v'_{i_j}\}$ and at least one such subsequence is such that $p \leqslant 0$. In relative product notations, this means that

$$a_0 R S_1 S_2 \cdots S_k a_0, \tag{40}$$

and the S_i satisfy the following conditions.

1. $S_i = R$ or $S_i = \bar{R}^{-1}$ for $1 \leqslant i \leqslant k$.
2. The number of cases $S_i = \bar{R}^{-1}$ cannot exceed the number of cases $S_i = R$ by more than one unit (otherwise $p > 0$ in (39)).

We prove that, in fact,

$$R S_1 S_2 \cdots S_k \cap I = \varnothing, \tag{41}$$

with I, the identity on A, contradicting (40) and establishing the theorem. We use induction on k. Suppose that $k = 1$. If $S_1 = \bar{R}^{-1}$ then (40) gives

$$a_0 R \bar{R}^{-1} a_0$$

that is,

$$a_0 R a_1 \quad \text{and} \quad a_0 \bar{R} a_1,$$

an absurdity. If $S_1 = R$, then

$$a_0 R R a_0,$$

yielding $a_0 R a_0$, by Condition (iv) in 1.44, which contradicts the irreflexivity of R. Suppose that (41) holds for $k = 1, 2, \ldots m$. We consider that $k = m + 1$, and prove that

$$R S_1 S_2 T \cap I = \varnothing,$$

with $T = S_3 \cdots S_{m+1}$ or possibly, $T = I$ (i.e., $m = 1$).

Case 1. $S_1 S_2 = \bar{R}^{-1} R$, then

$$R \bar{R}^{-1} R T \cap I \subset R T \cap I \quad \text{(by 1.44(i) and 1.43(ii))}$$
$$= \varnothing.$$

by the induction hypothesis.

Case 2. $S_1 S_2 = RR$. Then

$$R R R T \cap I \subset R T \cap I \quad \text{(by 1.44(iv) and 1.43(ii))}$$
$$= \varnothing.$$

Case 3. $S_1 S_2 = R \bar{R}^{-1}$. Then

$$R R \bar{R}^{-1} T \cap I \subset R T \cap I \quad \text{(by 1.44(iii) and 1.43(ii))}$$
$$= \varnothing.$$

Case 4. $S_1 S_2 = \bar{R}^{-1} \bar{R}^{-1}$. By Condition 2 above, we must have some index $j \leqslant k$ such that $S_{j-2} = \bar{R}^{-1}$, $S_{j-1} = \bar{R}^{-1}$, $S_j = R$; otherwise, the number of cases $S_i = \bar{R}^{-1}$ would exceed the number of cases $S_i = R$ by more than one unit.

We have thus

$$(R \cdots \bar{R}^{-1}\bar{R}^{-1}RS_{j+1} \cdots S_k) \cap I \subset (R \cdots \bar{R}^{-1}S_{j+1} \cdots S_k) \cap I = \emptyset,$$

by 1.44(v) and the induction hypothesis. This completes the proof of Theorem 1.41. ■

EXERCISES

1. List all the relations in $\{1,2\}$ that are reflexive on that set.
2. Which of the properties (a) to (h) of Definition 1.3 are satisfied by the relations R_1, R_2, R_3 defined by the following?

	a	b	c
a	R_1	—	—
b	R_1	R_1	R_1
c	—	—	R_1

$$R_2 = \{(c,a)\}, \quad R_3 = \{(x,y) \in \mathbb{R}^2 \mid |x - y| \leq 1\}$$

   (Draw a figure for R_3.)
3. Define $\mathcal{D}(R_1 \cap R_2)$, $\mathcal{D}(R_1 - R_2)$, and $\mathcal{R}(R_3)$ where R_1, R_2, and R_3 are as in Exercise 2.
4. How many relations are there in a set containing exactly n elements? Prove your answer.
5. Prove that $E_\mathbf{A}$ is an equivalence relation on A (complete the proof of Theorem 1.7).
6. Define $\bar{R}_1, \bar{R}_2$, and $\bar{R}_3$ where R_1, R_2, and R_3 are as in Exercise 2.
7. Under which conditions is an equivalence relation also a function? Under which conditions is the negation of a function also a function? Prove your answers.
8. How many functions are there mapping a set A containing n elements into a set B containing m elements? Give a proof. Use this result to provide a (new?) proof of the result of Exercise 4.
9. Show that the equipollence $\approx$ is an equivalence relation (Definition 1.12).
10. Let $\approx$ be the equipollence, as a relation in the set of all subsets of $\{1,2,3\}$. Define $\approx$ by extension (i.e., list the pairs in $\approx$).
11. Define a relation R such that $(\{a,b,c\}, R_1 \cup R)$ is a simple order where R_1 is as in Exercise 2.
12. (*The lexicographic ordering of* $\mathbb{R}^2$.) Define a relation $\precsim$ on $\mathbb{R}^2$ by

   $$(x,y) \precsim (x'y') \quad \text{iff} \quad \text{either } x < x' \quad \text{or} \quad (x = x' \quad \text{and} \quad y \leq y')$$

   Check that $(\mathbb{R}^2, \precsim)$ is a simple order.
13. For $x \in \mathbb{R}$, denote by $\langle x \rangle$ the largest integer smaller or equal to x. Define a relation $\succ$ on $\mathbb{R}$ by

   $$x \succ y \quad \text{iff} \quad \langle x \rangle \geq \langle y \rangle + 1.$$

   Prove that $\succ$ is a biorder from $\mathbb{R}$ to $\mathbb{R}$.

14. Let (A,R) be a simple order, with A a finite set. Show that there exists unique $a_1, a_2 \in A$ such that

   (i) $a_1 \bar{R} b$, for all $b \in A - \{a_1\}$.
   (ii) $b \bar{R} a_2$, for all $b \in A - \{a_2\}$.

   (*Hint.* Use Theorem 1.16.)

15. (*Continuation.*) Prove that, for any $a \in A$, we must have one of three possibilities.

   (i) $a \bar{R} b$, for all $b \in A - \{a\}$.
   (ii) $b \bar{R} a$, for all $b \in A - \{a\}$.
   (iii) $b \bar{R} a \bar{R} c$ for some $b, c \in A - \{a\}$, and there is no $d \in A$ satisfying $b \bar{R} d \bar{R} c$.

*16. Notice that if $(A, \precsim)$ is a weak order, then $\precsim$ is a biorder from A to A. Using this fact, prove that Condition (20), defining the biorder R, is not sufficient to ensure the existence of the functions h, g of Problem 1.25.

17. Construct a relation R in $A = \{a,b,c,d,e\}$, which is a biorder from A to A, irreflexive on A, but does not satisfy condition (iii) in Definition 1.40. Such construction constitutes a logical proof that condition (iii) is independent of conditions (i) and (ii) in Definition 1.40. Prove similarly that (i) is independent of (ii), (iii), and (ii) independent of (i) and (iii).

18. Consider the biorder

	x_1	x_2	x_3
a_1	R	—	—
a_2	R	R	—
a_3	R	R	—
a_4	R	R	R

   Construct two pairs of functions (h,g) and (h_0,g_0) satisfying aRx iff $h(a) \leqslant g(x)$ iff $h_0(a) \leqslant g_0(x)$, but $h(a_2) < h(a_3)$ and $h_0(a_3) < h_0(a_2)$. Discuss the implications of this fact on the uniqueness of the functions h, g satisfying (30) (cf. Ducamp & Falmagne, 1969).

*19. Let $\precsim$ be a relation in a set A. Assume either of conditions (i) and (ii) in Theorem 1.39. Thus, $(A, \precsim)$ is a weak order. Let $\mathbf{A}$ be the partition of A induced by $\precsim$. Define a relation $\|$ in $\mathbf{A}$ by $\mathbf{a} \| \mathbf{b}$ iff $b \succ a$ for some $a \in \mathbf{a}$, $b \in \mathbf{b}$, and there is no $c \in A$ satisfying $b \succ c \succ a$. Show that $\mathscr{F}(\|)$ is, at most, countable (Krantz et al., 1971).

*20. (*Continuation.*) Use this fact to prove that (ii) is equivalent to (i) in Theorem 1.39.

21. Prove that, if $(A, \precsim)$ is a weak order, then $(A, \succ)$ is a semiorder, but that the converse does not hold.

22. Prove Theorem 1.43. Show in particular that the reverse inclusion does not hold in 1.43(iv).

23. As observed in Remark 1.31, a biorder (A,X,R) induces two weak orders $(A,\precsim), (X,\precsim')$. It may be the case that these weak orders are, in fact, simple orders. From this observation define the notion of a simple biorder. (The biorder $(\mathbb{Q},\mathbb{R} - \mathbb{Q},\ll)$ of Example 1.27(a) is a "simple" biorder.)

*24. Let $(A, \precsim)$ be a low order and let $\{A_1,A_2\}$ be a partition of A. Consider the restriction R of $\precsim$ defined by $R = \precsim \cap (A_1 \times A_2)$. Characterize the structure (A_1,A_2,R) as a local weak biorder, or more simply, a low biorder.

*25. Adapt and prove Theorem 1.39 in the case where $(A,\precsim)$ is a low order.

*26. Let A be a finite set. Let $(a,b) \mapsto P_{a,b}$ be a mapping of $A \times A$ into the real interval $[0,1]$. Suppose that $P_{a,b} + P_{b,a} = 1$ for all $a,b \in A$. The interpretation is that $P_{a,b}$ is the probability that stimulus a subjectively exceeds b from the viewpoint of a sensory attribute under consideration. Find necessary and sufficient conditions on (A,P) for the existence of a function u mapping A into the reals, and a function F defined for all real numbers of the form $[u(a), u(b)]$ strictly increasing in the first variable and strictly decreasing in the second variable, satisfying $P_{a,b} = F[u(a), u(b)]$ for all $a,b \in A$. Krantz (1964) first investigated this representation. A solution to this problem can be found in Tversky and Russo (1969).

*27. A probabilistic version of a weak order is implicitly proposed in Exercise 26. This idea can be generalized to low orders. We define a *probabilistic low order* as a triple (A,C,P) in which C is a relation in A, P is a mapping of C in the closed interval $[0,1]$, and the following four conditions are satisfied for all $m \in \mathbb{N}$ and $a, b, c, b_1, b_2, \ldots, b_m \in A$.

(1) C is reflexive on A.
(2) If $P_{a,b} \leqslant \frac{1}{2} \leqslant P_{c,a}$ or $P_{b,a} \leqslant \frac{1}{2} \leqslant P_{a,c}$, then cCb.
(3) There exist $n \in \mathbb{N}$ and $a_1,a_2,\ldots,a_n \in A$ such that $a_1 = a$, $a_n = b$ and $a_i C a_{i+1}$ for $1 \leqslant i \leqslant n - 1$.
(4) If $P_{b_i,b_{i+1}} \leqslant \frac{1}{2}$ for $1 \leqslant i \leqslant m - 1$, *then* $P_{b_1,b_m} = \frac{1}{2}$ implies $P_{b_i,b_{i+1}} = \frac{1}{2}$ for $1 \leqslant i \leqslant m - 1$.
(5) $P_{a,b} + P_{b,a} = 1$, whenever aCb and bCa.

Reflect on these conditions and prove the following facts.

(i) $P_{a,a} = \frac{1}{2}$ for all $a \in A$.
(ii) C is symmetric on A.
(iii) *Weak stochastic transitivity* is satisfied, that is, $\max\{P_{a,b}, P_{b,c}\} \leqslant \frac{1}{2}$ implies $P_{a,c} \leqslant \frac{1}{2}$, whenever aCb, bCc, and aCc.
(iv) If $\min\{P_{a,b}, P_{b,c}\} < \max\{P_{a,b}, P_{b,c}\} \leqslant \frac{1}{2}$, then $P_{a,c} < \frac{1}{2}$, whenever aCb, bCc, and aCc.

28. *(Continuation.)* Define a relation $\precsim$ in A by $a \precsim b$ iff (aCb and $P_{a,b} \leqslant \frac{1}{2}$). Show that $\precsim$ is a low order on A. Using this result, prove that if A is at most countable, then there exists a function h mapping A into the reals, satisfying $h(a) \leqslant h(b)$ iff (aCb and $P_{a,b} \leqslant \frac{1}{2}$).

*29. Let A,X be two finite sets. Let $(a,x) \mapsto P_{a,x}$ be a mapping of $A \times X$ into the real interval $[0,1]$. Find necessary and sufficient conditions on (A,X,P) for the existence of two real-valued functions u,g, respectively, defined on A,X, and a function F, defined for all pairs of real numbers of the form $[u(a), g(x)]$ strictly increasing in the first argument, and strictly decreasing in the second argument, such that $P_{a,x} = F[u(a), g(x)]$ for all $a \in A$ and $x \in X$ (cf. Irtel & Schmalhofer, 1982).

2
Extensive Measurement

Extensive measurement means the measurement of fundamental physical quantities such as mass or length, using some qualitative devices. For mass, a typical example of such a device is the two-pan, equal-arm balance. The case of length is discussed in detail below. Since Helmholtz (1887), this type of measurement is recognized to involve two specific kinds of empirical procedures.

1. For any two objects a,b, a *comparison procedure* is used to decide which one of a,b has the greatest amount of the quantity or whether they have the same amount. In the case of mass, the procedure involves placing the two objects in the two pans of the balance and recording the equilibrium state of the balance.
2. A *concatenation procedure* is used to combine the two objects a,b into a new object ab of the same nature. For example, a and b can be placed in one pan of the balance and some other object c in the other pan. It can then be checked whether ab (i.e., a concatenated with b) has a greater mass than c.

There are compelling reasons to include extensive measurement as a topic in a discussion of psychophysical theory. Many scientists (especially physicists) maintain that the state of the art in a scientific discipline can be assessed by comparing its measurement procedures with those of physics. Whether this opinion is founded or not, the comparison is instructive—for the physicist as well as for the psychologist. One discovers that the algorithms for constructing fundamental scales are quite similar in physics and psychophysics. This similarity, which has not always been clearly recognized, has important implications. The theorems of this chapter are of general interest. Specifically, the key purpose of this chapter is the establishment of a result—Theorem 2.7—which will serve as the backbone of our theoretical developments (cf. Theorem 3.27).

We begin with a discussion of a number of algorithms for the construction of a physical scale of length. With this background in mind, we will then proceed to abstract the axioms required for such constructions.

Insofar as style is concerned, our developments will be fairly informal at first. In the first section, we rely heavily on the reader's experience of the "physical" world. Our arguments will often be intuitive, rather than based on axioms, definitions, and theorems. In addition, this section will familiarize the reader with our notations and prepare him or her for the more systematic developments of subsequent sections. The reader with a background in algebra will no doubt find this section redundant. (For instance, Method 2.4 is little else than a paraphrase of a part of the proof of Theorem 2.7.)

CONSTRUCTION OF A PHYSICAL SCALE FOR LENGTH

Consider a collection of thin rods. We want to measure the length of these rods, but no rulers or other devices are available. A natural way of measuring the length of a given rod would involve the following steps.

· Pick a given, fixed rod as a "unit."
· Count the maximum number of exact "copies" of this "unit," which can be placed along the rod to be measured without overlap.

The number thus obtained measures the length of the rod. If exact measurement is required, some refinements must be introduced. For the essential, however, this algorithm is the usual one. The intuition supporting it is so compelling that it is at first difficult to realize (1) that quite a number of assumptions about physical reality are implicitly made, and (2) that the algorithm involves a considerable amount of arbitrariness. Here, we analyze, in detail, this algorithm and some of its refinements. In the next section, we abstract the required assumptions, which we call axioms. Later (in 2.11), we consider an entirely different possibility of measuring length.

2.1. Notations. We denote by A the set of thin rods. The comparison procedure, for the rods a,b, involves placing the rods next to each other in such a way that they coincide at one end (see Figure 2.1). If they also coincide at the other end, we write $a \sim b$, If b covers a, but is not covered by it, we write $a \prec b$. A more compact notation is useful. Whenever either $a \prec b$ or $a \sim b$, we write $a \precsim b$. In the terminology of Chapter 1, $\sim$, $\prec$, and $\precsim$ are thus binary relations in A. The concatenation procedure, for rods a,b, involves placing a and b end to end along a straight line, forming a new object, which we denote ab. Using the comparison procedure, this new object can be placed along rod c to yield $ab \precsim c$, for example.

Where the rods of a sequence $a_1, a_2, \ldots, a_n$ are successively concatenated in the order a_1 with a_2, then $a_1 a_2$ with a_3, etc., the result is denoted as $a_1 a_2 \cdots a_n$.

A meaning will also be attached to expressions such as aa, aaa, aab, etc. At first, this might seem strange, since a rod cannot literally be placed end to end with itself. However, forbidding such expressions would render our developments more cumbersome without essential benefit. (To clarify this concept, the following empirical meaning can be given to aa. Suppose aa has to be compared to some rod b. Place a along b such that they coincide at one end. Make a mark at the other end of a. Remove a and place it so that one of its ends is on the mark, extending it in the other direction, etc.) By extension we say that aa is the result of the concatenation of a with itself. A convenient abbreviation will be

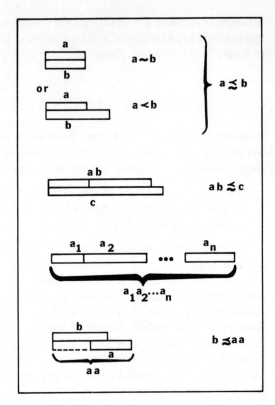

FIGURE 2.1. Measurement of length. Comparison and concatenation procedures. Notations.

used to denote the successive concatenation of *a* with itself. We write

$$n * a = \underbrace{aa \cdots a.}_{n \text{ times}}$$

Thus, in particular, $1 * a = a$, $2 * a = aa$, $b(3 * a) = baaa$, etc. By convention we admit that $n * a \sim n * a$, for $n = 1, 2, \dots$.

Another important concept must be introduced. Strictly speaking, *ab* or *aa* are not rods (i.e., *ab*, *aa* $\notin A$). However, the scale that we want to construct should also apply to objects such as *ab* or *aa*. This suggests the introduction of a set X, containing all the objects that can be formed, by concatenating the rods in A and including A itself. That is, X is precisely that set containing all the objects that we want to measure. Notice that there might be some limitations on X. For example, if a, b, and c are rods in A, it is conceivable that, in practice, *abc* cannot be constructed—due, say, to the physical limitations of the room. Defining exactly what kind of set X is will be one of the accomplishments of a correct theorization. For clarity, we denote the elements of X by the last letters of the alphabet $x, y, z \dots$. Thus $x \in X$ can either be a rod or an object resulting from the concatenation of two or more rods. In the sequel, it will be convenient to be slightly inaccurate and to refer to the elements of X also as rods. This ambiguous usage will not create difficulties. Extending the conventions introduced before for the elements of A, we define

$$n * x = \underbrace{xx \cdots x}_{n \text{ times}}, n * x \sim n * x, \text{ etc.}$$

The following interpretation might help the reader to grasp these conventions. Think of A as an "alphabet" and $a_1 a_2 \cdots a_n$ as a "word." The comparison procedure, then, involves comparing the "words" of the "language" X. Since we assume $A \subset X$, this "language" contains all the "one-letter-words."

2.2. First method. Take any $x \in X$. In order to measure its length, we arbitrarily pick a (small) rod $y \in X$ as a "unit." We also take a number of exact "copies" of y, which we denote $y_1, y_2, \ldots, y_n, y_{n+1}, \ldots$. We have thus $y \sim y_1 \sim y_2 \sim \cdots \sim y_n \sim y_{n+1} \cdots$. Next, we compare x successively with y, yy_1, yy_1y_2, etc., until the following situation is obtained.

$$yy_1y_2 \cdots y_{n-1} \precsim x \prec yy_1y_2 \cdots y_n. \tag{1}$$

We then assign the number n to x as its value on a scale measuring length, and we proceed similarly with the other elements of X. Another, equivalent method would involve forming the successive concatenations of y with itself, yielding

$$n * y \precsim x \prec (n + 1) * y. \tag{2}$$

Since (1) is somewhat more cumbersome to write than (2), we will discuss the latter method (our conclusions will apply to both). It seems reasonable, but in fact involves various difficulties.

To begin with, it is possible that $x \prec y$. In this case, we could assign the number zero to x. But this would not be very satisfying. For example, there might be another rod x', such that $x \sim x' \prec y$, but $y \precsim xx' \prec 2 * y$. In other words, both x and x' would have a scale value equal to zero, but xx' would have a scale value equal to 1—a very counterintuitive result! This shocking situation results from a general defect of the method: it is not very precise.

A second difficulty is that we have a priori no certainty that the method will work. Even if $y \prec x$, how can we be sure that, by successively concatenating y with itself, we will finally obtain (2) for some integer n? In the particular case analyzed here—considering the empirical signification of expressions such as $y \prec x, n * y$, etc.—it seems intuitively obvious that this will be the case. But where does this intuition come from? The answer is that we have learned from experience that the "physical" world around us satisfies a number of constraints or "laws." An instance of such a law, of immediate relevance to our discussion, is the following.

If $x, y \in X$, *either* $x \prec y$, *or there exists a positive integer* n *such that* $n * y \precsim x \prec (n + 1) * y$.

The method outlined above is based on the assumption that this law, and various others, are empirically true. In the rest of this chapter, such laws will be referred to as *axioms*. Another example of an axiom, intuitively consistent with the interpretation of the relation $\precsim$, as meaning "is not longer than," is

$$if \ z \precsim w \ and \ w \precsim t \ then \ z \precsim t.$$

(That is, $\precsim$ is transitive.) At this stage of our development, it would be tedious and probably not very enlightening to justify each step of the construction of the scale by the axiom or axioms on which it is based. It is sufficient for the moment to remember that the above method, or its refinement to which we turn in a moment, relies on axioms such as these. In the next section we review the required axioms systematically.

Finally, a third difficulty has to do with the possibility of errors. The errors we have in mind here are of a different nature than those arising in the first difficulty mentioned above because of the lack of precision of the method. A better term, perhaps, would be "inconsistencies." Suppose that we have to check whether some rod y' is an exact "copy" of y (i.e., whether $y' \sim y$). It is conceivable that if we were to repeat the test, say 20 times, we would end up with the following results.

$$y' \sim y \qquad y' \prec y \qquad y \prec y'.$$
$$11 \ \text{times} \qquad 4 \ \text{times} \qquad 5 \ \text{times}$$

We assume here that such inconsistencies do not occur. *In other words, the construction of the scale will be based on a deterministic theory.* This, of course, is a serious weakness since such inconsistencies are likely to be present in fair number in the data. Clearly, we require a probabilistic theory. One may wonder whether a deterministic theory has any interest. In fact, even though the theory that we describe in the next two sections is not realistic, it is nevertheless of central importance in that it provides the basic algebraic framework for probabilistic theories that one may wish to develop, in extensive measurement as well as in psychophysical measurement (cf. Chapter 4).[1]

Let us go back to the construction of the scale. Suppose that, as before, we take a rod y as a "unit," and we assign n as a scale value to a rod x, whenever $n*y \precsim x \prec (n+1)*y$. In this case, we are committing an error the size of which is smaller than the length of y, which by convention is equal to 1. The intuitive reason for this is the following. For any rod $z \in X$, let us denote $\ell(z)$ its length, as measured by this method. We assume that that for any $z,w \in X$

$$z \precsim w \qquad \text{iff} \qquad \ell(z) \leqslant \ell(w).$$

In the situation symbolized by the expression $n*y \precsim x \prec (n+1)*y$, we obtain

$$\ell(n*y) \leqslant \ell(x) < \ell[(n+1)*y]. \tag{3}$$

The natural interpretation of the concatenation procedure for rods leads us to require that whenever $zw \in X$, the length of zw must be the sum of the length of z

---

1. There are various directions that one might take in constructing probabilistic theories for extensive measurement. Such developments lie outside the scope of this book, however (see Falmagne, 1980).

and w, that is,

$$\ell(zw) = \ell(z) + \ell(w).$$

In general, for any sequence $z_1, z_2, \ldots, z_n \in X$ such that also $z_1 z_2 \cdots z_n \in X$, we must have

$$\ell(z_1 z_2 \cdots z_n) = \sum_{i=1}^{n} \ell(z_i).$$

In particular, if $z \in X$ and n is any positive integer such that $n * z \in X$, we must have

$$\ell(n * z) = n\ell(z). \tag{4}$$

Going back to (3), this gives

$$n\ell(y) \leqslant \ell(x) < (n+1)\ell(y),$$

which implies

$$\ell(x) = nl(y) + \gamma$$
$$= n + \gamma$$

with $0 \leqslant \gamma < 1$, since $\ell(y) = 1$. Consequently, when we assign the number n to x as a scale value, we are making an error the size of which is smaller than 1.

Methods minimizing such an error––making it as small as one wishes—are not hard to design. A simple possibility is considered as follows.

2.3. Second method. Take the successive concatenations of x with itself. Suppose, for example, that

$$m * y \precsim xx \prec (m+1) * y.$$

This leads to

$$\ell(m * y) \leqslant \ell(xx) < \ell[(m+1) * y],$$

which implies, by (4) and the fact that $\ell(y) = 1$,

$$m \leqslant 2\ell(x) < m + 1.$$

We conclude that

$$\ell(x) = (m/2) + \gamma$$

with $0 \leqslant \gamma < \frac{1}{2}$. This suggests to assign $m/2$ as a scale value to x, with an error smaller than $\frac{1}{2}$. Generalizing this argument, we see that if for some positive integers p, q

$$p * y \precsim q * x \prec (p+1) * y,$$

then

$$p/q \leqslant \ell(x) \leqslant (p+1)/q$$

and

$$\ell(x) = (p/q) + \gamma,$$

with $0 \leqslant \gamma < 1/q$. Assigning p/q as a scale value thus involves a positive error smaller than $1/q$. By concatenating x with itself a sufficiently large number of times, the error can be made as small as desired. In principle, this method is legitimate. It suffers, however, from some important practical limitations. For some rod x, making the error small will require concatenating x with itself many times. If x is large this may not be feasible in practice. In particular, the location in which these operations are carried out will always be of limited size. Realistically, it cannot be assumed that rods can be "multiplied" by n, where n is a positive integer as large as we please. The next and last method (2.4) does not make such an assumption. Incidentally, essentially the same objection could have been made earlier. In Method 2.2, we assumed that for any rod x strictly longer than the unit y, we would have $n * y \lesssim x \prec (n + 1) * y$. The following situation, however, is quite conceivable: $n * y \lesssim x$, but $(n + 1) * y$ is too long and cannot be constructed. It is thus impossible to check, using the comparison procedure, whether $x \prec (n + 1) * y$.

2.4. Third method.   Interestingly, this method is the natural counterpart of Method 2.3 in that it (almost) assumes that rods can be "divided" at will. Actually, the assumption that we will make is weaker but will serve the same purpose. More precisely, we assume that

For any rod z, there exists a rod w such that $ww \lesssim z$.

This method requires more work than the preceding ones. Notice that, in the above assumption, the rod w itself is such that for some rod w', $w'w' \lesssim w$. Using this idea, we first construct a "distinguished" sequence of shorter and shorter rods as follows. We choose w_1 arbitrarily. Next, we pick w_2 such that $w_2 w_2 \lesssim w_1$, etc. In general, we have $w_n w_n \lesssim w_{n-1}$. Thus, when n becomes large, w_n becomes shorter and shorter. In particular, if n is large enough we will have $w_n \lesssim x$ and $w_n \lesssim y$, where x and y are the rod to be measured and our "unit," respectively. Using a familiar argument, we also know that

$$p_n * w_n \lesssim x,$$

for some positive integer p_n, such that either $x \prec (p_n + 1) * w_n$ or possibly $(p_n + 1) * w_n$ cannot be constructed. Similarly, there exists a largest positive integer p'_n such that

$$p'_n * w_n \lesssim y.$$

(The index n in p_n, p'_n is a reminder that these integers depend on the term w_n in the sequence.) Considering the length of the rods involved in these expressions, we obtain

$$p_n \ell(w_n) \leqslant \ell(x) < (p_n + 1)\ell(w_n),$$
$$p'_n \ell(w_n) \leqslant 1 < (p'_n + 1)\ell(w_n).$$

The basic idea is to use these inequalities to approximate $\ell(x)$. Given w_n, the integers p_n, p'_n are empirically determined (we can "compute" them). A little algebra involving some of the above inequalities permits the elimination of the bothersome quantities $\ell(w_n)$; we obtain

$$p'_n\ell(x) < p_n + 1. \tag{5}$$

A similar computation on the remaining inequalities yields

$$p_n < \ell(x)(p'_n + 1). \tag{6}$$

Combining (5) and (6) and rearranging terms finally yields

$$p_n/(p'_n + 1) < \ell(x) < (p_n + 1)/p'_n, \tag{7}$$

providing two bounds for $\ell(x)$. Let us investigate the situation when n becomes large. As indicated earlier, this means that w_n gets shorter and shorter. In turn, p_n, p'_n must increase (a greater number of concatenations of w_n with itself is required to exceed x or y). In fact, when $n \to \infty$, we have both $p_n \to \infty$ and $p'_n \to \infty$. At this stage the consequences of this result on the two bounds in (7) are unclear. Fortunately, it can be shown that under the assumptions (axioms) underlying our discussion, the ratio p_n/p'_n converges to some limit ζ. This means, of course, that the two bounds in (7) converge to the same limit. That is, $p_n/(p'_n + 1) \to \zeta, (p_n + 1)/p'_n \to \zeta$, implying $\ell(x) = \zeta$. The outcome is clear: we can take either of the two bounds or p_n/p'_n itself as a scale value approximately $\ell(x)$, the approximation becoming increasingly accurate as n gets large. For example, we have

$$\ell(x) = (p_n/p'_n) + \gamma_n, \tag{8}$$

with

$$-(p_n/p'_n) \cdot (p'_n + 1)^{-1} < \gamma_n < 1/p'_n. \tag{9}$$

(We leave it to the reader to check our algebra; see Exercise 3.)

Taking p_n/p'_n as a scale value for x, involves thus an error γ_n, the absolute value of which can be as small as required by practical or scientific applications.

At this point, the reader probably feels somewhat uneasy about the foundations of these methods, especially the last one. A proof of the key results, such as the convergence of p_n/p'_n, requires a more precise apparatus than what is presently available. In particular, a precise statement of the axioms is required.

We had two aims in discussing these algorithms. First, we wanted to illustrate, with a minimum of formalism, the process by which qualitative observations — which are a typical outcome of an experiment — are progressively transformed into numerical statements regarding extensive measurement. This type of measurement is not only the most important example so far provided by science, but is also a cornerstone of various other types of measurement of interest to the psychologist. Not surprisingly, other algorithms analyzed in this book will appear to be germane to the methods we have discussed. Second, we wanted to permit the reader to handle our symbols in the concrete context of the comparison and the concatenation procedures for rods. Hopefully, she or he is now both motivated and prepared for a more systematic approach.

AXIOMS FOR EXTENSIVE MEASUREMENT

In this section our key empirical example remains the rods and the measurement of length by the procedures described in the preceding section. Our theory, however, is intended to apply in a variety of other cases. For this reason, we will adopt a neutral language, an illustration of which is given in the following definition.

2.5. Definition. Let A be a nonempty set; then x is a *string* of A iff there exists a positive integer n, and $a_1, a_2, \ldots, a_n \in A$, such that $x = a_1 a_2 \cdots a_n$. Thus, if x, y are strings of A, xy is also a string of A. A set Y of strings of some set is called *operant* iff there are $x, y \in Y$ such that also $xy \in Y$.

Our axioms concern thus a set A, a distinguished set X of strings of A, and a binary relation $\precsim$ in X. Definition 2.6 lists the axioms required to perform the construction of the scale, as outlined in 2.4. Comments on these axioms follow the definition.

2.6. Definition. Let A be a nonempty set; let X be an operant set of strings of A; let $\precsim$ be a binary relation in X. We write $x \prec y$ iff not $y \precsim x$, and $x \sim y$ iff both $x \precsim y$ and $y \precsim x$. Then, the triple $(A, X, \precsim)$ is *a measurement system for positive, extensive quantities*, or more briefly, *an extensive system* iff for all $x, y, x', y' \in X$:

1. $A \subset X$.
2. $(X, \precsim)$ is a weak order (transitive, connected, cf. Definition 1.3).
3. If $x' \precsim x$, $y' \precsim y$ and $xy \in X$, then $x'y' \in X$, with $x'y' \precsim xy$.
4. If $xy \in X$, then $x \prec xy$.
5. If $x \prec y$, then there exists $z \in X$, such that $xz \in X$ and $xz \sim y$.
6. $\{m \in \mathbb{N} \,|\, m * x \prec y\}$ is a finite set where $1 * x = x$ and for all integers $n > 1$, $n * x = [(n-1) * x]x$.

As indicated earlier, the notation $\mathbb{N}$ in Axiom 6 stands for the set of positive integers; this axiom also involves a definition of the expression $n * x$, for every $n \in \mathbb{N}$ and $x \in X$. Notice, for further reference, the immediate consequence of this definition (Exercise 5): if $n, m \in \mathbb{N}$ and $x \in X$, then $(n + m) * x = (n * x)(m * x)$ and $(nm) * x = n * (m * x)$.

In discussing each axiom in Definition 2.6, we ask ourselves two questions. (1) Is this axiom bound to be—at least approximately—satisfied in the case of length, as analyzed in the last section? (2) Is this axiom used, and how is it used, in Method 2.4? We consider question (1) first.

Axiom 1 is inescapable. We indicated earlier that if $\precsim$ is to be interpreted as "is not longer than", it was natural to assume it to be transitive. It is also clear that any two rods in X can be compared. That is, we can check whether $x \precsim y$ or $y \precsim x$

is true or whether both are true. In other words, $\precsim$ is connected. This means, of course (see Definition 1.14), that $(X,\precsim)$ is a weak order as asserted by Axiom 2. If x',y' are, respectively, not longer than x,y and if, in the condition of the experiment, x and y can be placed end to end, then $x'y'$ can also certainly be formed. Moreover, $x'y'$ cannot be longer than xy. Axiom 3 is a formalization of this idea. If we place rods x and y end to end we clearly obtain a rod longer than x itself. This yields Axiom 4. Axiom 5 is more demanding. It states that the set X is sufficiently rich that we can always find a rod exactly as long as the difference between two rods. Whereas the other axioms discussed so far are (approximately) true for any set X of rods, Axiom 5 will only apply in some cases. The restriction itself is not shocking, however. The following idea motivates Axiom 6. For any two rods $x,y \in X$, we must have either $y \precsim x$, or $x \prec y$, and in this last case, if we keep concatenating x with itself, forming successively $1 * x, 2 * x, \ldots$, there will be a largest $m \in \mathbb{N}$ such that $m * x \prec y$. Thus, if p is that largest positive integer, we will have either $y \precsim (p + 1) * x$, or possibly $(p + 1) * x$ does not exist (i.e., cannot be constructed). Axiom 6 is a compact formulation which, in the presence of other axioms, ensures that the above situation holds. In fact, p is simply the maximum of the set $\{m \in \mathbb{N} \mid m * x \prec y\}$. If $y \prec x$, this set is empty.

Discussing the axioms of Definitions 2.6 from the viewpoint of question (2) requires a more careful analysis. We will give one example involving Axioms 2, 3, and 5. Some other cases will be left for the exercises. In the third method the following key fact was used:

$$\text{any rod } z \in X \text{ is such that } ww \precsim z \text{ for some } w \in X. \tag{10}$$

In fact, the axioms of Definitions 2.6 do not rule out a particular rod z, which would be a minimal element of X (i.e., such that $x \prec z$ for no $x \in X$). For that particular rod z, we would not have $ww \precsim z$. This, however, is a special case for which an algorithm as elaborate as Method 2.4 is not needed. If such a z exists, it can be taken as a unit and Method 2.2 can be applied. This will lead to assign, as scale values, only the numbers $1,2,\ldots$, etc. but will involve no errors. (A proof of this fact is contained in 2.12.) Let us consider the other case. We assume that for all $z \in X$, $x \prec z$ for some $x \in X$. The simple argument below shows that under Axioms 1, 3, and 5 of Definition 2.6, proposition (10) must hold.

Take $z \in X$ arbitrarily. By hypothesis, $x \prec z$ for some $x \in X$. Using Axiom 5, there exists x' such that $xx' \in X$, with $xx' \sim z$. By Axiom 2, either $x \precsim x'$ or $x' \precsim x$ ($\precsim$ is connected). Suppose that $x \precsim x'$. We then have the following situation: $x \precsim x'$, $x \precsim x$ (since $\precsim$ is connected, it is also reflexive), and $xx' \in X$. From Axiom 3 we conclude that $xx \in X$ with $xx \precsim xx'$. But $xx' \sim z$. This implies, by the transitivity of $\precsim$ (Axiom 2), that $xx \precsim z$. Defining $w = x$ we see that (10) holds in this case. The other case, $x' \precsim x$, is similar and will be left to the reader. This piece of argument is a good illustration of how the axioms of Definition 2.6 are used to justify the steps of the method for constructing scales. In the next section we turn to a different approach to extensive measurement in which the emphasis is not on scale construction but rather on the very problem that the construction of a given scale is supposed to solve.

REPRESENTATION THEOREM

Reflecting on the position adopted so far in this chapter, it should be recognized that it is not devoid of some obscurities. In particular, we discussed in detail various methods for the construction of a scale for length, without ever making exactly clear which problems such a scale was supposed to solve. At each step of these constructions it was somehow natural or obvious that this was the right course to follow. This approach leaves too many questions unanswered to be satisfying. For example, what justifies the agreement existing in the scientific—as well as in the social—community that the scales obtained by such methods are appropriate? Is the agreement based on practical reasons, theoretical reasons, or both? Could we use a different scale? If yes, under which conditions?

Here, we take a more critical viewpoint regarding the methods of scale construction discussed earlier. Our empirical manipulations involve a set of objects, X, and two procedures: the comparison procedure (symbolized by the binary relation $\precsim$), and the concatenation procedure (symbolized by writing xy for the two objects x,y in X). A scale is essentially a device by which the objects in X are represented by numbers. *By which notions (operations, relations) of the real number system are we representing the two procedures?* Some hints were given earlier. In 2.2 we argued that a function ℓ mapping X into the positive reals and representing the true length of the rods should be such that

$$x \precsim y \quad \text{iff} \quad \ell(x) \le \ell(y). \tag{11}$$

In the same context we also maintained that a natural interpretation of the concatenation procedure for rods would lead to require that the length of xy should be equal to the length of x added to the length of y. Thus, whenever $xy \in X$,

$$\ell(xy) = \ell(x) + \ell(y). \tag{12}$$

In other words, the comparison procedure is represented by the ordering relation of the real numbers ($\le$), and the concatenation operation is represented by the addition of the real numbers ($+$). (Occasionally, we will say that a function ℓ satisfying (12) is *additive*.) Turning the question around leads us to ask the following question. *Under which conditions on $(A,X,\precsim)$ does there exist a mapping ℓ of X into the positive reals such that* (11) *and* (12) *are satisfied for all $x,y \in X$?* A typical answer to this problem is a list of axioms on $(A,X,\precsim)$. The following result will not come as a surprise.

2.7. Theorem.   *Let $(A,X,\precsim)$ be an extensive system. Then there exists a mapping ℓ of X into the positive reals such that, for all $x,y \in X$,*

   (i) $x \precsim y \quad iff \quad \ell(x) \le \ell(y)$.
   (ii) *if $xy \in X$, then $\ell(xy) = \ell(x) + \ell(y)$.*

Moreover, if k is another function satisfying these conditions then $k = \alpha\ell$ for some constant $\alpha > 0$.

The proof of this theorem is based on the following idea. We start by constructing the function ℓ essentially using Method 2.4. (Intuitively, the axioms are shown to imply that in Equation 8, p_n/p'_n converges and that $\gamma_n \to 0$. We define $\ell(x) = \lim_{n \to \infty} p_n/p'_n$; thus, in particular, $\ell(y) = 1$.) Next, we show that the conditions of the theorem are indeed satisfied. Notice the last proposition of the theorem: ℓ is a ratio scale, that is, ℓ is only defined up to a multiplication by a positive constant. The reader is not expected to study the details of this proof, which is rather long, at first reading. For this reason, the proof of Theorem 2.7 is relegated to the Complement section of this chapter (see 2.12).

2.8. Remarks. Since Helmholtz (1887), various axiom systems for extensive measurement have been proposed. Definition 2.6 is only one of the many possibilities. These axioms systems differ from each other in the emphasis placed on side conditions (e.g., some axiom systems do require that X contain all the strings of A) or in the representation involved (in some cases, the function ℓ of Theorem 2.7 satisfies a modified version of (i) or (ii), see Krantz (1967), Luce (1973), or Holman (1974)). Most of these axiom systems imply that ℓ is a ratio scale. For a more complete discussion of these developments, the reader is referred to the last section of this chapter. Theorem 2.7 and its proof are adapted from Krantz (1968). Some, more technical aspects of this theorem are found in the Complement section.

It must be realized that the representation of the concatenation procedure by the *addition* of real numbers is arbitrary to some extent. For instance, assuming that there is indeed a scale ℓ satisfying the conditions of the theorem, we can immediately deduce the following. There also exists a mapping g of X into the reals such that

$$x \precsim y \quad \text{iff} \quad g(x) \leqslant g(y),$$

and if $x, y, xy \in X$, then

$$g(xy) = g(x)g(y);$$

moreover, any function h satisfying these conditions is such that $h = g^\alpha$ for some $\alpha > 0$. It suffices indeed to define g on X by $g(x) = e^{\ell(x)}$. Thus, it seems that the choice of ℓ and addition over g and multiplication is essentially a matter of convention and justifiable only by considerations of convenience.

Finally, an important consequence of Theorem 2.7 is worth pointing out. In an extensive system, we must have

$$xy \sim yx \tag{13}$$

if both $xy, yx \in X$. This fact is empirically obvious in the case of the measurement of length by Method 2.4. Notice, however, that (13) was not explicitly assumed as part of the definition of an extensive system. It turns out that this property is derivable from Axioms 1 to 6 via Theorem 2.7. The argument is simple and relies on the commutativity of the addition of real numbers: suppose that $xy, yz \in X$

and let ℓ be the function of Theorem 2.7; successively,

$$\ell(xy) = \ell(x) + \ell(y) = \ell(y) + \ell(x) = \ell(yx),$$

yielding (13).

OTHER EMPIRICAL EXAMPLES

The theory developed in the preceding sections has a variety of other applications besides the measurement of length. Some of these applications are well known and involve current professional or scientific practices. One application is the measurement of mass, using the two-pan equal-arm balance. Other applications are less familiar. Some are even rather bizarre. This section is devoted to a brief discussion of some of these examples. We will successively consider the cases of mass, time, and a different, somewhat unusual, alternative for the measurement of length. This material can be skipped without any loss of continuity. However, we advise the novice reader to take the time for reflection on these examples. This exercise will give him or her useful insight on the surprisingly arbitrary character of the most commonly used measurement procedures of physical phenomena.

2.9. Example: Mass.   This case was briefly considered earlier but is given more critical discussion here. An experimenter has, at his or her disposal, a two-pan equal-arm balance, which he or she uses to measure the mass of a collection A of objects. Formalizing this procedure, we write ab when $a,b \in A$ are placed in the same pan and $ab \precsim cde$ if the pan containing $c, d,$ and e does not stabilize itself at a higher level than the pan containing a,b. We then define a set X of strings of A, such that $x = a_1 a_2 \cdots a_n \in X$ whenever all the objects $a_1, a_2, \ldots, a_n \in A$ can be placed simultaneously in one of the pans. Examining Definition 2.6 of a measurement structure for extensive quantities, we might hastily conclude that the formalization is adequate and that the axioms will probably be satisfied to a reasonable approximation. In fact, some adaptation of the axioms is required. The difficulty—a fairly trivial one—comes from expressions such as aa, xxy, etc., that is, expressions involving one or more repetitions of a symbol in a string. Such expressions are unavoidable if Definition 2.6 is used. Indeed, suppose that X contains three elements $x,y,$ and z with $x \precsim y$, $x \precsim z$, and $yz \in X$. An application of Axiom 3 immediately yields $xx \in X$. In the case of the measurement of length using, say, Method 2.4, such an expression corresponded to a specific experimental device and made sense. No such device seems to be available in the present case. Definition 2.6 is easy to correct, however. For example, Axiom 3 could be generalized as follows.

> If $x' \precsim x, y' \precsim y, xy \in X,$ and x',y' have no common term, then $x'y' \in X$ and $x'y' \precsim xy.$ (Where $x' = a_1 a_2 \cdots a_n$, $y = b_1 b_2 \cdots b_m$ have a common term if $a_i = b_j$ for some i, $1 \leqslant i \leqslant n$ and $j, 1 \leqslant j \leqslant m$.)

Clearly, the derivation of $xx \in X$ using the above argument is now blocked. Note, however, that this modified axiom does *not* preclude expressions such as

$xx \in X$. This axiom is neutral in that respect: it neither implies nor prevents the fact that $xx \in X$ for some $x \in X$. Other axioms of Definition 2.6 could be modified along the same lines. The resulting axiomatic system is heavier, but may be judged preferable in some cases. These developments have no impact on later topics and will not be pursued here. (See, however, Exercises 16, 17, and 18.) Incidentally, similar criticisms could be made about expressions such as $x \precsim x$ or $x \precsim yxz$. These expressions involve the same string on both sides of the relational symbol $\precsim$, which may occasionally be puzzling from an empirical standpoint. (An object cannot literally be placed on the two pans of the balance at the same time.) If one wishes, Definition 2.6 can be reformulated in order to eliminate the need for such expressions. This task will be left to the interested reader (Exercise 17).

2.10. Example: Time duration.   This example is attributed to Campbell (1957, pp. 550–553). The elements of A are pendulums. The experimenter's aim is to assign a number to each pendulum, measuring the duration of its period. Appropriate devices have been constructed permitting the following operation on two pendulums a,b: they can be started at exactly the same time; b can be started at the exact moment when a completes a full period; and it can be checked whether a completes a full period before b does. We write $ab \precsim c$ whenever a and c are started at the same time, b is started at the end of the first full period of a, and c does not terminate its first full period before b does. Notice that expressions such as $n * a$ and aba can be given a natural empirical meaning here. For instance, we write $n * a \prec b$ if pendulum a completes n consecutive full periods before pendulum b completes one full period. The specification of the set X in this context is now clear. With these conventions, the triple $(A,X,\precsim)$ should satisfy, at least approximately, the axioms of a measurement structure for extensive quantities. The physics of the pendulum is at the basis of some of our most traditional time-measuring devices. It is interesting to discover that these devices are justified in Theorem 2.7.

2.11. Example: Length, an alternative.   Few people realize exactly how arbitrary the basic physical scales are. Length, for example, could be measured by procedures essentially different from those discussed so far in this chapter, with no other consequences than that of rendering the writing of some physical laws more cumbersome and the actual application of the procedures more painful. I am not suggesting that mathematical or practical convenience are matters to be taken lightly. Clearly, however, they have no bearing on "physical reality." It is of some importance for a psychophysicist to have a clear understanding of such facts. Ultimately, the measurement of sensation will rely on an agreement in the psychophysical community, based essentially on considerations of convenience. The alternative procedure for measuring length discussed in this paragraph illustrates these remarks.

The experimenter is in a circular room. His or her task is to measure a collection A of rods. Rather than using the traditional procedures, the experimenter decides to compare the length of the rods by laying them against the wall with one end coinciding with a point p on the wall and extending to the right. (See Figure 2.2.)

For example, in order to check $ab \lesssim c$, rods a and c are placed with their left ends on point p and their right ends against the wall. Rod b is then laid against the wall with its left end coinciding with the right end of a. If the right end of b does not exceed the right end of c, one writes $ab \lesssim c$. Thus the set X is then the set of all strings of rods in A, which can be formed by laying down the rods end to end against the wall, as specified in Figure 2.2, without exceeding point p'. Points p and p' are on the same diameter. It should be clear that these procedures cannot yield the same scale as the usual one. However, it is not difficult to convince oneself that all the axioms of Definition 2.6 are approximately satisfied. (I am assuming that factors such as the width of the rods are negligible or have been appropriately taken care of by such devices as making marks on the wall.) Thus, we can apply Theorem 2.7 and claim that there is some function f such that for all rods $x, y \in X, x \lesssim y$ iff $f(x) \leqslant f(y)$, and if $xy \in X$ then $f(xy) = f(x) + f(y)$. Remember that this concatenation is different from the usual one. We do not have $\ell(xy) = \ell(x) + \ell(y)$, where ℓ is the function constructed —or approximated—using Method 3.4. (A different notation could have been used to stress the fact that the two concatenations under consideration involve distinct empirical operations. We could have written, for example, $f(\widehat{xy}) = f(x) + f(y)$.)

Nevertheless, from the viewpoint of "physical reality," f is as defensible as ℓ as a possible scale for length. The choice between ℓ and f—or between the two concatenations—is in no way based on empirical data. It is clear that ℓ is preferable but for the following practical reasons: it is easier to construct empirically and renders the writing of physical laws somewhat easier. For a more detailed discussion of this practically minded, or positivistic, attitude toward measurement, the reader is referred to Ellis (1966), where several other empirical examples of extensive measurement will also be found. This paragraph raises the question of the relation between ℓ and f. The answer is simple enough:

$$\ell(x) = \sin \left[\alpha f(x) \right] \tag{14}$$

for some constant $\alpha > 0$. We might perhaps have guessed this result. The

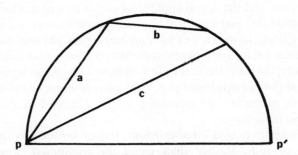

FIGURE 2.2. Alternative procedures for measuring the length of rods: $ab \lesssim c$.

procedure discussed here amounts, in fact, to the concatenation of the angles—from the center of the circle—subtended by the rods; $f(x)$ in Equation 14 is a measure of the angle subtended by x. A proof that Equation 14 is correct is contained in Exercises 21 to 24 at the end of the chapter. The importance, in the above discussion, of the shape of the wall along which the rods are laid, should be clearly recognized: a circular shape is critical. The measurement procedure outlined above could not be carried out if the wall had a different shape, say elliptic or parabolic. This may be puzzling since it is far from obvious which of the axioms of Definition 2.6 would fail to hold (see Exercise 27). A quick way of convincing oneself that at least one of these axioms must fail is to show that the "commutativity" relation

$$xy \sim yx$$

would not hold in these cases (cf. Remark 2.8). It turns out that the straight line and the circle are the only curves with this property.

In the next section, we turn to more technical matters. First, we return to Theorem 2.7 and provide a proof. We also show that, under the assumptions of this theorem, the set $\ell(X)$ of scale values must, in some sense, be "regularly spaced." One example of such a regularly spaced set is the set of positive integers $\mathbb{N}$. That is, we assign the number 1 to the smallest rod, the number 2 to the next smallest rod, and so on. Another example is an open or half open interval; that is $\ell(X) = (0,\zeta)$ or $\ell(X) = (0,\zeta)$, for some positive number ζ. In this second example there is no smallest rod. These are only two cases of a very general situation that is analyzed precisely in Theorem 2.13. The case where $\ell(X)$ is an interval is then investigated in detail. We ask and answer the following question. Under which additional axiom on an extensive system is the function ℓ of Theorem 2.7 a mapping onto a real interval? This section is written in a mathematically more compact style than the preceding ones. To stress this fact, we star the whole section.

*COMPLEMENTS AND PROOFS

2.12. Proof of Theorem 2.7. We recall that if $n,m \in \mathbb{N}$ and $x \in X$, then $(n + m) * x = (n * x)(m * x)$ and $nm * x = n * (m * x)$. Let us first state several lemmas.

Lemma 1. If $n,m \in \mathbb{N}, n * x \in X$, and $m * x \in X$, then $n * x \precsim m * x$ iff $n \leqslant m$ (see Exercise 7).

Define

$$S(x,y) = \{m \in \mathbb{N} \mid m * x \prec y\},$$

$$S'(x,y) = \{m \in \mathbb{N} \mid m * x \precsim y\}.$$

Lemma 2. For any $x,y \in X, S'(x,y)$ is a finite set.

Proof.   Take $x, y \in X$ arbitrarily and suppose that $x \prec y$. By Axiom 6, there is a positive integer $q = \max S(x,y)$. If $(q + k)$, $(q + k + j) \in S'(x,y)$ for some $k, j \in \mathbb{N}$, we obtain $(q + k + j) * x \precsim y \precsim (q + k) * x$, since $(q + k) \notin S(x,y)$, by definition of q. Since $\precsim$ is transitive, this yields $(q + k + j) * x \precsim (q + k) * x$, a contradiction of Lemma 1. Thus, $S'(x,y)$ contains at most one integer not contained in $S(x,y)$. In the case $y \precsim x$, it follows easily that $S'(x,y) = \{1\}$. ∎

Lemma 3.   *If $y \in X$ is such that $z \prec y$ for no $z \in X$, then for all $x \in X$, there exists a unique, positive integer $p(x)$ such that $p(x) * y \sim x$.*

Proof.   Using Lemma 2, define $p(x) = \max S'(y,x)$. We have thus $p(x) * y \precsim x$. Suppose that $p(x) * y \prec x$. By Axiom 5 we have, for some $z \in X$, $[p(x)*y]z \sim x$ with $y \precsim z$ by hypothesis. From Axiom 3 we derive

$$[p(x) * y] y \in X$$

with $[p(x) * y] y = [p(x) + 1] y \precsim [p(x) * y] z \sim x$. Using Axiom 2 again (transitivity), this gives $[p(x) + 1] \in S'(y,x)$, a contradiction. The uniqueness of $p(x)$ follows from Lemma 1.

We consider two cases.

Case 1.   There exists $y \in X$ such that $z \prec y$ for no $z \in X$. Define $\ell(x) = p(x)$ for all $x \in X$ (Lemma 3). Suppose that $xz \in X$. Then, successively,

$$\ell(xz) * y \sim xz \qquad\qquad \text{(by Lemma 3)}$$
$$\sim [\ell(x) * y][\ell(z) * y] \qquad \text{(by Axioms 2, 3 and Lemma 3)}$$
$$= [\ell(x) + \ell(z)] * y$$

yielding $\ell(xz) = \ell(x) + \ell(z)$ by Lemma 1. This proves (ii). By Axiom 2 and Lemmas 1 and 3, for any $x, z \in X$, $x \precsim z$ iff $\ell(x) * y \precsim \ell(z) * y$ iff $\ell(x) \leqslant \ell(z)$, establishing (i). This also shows that $\ell > 0$ since $1 * y \sim y$ implies that $1 = \ell(y) \leqslant \ell(x)$ for all $x \in X$. Finally, we turn to the uniqueness. Let k be another function satisfying the conditions of the theorem. Since X is operant, we have $yx \in X$ for some $x \in X$; this implies that $yy \in X$, $y \prec yy$ by Axioms 3 and 4. Thus, $k(y) < 2 k(y)$, yielding $k(y) = \alpha$ for some $\alpha > 0$. For every $x \in X$, we have $k(x) = k[p(x) * y] = p(x)k(y) = \ell(x)\alpha$.

Case 2.   For all $x \in X$ there exists $w \in X$ such that $w \prec x$. As a first step, we construct a sequence (w_n) in X inductively as follows. Choose w_1 arbitrarily. Next, take w'_1, w''_1 such that $w'_1 \prec w_1$, $w'_1 w''_1 \sim w_1$. (This is possible by hypothesis and Axiom 5.) If $w'_1 \precsim w''_1$, define $w_2 = w'_1$; otherwise define $w_2 = w''_1$. Thus, $w_2 \sim \min_{\precsim} \{w'_1, w''_1\}$ (where this minimum is arbitrary if $w'_1 \sim w''_1$). If $w'_n w''_n \sim w_n$, similarly define $w_{n+1} \sim \min_{\precsim} \{w'_n, w''_n\}$. Clearly, w_n is well defined for every $n \in \mathbb{N}$, with $w_{n+1} \prec 2 * w_{n+1} \precsim w_n$ (Axioms 4, 3, and 2). By induction, we obtain for all $n, m \in \mathbb{N}$, $2^m * w_{n+m} \precsim w_n$. Notice that for all $x \in X$, we must have $w_n \precsim x$ if n is large enough. (Indeed, if $x \prec w_n$ for all $n \in \mathbb{N}$, we have $2^m * x \precsim 2^m * w_{m+1} \precsim w_1$ for all $m \in \mathbb{N}$. In other words, $S'(x,w_1)$ is an infinite set contradicting Lemma 2.) For any $x \in X$ and $w_n \precsim x$, define $p_n(x) = \max S'(w_n,x)$. By definition,

$p_n(x) * w_n \lesssim x$. Successively,

$$[2^m p_n(x)] * w_{n+m} = p_n(x) * (2^m * w_{n+m}) \lesssim p_n(x) * w_n \lesssim x,$$

hence

$$2^m p_n(x) \leqslant \max S'(w_{n+m}, x)$$
$$= p_{n+m}(x).$$

This argument shows that for every $x \in X$, $p_n(x) \to \infty$. We establish the following key facts.

(a) For every $x, z \in X, (p_n(x)/p_n(z))$ converges.
(b) If we fix $y \in X$ and define for all $x \in X, \ell(x) = \lim_{n \to \infty} [p_n(x)/p_n(y)]$, then ℓ satisfies conditions (i) and (ii) of the theorem.

We use two basic inequalities: if $n \geqslant m$, and m is large enough that $w_m \lesssim x$, then

$$p_m(x) p_n(w_m) \leqslant p_n(x) < [p_m(x) + 1][p_n(w_m) + 1]. \tag{15}$$

To prove (15) observe that, since $p_n(w_m) * w_n \lesssim w_m$, we have, by Axiom 3,

$$[p_m(x) p_n(w_m)] * w_n = p_m(x) * [p_n(w_m) * w_n]$$
$$\lesssim p_m(x) * w_m$$
$$\lesssim x,$$

yielding the left inequality by Axiom 2 and the definition of $p_n(x)$. Suppose that $[p_m(x) + 1][p_n(w_m) + 1] \leqslant p_n(x)$. Then $\{[p_m(x) + 1][p_n(w_m) + 1]\} * w_n \lesssim x$. From $w_m < [p_n(w_m) + 1) * w_n$, we obtain $[p_m(x) + 1] * w_m \lesssim x$, a contradiction. We conclude that (15) holds. In particular

$$p_n(x) < [p_n(w_m) + 1][p_m(x) + 1]$$

and

$$p_n(w_m) p_m(z) \leqslant p_n(z),$$

for any $x, z \in X$ with $w_n, w_m \lesssim x, z$. Multiplying these two inequalities and rearranging terms, yields

$$\frac{p_n(x)}{p_n(z)} < \frac{[p_n(w_m) + 1][p_m(x) + 1]}{p_n(w_m) p_m(z)}$$

which leads to

$$\limsup_{n \to \infty} \frac{p_n(x)}{p_n(z)} < \frac{p_m(x) + 1}{p_m(z)}. \tag{16}$$

Let $\bar{L}, \underline{L}$ be respectively the lim sup and lim inf of the sequence $[p_n(x)/p_n(z)]$. From (16), we obtain

$$\bar{L} \leqslant \liminf_{m \to \infty} \frac{p_m(x) + 1}{p_m(z)} = \underline{L},$$

since $p_m(z) \to \infty$.

We conclude that $0 < \bar{L} \leqslant L$. In other words, for any $x, z \in X$ the sequence $[p_n(x)/p_n(z)]$ converges to a positive real number. Fix $y \in X$ arbitrarily and define for any $x \in X$, $\ell(x) = \lim_{n \to \infty} [p_n(x)/p_n(y)]$. Then $0 < \ell(x)$ and, in particular, $\ell(y) = 1$. Suppose that $xz \in X$. Since $p_n(x) * w_n \precsim x, p_n(z) * w_n \precsim z$ as soon as n is large enough, we have, by Axiom 3,

$$[p_n(x) * w_n][p_n(z) * w_n] = [p_n(x) + p_n(z)] * w_n \precsim xz,$$

from which we immediately derive

$$p_n(x) + p_n(z) \leqslant p_n(xz) < p_n(x) + p_n(z) + 2. \tag{17}$$

(Indeed, if $p_n(x) + p_n(z) + 2 \leqslant p_n(xz)$, then

$$xz \prec \{[p_n(x) + 1] * w_n\}\{[p_n(z) + 1] * w_n\} = [p_n(x) + p_n(z) + 2] * w_n \precsim xz.)$$

Dividing in (17) by $p_n(y)$, and letting $n \to \infty$, yields $\ell(xz) = \ell(x) + \ell(z)$. In other words, Property (ii) of the theorem holds. Suppose that $x \prec z$; then $xw \sim z$ for some $w \in X$, by Axiom 5. This leads to $p_n(xw) = p_n(z)$. Dividing by $p_n(y)$ and letting $n \to \infty$ yields $\ell(xw) = \ell(x) + \ell(w) = \ell(z)$, which implies $\ell(x) < \ell(z)$. Thus Property (i) also holds. We consider uniqueness. Take any $x \in X$. Suppose that $x \prec z$ for some z. Then $xw \sim z$, with $w_n \precsim w$ for some $w \in X$ and some $n \in \mathbb{N}$. By Axiom 3 this leads to $xw_n \in X$. Hence $[p_n(x) + 1] * w_n \in X$. We have thus

$$p_n(x) * w_n \precsim x \prec [p_n(x) + 1] * w_n. \tag{18}$$

Similarly,

$$p_n(w_2) * w_n \precsim w_2 \prec [p_n(w_2) + 1] * w_n. \tag{19}$$

If some function k exists, mapping X into the positive reals, and satisfying (i) and (ii), then (18) and (19) yields, respectively,

$$p_n(x)k(w_n) \leqslant k(x) < [p_n(x) + 1]k(w_n)$$

$$p_n(w_2)k(w_n) \leqslant k(w_2) < [p_n(w_2) + 1]k(w_n).$$

Dividing these inequalities appropriately, we obtain

$$\frac{p_n(x)}{p_n(w_2) + 1} < \frac{k(x)}{k(w_2)} < \frac{p_n(x) + 1}{p_n(w_2)}.$$

If $n \to \infty$, this gives $\ell(x)/\ell(w_2) = k(x)/k(w_2)$, that is, $k(x) = \alpha\ell(x)$, with $\alpha = k(w_2)/\ell(w_2) > 0$. If $z \precsim x$ for all $z \in X$, then in particular, $z'z'' \sim x$ for some z', z'', yielding $k(x) = k(z'z'') = k(z') + k(z'') = \alpha\ell(z') + \alpha\ell(z'') = \alpha\ell(x)$. ∎

Under the assumptions of Theorem 2.7, the set of scale values assigned to the rods by the function ℓ can be described as "regularly spaced." This notion is made precise in the next theorem (Falmagne, 1971a, 1975).

2.13. Theorem.   Let $(A, X, \precsim)$ be an extensive system, then $\ell(X) = G \cap I$, where ℓ is the function of Theorem 2.7, G is a subgroup of the additive reals, and I is a real, positive interval having 0 as a limit point.

(We recall that a number ξ is a limit point of a set S of real numbers iff every neighborhood of ξ contains a point $p \neq \xi$ such that $p \in S$.)

For example, we can have $\ell(X) = \mathbb{Z} \cap (0,\zeta)$ or $\ell(X) = \mathbb{Q} \cap (0,\zeta)$, ζ being some positive constant. In the proof of this theorem, we will use the following two facts: (i) if $r,s,t \in \ell(X)$, with $r + s \leqslant t$, then $(r + s) \in \ell(X)$; (ii) if $s,t \in \ell(X)$, with $s < t$, then $(t - s) \in \ell(X)$. The proofs are almost immediate (Exercise 25).

Proof.   Let G be the subgroup of the additive reals generated by $\ell(X)$. Take $s \in \ell(X), t \in G$, and $0 < t < s$. The theorem follows if we show that $t \in \ell(X)$. Since $\ell(X)$ generates G,

$$t = \sum_{i \in J} s_i - \sum_{j \in J'} s_j \tag{20}$$

for two finite index sets J,J' and $s_i, s_j \in \ell(X)$ for all $i \in J, j \in J'$. In fact, we can assume without loss of generality that J' is empty. Indeed, suppose this is not the case but that appropriate cancellations have been made in (20), that is, $s_i \neq s_j$ for all $i \in J, j \in J'$. Let $s_n = \max\{s_k \,|\, k \in J \cup J'\}$. If $n \in J$, then $s_n > s_m$ for some $m \in J'$ and we have $s_n = s'_m + s_m$ for some $s'_m \in \ell(X)$. Thus t can be rewritten as follows.

$$t = \sum_{i \in J - \{n\}} s_i + s'_m - \sum_{j \in J' - \{m\}} s_j.$$

Notice that the number of terms has been reduced by one. Suppose that $n \in J'$. Then $s_n > s_m$ for some $m \in J$, with $s_n + s'_m + s_m$ for some $s'_m \in \ell(X)$. We write t as

$$t = \sum_{i \in J - \{m\}} s_i - \sum_{j \in J' - \{n\}} s_j - s'_m,$$

and again, the number of terms has been reduced by one. At each step of this reduction process, either a positive or negative term is eliminated in the expression of t. Then, some further cancellation takes place if appropriate. (For instance, s'_m in the above equation may be equal to one of the s_i, $i \in J$.) Observing that $t > 0$, we see that this reduction process must lead to the exhaustion of the negative terms before the positive terms. Without loss of generality, we can thus simply assume that $t = \sum_{i \in J} s_i, s_i \in \ell(X)$ for all $i \in J$. If $J = \{i\}$, then $s_i = t \in \ell(X)$. Otherwise for $i,j \in J$, we have $s_i + s_j \leqslant t < s$, and fact (i) gives us $(s_i + s_j) \in \ell(X)$. By induction we conclude that $\sum_{i \in J} s_i = t \in \ell(X)$.

2.14. Example.   This case was already analyzed in 2.12 (the proof of Theorem 2.7). We discuss it here from the viewpoint of Theorem 2.13. Let $(A,X,\precsim)$ be an extensive system with a distinguished element $\zeta \in X$ satisfying the following: for all $x \in X$, $x \sim n * \zeta$ for some $n \in \mathbb{N}$. Let ℓ be the function of Theorem 2.7. We can assume that $\ell(\zeta) = 1$. Then if $x \sim n * \zeta$, we have $\ell(x) = \ell(n * \zeta) = n\ell(\zeta) = n$. We have thus either $\ell(X) = \mathbb{N}$ or $\ell(X) = \{n \in \mathbb{N} \,|\, n < m\}$ for some $m \in \mathbb{N}$. In other words, $G = \mathbb{Z}$.

By far the most interesting case from an empirical standpoint in Theorem 2.13 arises when $G = \mathbb{R}$ that is, $\ell(X)$ itself is a real interval. The above example shows that some additional axiom on $(A,X,\precsim)$ is needed. Theorem 2.15 and Definition 2.16 pave the way for Theorem 2.17, where an appropriate axiom is introduced.

2.15. Theorem. *Let G be a subgroup of the additive group of the reals such that* $G \cap I = \phi$ *for some open, nondegenerate interval I; then G is a discrete subgroup, namely* $G = \{s \in \mathbb{R} \mid s = n\zeta, n \in \mathbb{Z}\}$ *for some real number* ζ.

This is a well-known result (e.g., Choquet, 1966, p. 56).

Proof. Under the conditions of the theorem, 0 is an isolated point of G. (Otherwise, we can find $t \in G$ and $m \in \mathbb{Z}$ such that $mt \in I$, a contradiction.) Let $\zeta = \inf \{s \in G \mid s > 0\}, \zeta > 0$. Suppose that $\zeta \notin G$. Then ζ is a limit point of G and there exists a strictly decreasing sequence (t_n) in G converging to ζ. If n is large enough, $\zeta > (t_n - t_{n-1}) \in G$, a contradiction. Thus $\zeta \in G$ and

$$G_0 = \{s \in \mathbb{R} \mid s = n\zeta, n \in \mathbb{Z}\} \subset G.$$

Suppose that $G - G_0$ is not empty. Then $n\zeta < r < (n + 1)\zeta$ for some $r \in G$ and $n \in \mathbb{Z}$. The element $(r - n\zeta) \in G$ would satisfy $0 < r - n\zeta < \zeta$, which is impossible by the definition of ζ. ∎

2.16. Definition. Let $(X, \precsim)$ be a weak order. A partition $\{X', X''\}$ of X is a *cut* iff $x' \prec x''$ for all $x' \in X'$, $x'' \in X''$. A point $x \in X$ is a *separating point* of a cut $\{X', X''\}$ iff $x' \precsim x \precsim x''$ for all $x' \in X'$, $x'' \in X''$. A weak order is *Dedekind complete* iff all its cuts have separating points, and moreover $x \sim y$ whenever x and y are separating points of the same cut. An extensive system $(A, X, \precsim)$ is *Dedekind complete* iff $(X, \precsim)$ is Dedekind complete.

2.17. Theorem. *Let* $(A, X, \precsim)$ *be a Dedekind complete, extensive system. Then, the function* ℓ *of Theorem 2.7 maps X on a real, positive interval, having 0 as a limit point.*

Proof. Since X is operant, $\ell(X)$ contains at least two points, say $\ell(x_1) < \ell(x_2)$. By Theorem 2.13, $\ell(X) = G \cap I$ for some subgroup G of the additive reals and some real, positive interval I having zero as a limit point. Observe that G cannot be a discrete subgroup of the form $G = \{s \in \mathbb{R} \mid s = n\zeta, n \in \mathbb{Z}\}$, for some positive real number ζ. (Indeed, if this were the case we would have $\ell(x_1) = n\zeta < (n + 1)\zeta = \ell(z) \leqslant \ell(x_2)$ for some $z \in X, x_1 \prec z \precsim x_2$. Defining $W' = \{w \in X \mid w \precsim x_1\}$, $W'' = \{w \in X \mid z \precsim w\}$, we would have a cut $\{W', W''\}$ with two separating points x, z satisfying $x \prec z$, a contradiction of the hypothesis.) Take $s \leqslant r \leqslant t$, for some $s, t \in \ell(X)$ and assume that $r \notin \ell(X)$. Define $X' = \{x \in X \mid \ell(x) < r\}$, $X'' = \{x \in X \mid \ell(x) > r\}$. Then $\{X', X''\}$ is a cut that, by hypothesis, has a separating point y, with say $\ell(y) = r_0$. We must have either $r_0 < r$ or $r < r_0$. If $r_0 < r$, then $[(r_0, r) \cap G] \subset [(r_0, r) \cap \ell(X)] = \varnothing$. By Theorem 2.15, G is discrete, a contradiction. The argument in the case $r < r_0$ is similar. We conclude that $G = \mathbb{R}$, that is, $\ell(X) = I$. ∎

2.18. Example. Suppose that a spring balance is used to measure the mass of a set X (of strings of a set A) of objects rather than the two-pan equal-arm balance of Example 2.9. Let the number $H(x)$ be the reading of the spring balance when the string x is placed in the pan. We do not assume that the balance has been calibrated, or that Hooke's law holds perfectly.[2] In other terms $H(x)$ need not be an accurate assessment of the mass of x. We assume, however, that the set X is so finely graded that if $H(x) < t < H(y)$ for some strings x, y and some real number t, then it is possible to find some string $z \in X$ such that $H(z) = t$. Define a binary relation $\precsim$ on X by $x \precsim y$ iff $H(x) \leqslant H(y)$. Then $(X, \precsim)$ is a weak order. It is easy to see that all cuts $\{X', X''\}$ of X have separating points; and that if x, y are two separating points of $\{X', X''\}$, then $\sup H(X') \leqslant H(x) \leqslant H(y) \leqslant \inf H(X'')$. That is, $x \sim y$. If the triple $(A, X, \precsim)$ also satisfies the other axioms of an extensive system (Definition 2.6), then the function ℓ of Theorem 2.7 maps X onto a real interval.

REFERENCE NOTES—FURTHER DEVELOPMENTS

The first attempt to theorize extensive measurement seems to have been made by Helmholtz (1887). The first correct axiomatization is due to Hölder (1901), (see Exercise 15). Both Helmholtz and Hölder formalized the concatenation procedure by a binary operation $(a, b) \mapsto a \nabla b$ on a set A; the comparison procedure is formalized by a binary relation $\precsim$. This viewpoint has prevailed in all works published since then. The notations in this chapter are slightly different, the concatenation being formalized by the notion of a string. A possible objection to the language of strings—which was adopted here mainly for expository reasons—is that it deemphasizes the associativity of the concatenation. Indeed, if the binary operation ∇ is used, one has to state formally that

$$a \nabla (b \nabla c) = (a \nabla b) \nabla c,$$

that is, forming $b \nabla c$, then $a \nabla (b \nabla c)$, results in the same object as when forming $a \nabla b$ first, then $(a \nabla b) \nabla c$. In the language of strings, this holds automatically since both objects are denoted by the same string abc. The impact of this objection seems minor. For example, in the cases of mass or length, as measured by the usual methods (those discussed in this chapter), associativity is automatically satisfied by the very nature of the empirical manipulations involved and should not be regarded as a substantive axiom. In such cases, it seems proper to deemphasize this condition in the axiom system.[3]

The progress made since Hölder's work has been toward a greater realism of the axiom systems. For instance, Hölder assumes that the binary relation ∇ is closed (i.e., $a \nabla b$ is defined for all $a, b \in A$). This, of course, leads us to postulate the existence of arbitrarily long rods (or of objects of arbitrarily large mass). This

---

2. Hooke's law: the extension of a piece of uniform material is proportional to the force applied to it. In this example, we only require the extension—measured in usual length unit—to be strictly increasing with the force. This assumption is reasonable since Hooke's law only holds approximately.

3. In fact, one can object to the binary operation ∇ when used in conjunction with a weak order $\precsim$. The difficulty comes from expressions such as $a \nabla b = c$. If we can ascertain that the composite object $a \nabla b$—for instance, a and b placed in the same pan of the balance—is *identical* to some object c, the relation $\precsim$ might as well be a simple order (an antisymmetric weak order). On the whole, the language of strings seems preferable, at least in some experimental situations.

assumption is relaxed in the axiom systems of Krantz (1968), Luce and Marley (1969), and Falmagne (1971a, 1975). In the last two papers, another assumption is also relaxed. As indicated in Theorem 2.17, Definition 2.6 implies that, in the Dedekind complete case, objects with arbitrarily small (positive) scale values exist. The key axiom responsible for this situation is Axiom 5, which states that if $x \prec y$ there exists z such that $xz \sim y$. The axiom systems in Falmagne (1971a, 1975) do not involve such assumptions. In the Dedekind complete case, the scale ℓ maps the set of empirical objects onto a real, positive interval that may or may not have 0 as a limit point. Incidentally, the assumption that arbitrarily small (or large) elements exist in the empirical set should not be considered as an innocuous mathematical idealization. For example, if Axiom 5 is dropped in Definition 2.6, the following condition cannot be derived: if $xy \sim zw$, $y'w \sim xz'$ and $y'y, zz' \in X$, then $y'y \sim zz'$ (Exercise 20). The empirical importance of this last condition is clear. The associativity of the concatenation can also be relaxed. Cohen and Narens (1979) explored in depth the consequences of a condition generalizing associativity.

Another direction of progress involves the binary relation formalizing the comparison procedure. Krantz (1967), Luce (1973), and Holman (1974) considered the case where the comparison procedure lacks sensitivity: if $x \sim y$, it may, in fact, be that x has a little less or a little more of the attribute to be measured than y has. This idea was encountered in Chapter 1 (1.40, 1.41), where it was formalized as a binary relation called semiorder. In the context of extensive measurement, this leads to a theory of approximate measurement. For other developments on the algebraic theory of extensive measurement, see Krantz et al. (1971, Chapter 3; a second volume is in preparation), where further references can also be found.

Finally, probabilistic axiomatizations of extensive measurement were investigated by the author (Falmagne, 1980).

EXERCISES

1. Suppose that the construction of an extensive scale for length is carried out in a room, the size of which is exactly equal to that of $24 * y$, where y is the "unit." What is the least upper bound on the error committed in measuring a rod x, such that $6 * y \precsim x \prec 7 * y$, using Method 2.3?
2. Give a detailed derivation of (5), (6), and (7).
3. Give a detailed derivation of (9).
4. Let (w_n) be the sequence of smaller and smaller rods used in Method 2.4.

   (i) Give an informal argument showing that $2^m * w_{n+m} \precsim w_n$.
   (ii) Let x be any rod such that $w_{18} \precsim x \precsim y$, where y is the unit; assume that $w_1 \precsim y$. Show that the absolute value of the error committed in assigning p_{18}/p'_{18} as a scale value to x is smaller than 2^{-17}. That is, prove that $|\gamma_{18}| < 2^{-17}$. (*Hint.* Use Formula 9 and (i) above.)

5. Using Definition 2.6, give an inductive proof of the following facts: if $n,m \in \mathbb{N}$ and $x \in X$, then $(n + m) * x = (n * x)(m * x)$ and $(nm) * x = n * (m * x)$.
6. Give an instance of application for Axioms 4 and 6 of Definition 2.6 when using Method 2.4.
7. Prove Lemma 1 in 2.12.
8. Prove that an extensive system (Definition 2.6) satisfies the following properties.

   For all $x,y \in X$:

   (i) $y \prec xy$.
   (ii) $xy \in X$ iff $yx \in X$, and when both hold, then $xy \sim yx$.

   (*Hint.* Use (i) and Theorem 2.7 to prove (ii); only Axioms 2 to 5 are needed to prove (i).)
9. Verify that Axiom 1 of Definition 2.6 is not satisfied by the following triple $(A,X,\precsim)$ but that all the others are: $A = \{a,b,c\}$; $X = \{a,b,aa\}$; $a \precsim b \sim aa$. (In this and the following four exercises, we assume that $\precsim$ is a reflexive, transitive, binary relation with $a \prec b$ iff ($a \precsim b$ and not $b \precsim a$); $a \sim b$ iff ($a \precsim b$ and $b \precsim a$). This example shows that Axiom 1 is *independent* of the other five axioms of Definition 2.6, in the sense that it cannot be derived from them. It can be shown that, in fact, each of the six axioms of Definition 2.6 is independent of the remaining ones. The following five exercises establish this fact. Each one involves an example satisfying all the axioms except one. The reader should discover the failing axiom, provide an explicit counterexample showing that it does indeed fail, and verify that the other axioms are satisfied.
10. (*Continuation.*) $A = \{a,b,c\}$; $X = A \cup \{aa\}$; $a \prec b \sim aa$.
11. (*Continuation.*) $A = \{a,b,c\}$; $X = A \cup \{aa, bc, cb\}$; $a \sim b \sim c \prec aa \sim bc \sim cb$.
12. (*Continuation.*) $A = \{a\}$; $X = \{n * a \mid n \in \mathbb{N}\}$; $n * a \sim m * a$ for all $n,m \in \mathbb{N}$.
13. (*Continuation.*) $A = \{a,b\}$; $X = A$; $a \prec b$.
*14. (*Continuation.*) This example is more difficult to state than the preceding ones. We set $A = \{(r,s) \in \mathbb{R} \times \mathbb{R} \mid r > 0 \text{ or } (r = 0, s > 0)\}$; let X be the set of all strings of A. To define $\precsim$ on X we first define a simple order $\leqslant$ on A as follows: $(r,s) \leqslant (r',s')$ iff either $r < r'$ or ($r = r'$ and $s \leqslant s'$). (This type of ordering is called a *lexicographic ordering*. It is easy to prove that $\leqslant$ is reflexive, transitive, connected, and antisymmetric on A; cf. Exercise 12 in Chapter 1.) Next, for $x,y \in X$ with $x = a_1 a_2 \cdots a_n$, $y = b_1 b_2 \cdots b_m$ $(a_i \in A, 1 \leqslant i \leqslant n; b_j \in A, 1 \leqslant j \leqslant m)$, we define $x \precsim y$ iff $\sum_{i=1}^{n} a_i \leqslant \sum_{j=1}^{m} b_j$ (where $\sum$ represents the vector addition on the real plane).
*15. Show that the following result, known as Hölder's theorem (1901), is a corollary of Theorem 2.7: Any Archimedean, simply ordered group is isomorphic to an ordered subgroup of the additive real numbers. We recall that $(G,\nabla,\leqslant)$ is *an ordered group* iff (i) (G,∇) is a group, (ii) $(G,\leqslant)$ is a simple order, and (iii) if $a,b,c \in G$, then $a \leqslant b$ implies both $a \nabla c \leqslant b \nabla c$ and $c \nabla a \leqslant c \nabla b$. The ordered group $(G,\nabla,\leqslant)$ is *Archimedean* iff whenever $e < a$ and $b \in G$, then $b < na$ for some $n \in \mathbb{N}$, where e is the identity of the group.
16. Rewrite Axiom 6 of Definition 2.6 avoiding expressions such as $m * x$. Which

other axioms of this definition involves such expressions? If there are any, modify them accordingly.

17. Rewrite Definition 2.6 avoiding expressions such as $x \lesssim x$, $ab \lesssim bac$, etc. (Such expressions should not be derivable from the axioms.)

*18. Is the axiom system modified as in the two preceding exercises such that a version of Theorem 2.7 still holds? If this is the case, state the result exactly and sketch a proof.

19. Let A be a set of resistors: for $a_1, a_2, \ldots, a_n \in A$ denote $a_1 a_2 \cdots a_n$ the sequence of resistors wired in series; write $a_1 a_2 \cdots a_n \lesssim b_1 b_2 \cdots b_m$ if the resistance of $a_1 a_2 \cdots a_n$ does not exceed that of $b_1 b_2 \cdots b_m$. Discuss this example from the viewpoint of Definition 2.6 (Krantz et al., 1971).

20. Show that the following condition is independent of Axioms 1, 2, 3, 4, and 6 of Definition 2.6: if $xy \sim zw$, $y'w \sim xz'$ and $y'y$, $zz' \in X$, then $y'y \sim zz'$. (Construct an example in which this axiom is not satisfied but Axioms 1 to 4 and 6 are; see Falmagne, 1975.)

21. Let $(A, X, \lesssim)$ be an extensive system. Let ℓ be a mapping of A into some arbitrary set. Let X_ℓ be the set of strings of $\ell(A)$, defined by $\ell(a_1)\ell(a_2)\cdots \ell(a_n) \in X_\ell$ iff $a_1 a_2 \cdots a_n \in X$. Define a binary relation $\lesssim_\ell$ on X_ℓ by $\ell(a_1)\ell(a_2)\cdots \ell(a_n) \lesssim_\ell \ell(b_1)\ell(b_2)\cdots \ell(b_m)$ iff $a_1 a_2 \cdots a_n \lesssim b_1 b_2 \cdots b_m$. Sketch a proof showing that $(\ell(A), X_\ell, \lesssim_\ell)$ is an extensive system.

22. Let $(A, X, \lesssim)$ be as in 2.11; let $\ell(x)$ denote the usual length of x; let $f(x)$ denote the length of x as measured by the method of 2.11. Suppose that $ab \sim c$ (thus $f(c) = f(a) + f(b)$). Assume that the diameter of the room has a usual length equal to 1 ($\ell(d) = 1$). Using basic trigonometric formulas, prove that

$$\ell(c) = \{\ell(a)^2 + \ell(b)^2 - 2\ell(a)^2\ell(b)^2 + 2\ell(a)\ell(b)[1 - \ell(a)^2]^{1/2} \cdot [1 - \ell(b)^2]^{1/2}\}^{1/2}.$$

*23. (*Continuation.*) Using the result of Exercise 21 to prove that there exists some function ψ, the domain of which includes the range of ℓ, such that for some constant $\zeta > 0$, $\zeta f(a) = \psi[\ell(a)]$, for all $a \in A$ with, in particular, if $ab \sim c$, $\zeta f(ab) = \psi[\ell(c)] = \psi[\ell(a)] + \psi[\ell(b)] = \zeta f(a) + \zeta f(b)$.

*24. (*Continuation.*) Show that

$$\psi\{[s^2 + t^2 - 2s^2 t^2 (1 - s^2)^{1/2} (1 - t)^{1/2}]^{1/2}\} = \psi(s) + \psi(t).$$

Assume that ψ is differentiable with $\psi'(0) \neq 0$. Show that $\psi(s) = \alpha \sin^{-1}(s)$ for some $\alpha > 0$. (*Hint.* Compute $\psi'(s)/\psi'(t)$, set $t = 0$ and integrate.) Argue that this and the preceding two exercises constitute a proof that Equation 18 is indeed correct.

25. Let $(A, X, \lesssim)$ be an extensive system with a function $\ell \colon X \to \mathbb{R}$, satisfying the condition of Theorem 2.7. Prove that (i) if $r, s, t \in \ell(X)$ with $r + s \leqslant t$, then $(r + s) \in \ell(X)$; (ii) if $s, t \in \ell(X)$ with $s < t$, then $(t - s) \in \ell(X)$.

26. This exercise involves an incursion in acoustic theory. Consider a collection of cophasics, 2000 Hz pure tones, of 0.5 sec duration, varying in intensity. Pairs (a, b) of such tones are selected and presented to the subject, using

earphones: tone *a* in the left auditory channel, tone *b* in the right auditory channel. Such stimuli are known to fuse, including a unique sensation of loudness, fairly sharply localized in the head. The locus of the sensation seems to vary systematically with the intensities (Mills, 1972, Chapter 8). Write $a \lesssim b$ if the pair (a,b) gives rise to a sensation localized in the median plane between the ears, or to the right of this plane; write *ab* for the tone resulting from the physical superposition of *a* and *b*. (Thus, for example, *ab* can be presented in the left auditory channel and *cde* in the right.)

   Which axioms of extensive measurement could possibly be violated? (Assume symmetry of the two auditory channels.)

27. Suppose that the extensive measurement procedures are carried out as outlined in Example 2.11, except that the shape of the room is elliptical rather than circular. Which of the axiom(s) of Definition 2.6 if any, would be violated? Prove your answer.

3
Functional Equations

It sometimes happens that theories in psychology or other empirical sciences are formalized by equations involving unknown functions. For instance, the theorist may be reluctant to make specific assumptions regarding the form of the functions involved in a mathematical model. The equations themselves often reduce the possibilities, however, and occasionally the restrictions are so severe as to restrict all forms to but a few. The most celebrated case in psychophysics involves the connection between Weber's law and the so-called Fechner's problem. The restrictions there are such as to yield a logarithm as the only possible form for a function, which Fechner interpreted as measuring the magnitude of the sensation evoked by a stimulus (cf. Chapters 4 and 5). Many other examples will be encountered in this book. This chapter discusses some useful results for analyzing such questions. The term functional equations describes the part of mathematics devoted to the discussion of problems of this kind, in which the unknowns are not numbers, but the form of the functions entering in an equation, or a system of equations. For a systematic treatment of functional equations, see for example, Aczél (1966).

With the exception of a basic result (Theorem 3.27, the proof of which relies on Theorems 2.7 and 2.17 established in Chapter 2), this chapter is self-contained. The techniques used in the proofs of the other theorems are elementary, and should be accessible to a reader armed with patience and only a limited amount of mathematical training. We further motivate our developments by a discussion of a few examples.

3.1. Examples. (a) *Plateau's experiment.* In a classical study, Plateau (1872) gave a pair of painted disks—one white, one black—to each of eight artists and instructed them to return to their respective studios and paint a gray disk midway between the two. The resulting gray disks, reported Plateau, were virtually identical for all eight artists, in spite of the variation in the illumination conditions. Let us suppose that such results would hold for any pair of gray disks. A possible formalization of this data would be as follows. We label the disks by their luminance in conventional units (lux). In particular, let (a,b) be a pair of gray disks in a specified viewing condition in Plateau's lab. We denote by $M(a,b)$ the resulting gray disk, under the same viewing conditions. Thus, M is a function of two variables, with values in the same (lux) scale. The artist, however, has performed the task in his studio, in different illumination conditions; that is, with the pair (ca,cb) (where c is some positive constant equal to the ratio of the illumination in the artist's studio to that of Plateau's lab). Formalizing Plateau's empirical finding, we hypothesize the resulting disk to be independent of the illumination. Consequently, the following equation must hold.

$$cM(a,b) = M(ca,cb). \tag{1}$$

Indeed, this equation means that the gray disk obtained in Plateau's lab is identical to that obtained in the artist's studio when seen under the same conditions. We still need to explain how the artist performs the task. A simple idea is that the gray disk is obtained from averaging the values of the two disks in the pair. This averaging, however, is not necessarily carried out on the lux scale. More precisely, we postulate the existence of a function u, a psychophysical scale, mapping the lux scale into the reals, and such that for any pair (a,b) of gray disks,

$$u[M(a,b)] = \frac{u(a) + u(b)}{2}. \tag{2}$$

Even though the function u is left unspecified, the above equation puts stringent constraints on the data and is quite testable (cf. Chapter 11). In fact, if both (1) and (2) are assumed to hold, the possible forms of u are limited to just two. Using the techniques of this chapter, it can be shown that under mild side conditions, u must be either a power function,

$$u(a) = \alpha a^\beta + \gamma;$$

or a logarithmic function

$$u(a) = \alpha \log a + \beta,$$

(α, β, γ being constants). *No other forms exist that would satisfy both (1) and (2)* (Theorem 3.12). This was noted by Krantz (personal communication, 1978), who also remarked that essentially the same argument applies to the basic "equal spacing" principle underlying the construction of the Munsell system (Munsell Book of Color, 1929).

(b) *Sound localization.* A subject is in a soundproof room wearing earphones. At each trial of an experiment, a pure tone of a given frequency (say, 1000 cps) is presented to him or her, with different intensities in the two auditory channels. Typically, the two components of the stimulus will fuse, and determine a sensation of loudness, fairly sharply localized in the head, at a point somewhere between the two ears. If one intensity is changed, the other remaining constant, the point of fusion (sound image) appears to move in the direction of 'the increased intensity. If both intensities are increased, their ratio remaining constant, no change in localization is experienced.[1]

In a well-known version of this study, the locus of the sensation was determined by a pointer attached to a mechanism delivering a puff of air on

---

1. This is not surprising. This experiment mimics a more realistic situation, in which a sound source located at some distance is moved toward a listener. It is of obvious biological importance that, in a free field, the perceived direction of the sound remains invariant.

subject's forehead (Békésy, 1960). The subject thus was required to move the mechanism until the direction of the puff seemed to coincide with the locus of the sensation evoked by the stimulus. The position of the pointer was recorded. It is generally believed that, in this situation, the locus of the sensation depends on the "difference between the intensities" of the tone in the two auditory channels (Mills, 1972). The quotes are ours and are meant to suggest a nonliteral intepretation. The difference in question is not necessarily to be taken in the standard physical units of intensities (i.e., sound pressure).

Conceivably, some transformation of these units may take place. Let us formalize this idea. We denote $M(a,b)$ to be the locus of the sensation evoked by the stimulus (a,b). Thus, a,b are in standard units of intensity and correspond to the left and right auditory channel, respectively, and $M(a,b)$ is a number indicating position (on the forehead, in Békésy's situation). The invariance of the locus for a constant ratio of the intensities implies.

$$M(a,b) = M(ca,cb), \tag{3}$$

where c is a positive constant. The assumption that the locus of the sensation depends on the "difference between the intensities" in the two auditory channels seems naturally captured by the equation

$$M(a,b) = F[\ell(a) - r(b)]. \tag{4}$$

The functions ℓ,r correspond to the left and right auditory channels (there is no *a priori* reason to assume symmetry); the function F maps the differences into the particular measure of location adopted in the experiment, for instance, the reading of the pointer in Békésy's situation. Equations 3 and 4 can each be tested empirically. If (3) is true, however, (4) is also true, and the analytical form of the functions ℓ, r is practically determined. We must have

$$\ell(a) = \alpha \log a + \beta,$$

$r(a) = \alpha \log a + \beta'$ for some constants α,β,β' (Exercise 15). No explicit error models were involved in this and the preceding example. We consider probabilistic models in our last four examples.

(c) *Normal distribution of sensory variables.* This example is perhaps less realistic than the preceding ones but quite in line with traditional assumptions. We use it here mainly to illustrate a startling result. The subject's task is similar to that of Plateau's experiment, in Example (a). At each trial of an experiment, two monochromatic patches of light, a,b differing in intensity, are flashed on a screen. By appropriately controlling two knobs, the subject must produce two new patches of light, z_1,z_2, according to two rules: (i) a must be midway between z_1 and b; (ii) z_2 must be between a and b and such that the "subjective distance" between z_2 and a is twice that between b and z_2. We symbolize these two rules by the following mnemonics (which have no arithmetical meaning).

$$a \cong \tfrac{1}{2}z_1 \oplus \tfrac{1}{2}b, \tag{5}$$

$$z_2 \cong \tfrac{1}{3}a \oplus \tfrac{2}{3}b. \tag{6}$$

Suppose that the presentation of a,b determines two (unobservable) sensory impressions, x_a,x_b, which we regard as values of two random variables $\mathbf{X}_a,\mathbf{X}_b$. The subject manipulates the knobs until two patches of light are obtained, determining two new impressions, w_1,w_2, satisfying

$$x_a = \frac{w_1 + x_b}{2}$$

$$w_2 = \frac{x_a + 2x_b}{3}$$

(compare with (5) and (6)). We assume thus that x_a, x_b, w_1, w_2 are real numbers. To w_1,w_2 correspond two observable intensities $z_1 = G(w_1), z_2 = G(w_2)$; the function G is strictly increasing and maps the set of impressions into the physical intensity scale. This model implicitly postulates the existence of two observable random variables, $\mathbf{Z}_1,\mathbf{Z}_2$, such that

$$\mathbf{Z}_1 = G(2\mathbf{X}_a - \mathbf{X}_b) \tag{7}$$

$$\mathbf{Z}_2 = G\left[\frac{\mathbf{X}_a + 2\mathbf{X}_b}{3}\right] \tag{8}$$

Two frequent assumptions in phychophysics concerning such sensory random variables $\mathbf{X}_a$ and $\mathbf{X}_b$ is that they are independent and normally distributed. If we also assume that they have equal variance, it can be derived without much difficulty that Z_1 and Z_2 must be independent (Exercise 17). A converse of this proposition is more surprising. If $\mathbf{Z}_1$ and $\mathbf{Z}_2$ are independent, and $\mathbf{X}_a$ and $\mathbf{X}_b$ are also independent, then $\mathbf{X}_a$ and $\mathbf{X}_b$ must be normally distributed (Theorem 3.17)! The proof depends on a couple of functional equation results.

(d) *Rating the number of excitations.* A suitably dark adapted subject is continuously (say, for 1 min) fixating a faint red light on a dark background. The subject's head is kept fixed. At time τ, a dim, small patch of monochromatic light, of short duration $t - \tau$ ($<50\,\text{msec}$) is presented in a fixed location on the temporal retina. Several stimuli of different durations can be presented successively on any trial. The presentation of each stimulus may be indicated by a brief tone. The subject is requested to rate the sensory impression evoked by each stimulus on a scale from 0 to 100 (0 means no perceptible stimulus; 100 means very intense stimulus; this last value is an upper bound, not to be used in practice). In line with Sakitt (1972), it may be hypothesized that, in a situation of this type, the rating $\mathbf{R}(\tau,t)$ is strictly increasing with the number $\mathbf{L}(\tau,t) = \mathbf{M}(\tau,t) + \mathbf{N}(\tau,t)$ of nervous excitations, where $M(\tau,t)$ denotes the number of photons absorbed by the retina, or more precisely, the number of rod signals, and $\mathbf{N}(\tau,t)$ is the number of signals resulting from the spontaneous activity of the nervous system. We have thus

$$\mathbf{R}(\tau,t) = G[\mathbf{L}(\tau,t)] \tag{9}$$

for some strictly increasing function G. Notice that $\mathbf{L}(\tau,t)$, and thus $\mathbf{R}(\tau,t)$ are random variables. The sources of variability are the Poisson distribution of the number of photons reaching the eye between time τ and t, and the random character of the absorption process and of the spontaneous activity. In fact, for a fixed τ, $\Lambda_\tau = \{L(\tau,t)|t > \tau\}$ is a stochastic process. Even though the arrival of the photons is governed by a Poisson process, it is not clear that Λ_τ will be Poisson. If, however, as is often assumed (Hecht, Shlear, & Pirenne, 1942; Sakitt, 1972), Λ_τ is Poisson, then some interesting consequences follow from the observable random variables $R(\tau,t)$. Any two random variables $R(\tau,t)$, $R(\tau',t')$, $(\tau < t \leqslant \tau' < t')$ are independent. A reverse implication also holds. Suppose that (i) Equation 9 holds; (ii) whenever $\tau < t \leqslant \tau' < t'$ the random variables $R(\tau,t)$, $R(\tau',t')$ are independent; (iii) whenever $\tau < t$ and $0 \leqslant r < 100$, the probability that $R(\tau,t)$ is equal to r only depends on $t - \tau$. Then the (unobservable) random variables $L(\tau,t)$ have a "homogeneous compound" Poisson distribution (Exercises 6 and 7).

(e) *A memoryless phenomenon.* An observer is watching a display. His or her task is to detect the realization of an event. The phenomenon is memoryless in the following sense: if the event does not occur between times 0 and t, the probability that it does not occur between times 0 and $t + s$ only depends on s. Formally, let T be a random variable respresenting the time elapsed until the occurrence of the event. The lack of memory is then represented by the equation

$$\mathbb{P}\{T > t + s | T > t\} = g(s),$$

where $\mathbb{P}$ represents the probability measure, and g is a strictly decreasing function. It can be shown that, under those conditions, T must be distributed exponentially: $\mathbb{P}(T \leq t) = 1 - e^{-\alpha t}$, for some constant $\alpha > 0$ (Exercise 4).

(f) *Weber's inequality.* In all five examples discussed so far, the conditions constraining the form of the unknown function(s) consisted of one or more functional equations. However, functional inequalities also turn out occasionally to yield useful information regarding the unknown function(s). An example is given here. Let $P_{a,b}$ be a choice probability in a psychophysical experiment; thus, a,b are numbers representing the intensities of two stimuli. Weber's law states that for any positive numbers a, b, and ξ,

$$P_{a,b} = P_{\xi a, \xi b}. \tag{10}$$

(This is essentially equivalent to the more usual statement that the Weber fraction does not vary with the intensity of the stimulus. For a detailed discussion of (10) and related topics, see Chapter 8.) Fechner's problem, which is discussed in detail in Chapter 4, involves finding a pair g,G of (strictly) increasing functions satisfying[2]

$$P_{a,b} = G[g(a)/g(b)]. \tag{11}$$

It is clear that Fechner's problem has a solution if Weber's law holds. Indeed, setting $\xi = 1/b$ in (10), we obtain

$$P_{a,b} = P_{a/b,1},$$

---

2. Equation 11 is usually written under the equivalent form $P_{a,b} = F[u(a) - u(b)]$, which yields $u(a) = \delta \log a + \gamma$.

a particular case of (11), with $g(a) = a$, $G(s) = P_{s,1}$. The trouble is that, as a rule, Weber's law fails to hold at low intensities. The typical data strongly supports the assumption

$$P_{\xi a, \xi b} \geqslant P_{a,b} \tag{12}$$

whenever $a \geqslant b, \xi \geqslant 1$. We will refer to (12) as *Weber's inequality*. It is equivalent to stating that the Weber fraction is decreasing with intensity. (This is shown in Chapter 8.) A tempting conjecture is that, if Weber's inequality holds, then (11) is approximately true provided that a,b are large enough. This conjecture, which we translate into the equation

$$\lim_{\xi \to \infty} P_{\xi a, \xi b} = G(a^\beta / b^\beta) \tag{13}$$

is false. For example,

$$P_{a,b} = G(e^a / e^b) \tag{14}$$

is consistent with (12) but contradicts (13), as can be checked easily. However, if we assume that g in (11) is dominated by *some* power function, then (14) can be derived (Falmagne, 1977; Iverson, 1983).

In the next section, we discuss in detail a class of well-known functional equations, which are perhaps the most useful ones in psychophysical applications.

CAUCHY AND RELATED EQUATIONS[3]

We begin with a simple example. Consider a function f, real valued, defined on the set $\mathbb{N}$ of all positive integers, and such that

$$f(a + b) = f(a) + f(b), \tag{15}$$

for all $a,b \in \mathbb{N}$. It is easy to show that f can only be of the form,

$$f(a) = \beta a, \tag{16}$$

for some constant β. Indeed, if $f(1) = \beta$, then $f(2) = f(1) + f(1) = \beta 2$, and if for some $a \in \mathbb{N}, f(a) = \beta a$, then $f(a + 1) = f(a) + f(1) = \beta(a + 1)$. The result follows by induction. With a little ingenuity, we can extend this result to a more complicated situation. Suppose, for example, that f is defined on the positive rational numbers. Using essentially the same argument as above, we derive

$$f(na) = nf(a) \tag{17}$$

for any $n \in \mathbb{N}$ and $a \in \mathbb{Q}^+$. (We recall that $\mathbb{Q}^+$ denotes the set of positive rational numbers.) Successively,

$$f(a) = f[n(a/n)] = nf(a/n)$$

3. Equation 15 is usually associated with the name of Cauchy, who investigated it in 1821.

by (17), yielding

$$f(a/n) = (1/n) f(a) \tag{18}$$

for any $n \in \mathbb{N}$ and $a \in \mathbb{Q}^+$. This means that (16) must hold in this case, since for any positive rational $r = n/m$,

$$
\begin{aligned}
f(r) &= f(n/m) \\
&= f(1/m)n & \text{(by (17))} \\
&= f(1)(n/m) & \text{(by (18))} \\
&= \beta r,
\end{aligned}
$$

with $\beta = f(1)$. We conclude that (16) also holds if f is continuous and defined on the positive reals. The theorem below generalizes this result. Note that the continuity assumption can be replaced by that of strict monotonicity.

3.2. Theorem.   *Let I be a real, open interval, having 0 as a limit point; let f be a real-valued, continuous (or strictly monotonic) function defined on I, such that whenever $a, b, a + b \in I$, then*

$$f(a + b) = f(a) + f(b).$$

Then, necessarily $f(a) = \beta a$ for some constant β and all $a \in I$.

The full proof of this result will be deferred to the last section of this chapter (see 3.30).

3.3. Remark.   In this and later theorems, the side assumptions are critical. For instance, Theorem 3.2 does not hold if the Provision that 0 is a limit point of I is dropped (Exercise 8). Notice also that the continuity condition can be weakened: only semicontinuity (i.e., one-sided continuity) is sufficient to yield the result. This remark holds for all the theorems of this section where a continuity condition is used.

Notice an immediate consequence of this result. Suppose that I is defined as in Theorem 3.2, and let g be a real-valued continuous or strictly monotonic function on I, satisfying

$$g(s + t) = g(s)g(t),$$

whenever $s, t, s + t \in I$. Then g is necessarily of the form $g(s) = \exp \beta s$, for some constant β. Indeed, we must have $g > 0$. (Why? See Exercise 2.) Taking logarithms on both sides of the above equation reduces it to a case of Theorem 3.2 and the following result follows. Some other consequences are listed in Theorem 3.4.

3.4. Theorem.   *Let I be a real, positive interval having 1 as a limit point and let g be a real-valued, continuous (or strictly monotonic) function defined on I. Suppose that*

$$g(st) = g(s) + g(t) \tag{19}$$

whenever $s, t, st \in I$. Then, necessarily $g(s) = \beta \ln s$ for some constant β. If, under the same conditions,

$$g(st) = g(s)g(t) \tag{20}$$

whenever $s, t, st \in I$, then $g(s) = s^\beta$ for some constant β.

The proof of this result is left to the reader (Exercise 3). Next, we consider the case where the function in (19) and (20) is defined on the positive integers (cf. Erdös, 1946).

3.5. Theorem. *Let k be a strictly monotonic function defined on $\mathbb{N}$. If*

$$k(nm) = k(n) + k(m) \tag{21}$$

for all $n, m \in \mathbb{N}$, then, necessarily, $k(n) = \beta \ln n$ for some constant $\beta \neq 0$. If

$$k(nm) = k(n)k(m), \tag{22}$$

then necessarily $k(n) = n^\beta$ for some constant $\beta \neq 0$.

The basic idea of the proof is simple: we extend the function k to a function $\bar{k}$, defined on the set of all positive real numbers, and satisfying (19) or (20), and we use Theorem 3.4 to yield the result.

Proof. We first establish the result involving Equation 21. For concreteness, assume that k is strictly increasing. As a first step, we define $\bar{k}$ on the set of positive rational numbers by

$$\bar{k}(n/m) = k(n) - k(m)$$

for all $n, m \in \mathbb{N}$. The function $\bar{k}$ is a well-defined extension of k. Indeed, $k(1 \cdot 1) = 2k(1)$ yields $k(1) = 0$. Thus, $\bar{k}(n/1) = k(n) - k(1) = k(n)$, and if $n/m = n'/m'$ for $n, m, n', m' \in \mathbb{N}$, then $nm' = mn'$, $k(nm') = k(n) + k(m') = k(mn') = k(m) + k(n')$, implying that $k(n) - k(m) = k(n') - k(m')$. A slight modification of the above argument shows that $\bar{k}$ is strictly increasing on $\{p \in \mathbb{Q} | p > 0\}$ ($n/m < n'/m'$ implies that $nm' < mn'$, etc.). Moreover, $\bar{k}$ satisfies Equation 19 for all positive rationals $s = n/m$, $t = n'/m'$, since

$$\bar{k}\left(\frac{n}{m} \cdot \frac{n'}{m'}\right) = k(nn') - k(mm')$$

$$= k(n) + k(n') - k(m) - k(m')$$

$$= \bar{k}\left(\frac{n}{m}\right) + \bar{k}\left(\frac{n'}{m'}\right).$$

For the positive real numbers, we define

$$\bar{k}(s) = \sup\{\bar{k}(p) | p \in \mathbb{Q}, 0 < p \leqslant s\}.$$

(Thus, s is rational or irrational.) Let us show that Equation 19, with $g = \bar{k}$ holds for all positive real numbers s,t. Define

$$S(s,t) = \{\bar{k}(r) \,|\, r \in \mathbb{Q}, 0 < r \leqslant st\}$$

$$S'(s,t) = \{\bar{k}(pq) \,|\, p,q \in \mathbb{Q}, 0 < p \leqslant s, 0 < q \leqslant t\}.$$

Sup $S(s,t) = \bar{k}(st)$, sup $S'(s,t) = \bar{k}(s) + \bar{k}(t)$. We must prove that sup $S(s,t) =$ sup $S'(s,t)$. Since for any $p,q \in \mathbb{Q}$, $0 < p \leqslant s$, $0 < q \leqslant t$ imply $0 < pq \leqslant st$, we have $S'(s,t) \subset S(s,t)$. This yields sup $S'(s,t) \leqslant$ sup $S(s,t)$, the equality holding if $st \in \mathbb{Q}$. To prove the reverse inequality, take $\bar{k}(r) \in S(s,t)$ arbitrarily with $st \notin \mathbb{Q}$. Then we can choose, successively, two rational numbers p,q such that $r/t \leqslant p < s$, $r/p \leqslant q < t$; that is, $0 < p < s$, $0 < q < t$, $r < pq$. Thus, we have sup $S(s,t) \leqslant$ sup $S'(s,t)$. We conclude that $\bar{k}(st) = \bar{k}(s) + \bar{k}(t)$, as asserted. Using Theorem 3.4, we obtain

$$\bar{k}(n) = k(n) = \beta \ln n$$

for some constant $\beta > 0$ and all $n \in \mathbb{N}$. If k is strictly decreasing, the same result holds with $\beta > 0$. In the case of Equation 22, we must have $k > 0$. Taking logarithms on both sides of (22) gives an equation of the form of (21), and the result follows. ∎

We are now equipped to investigate a couple of more general forms. Consider, for instance, the equation

$$h(a + b) = v(a) + g(b), \tag{23}$$

generalizing the basic Cauchy equation (15), and involving three unknown functions h, v, and g. We assume that these three functions are real valued, continuous, and defined on the real numbers. A couple of simple substitutions permits recasting this equation under the basic form (15). Fixing $b = 0$ in (23), we obtain

$$h(a) = v(a) + g(0), \tag{24}$$

which, together with (23), yields

$$v(a + b) = v(a) + g(b) - g(0). \tag{25}$$

We define

$$g_0(a) = g(a) - g(0). \tag{26}$$

Notice that the function g_0 is continuous, with $g_0(0) = 0$. Combining (25) and (26), we have

$$v(a + b) = v(a) + g_0(b) \tag{27}$$

a form intermediate between (15) and (23), involving two unknown functions v and g_0. The function v in (27) can be handled by a similar method. From (27)

$$v(a) + g_0(b) = v(b) + g_0(a);$$

with $b = 0$,

$$v(a) = v(0) + g_0(a). \tag{28}$$

Substituting in (25), we get

$$v(0) + g_0(a + b) = v(0) + g_0(a) + g_0(b);$$

that is,

$$g_0(a + b) = g_0(a) + g_0(b).$$

Using Theorem 3.2, we derive

$$g_0(a) = \beta a$$

for some constant β. From (26), (28), and (24), we conclude successively that

$$g(a) = \alpha + \beta a,$$
$$v(a) = \gamma + \beta a,$$
$$h(a) = \gamma + \alpha + \beta a,$$

with $\alpha = g(0)$ and $\gamma = v(0)$.

This substitution technique is used repeatedly in the proof of the theorem below, which involves four unknown functions, and includes (23) as a special case. This result may come as a surprise.

3.6. Theorem. *Let h, v, g, and k be real-valued functions defined on an open interval I having 0 as a limit point, with h and g strictly monotonic (or nonconstant, continuous); suppose that*

$$h(a + b) = v(a) + k(a)g(b) \tag{29}$$

whenever $a, b, a + b \in I$. Then either k is a constant function and there are constants $\beta_0, \beta_1, \beta_2,$ and β_3, with $\beta_3 \neq 0$, such that for all $a \in I$

$$h(a) = \beta_0 a + \beta_1 + \beta_2,$$
$$v(a) = \beta_0 a + \beta_2,$$
$$g(a) = (\beta_0/\beta_3)a + (\beta_1/\beta_3),$$
$$k(a) = \beta_3;$$

or k takes at least two distinct values and there are constants $\beta_0, \beta_1, \beta_2, \beta_3,$ and λ with $\beta_3 \neq 0$ such that for all $a \in I$

$$h(a) = \beta_0(1 - e^{\lambda a}) + \beta_1 + \beta_2,$$
$$v(a) = (\beta_0 + \beta_1)(1 - e^{\lambda a}) + \beta_2,$$
$$g(a) = (\beta_0/\beta_3)(1 - e^{\lambda a}) + (\beta_1/\beta_3),$$
$$k(a) = \beta_3 e^{\lambda a}.$$

In short, but less precisely, Equation 29 implies that the four functions, $h, v, k,$ and g must be either all linear or all exponential.

Proof. Suppose that the functions h and g are strictly monotonic; for concreteness say, strictly increasing. This implies that $k(a) > 0$ for all $a \in I$. Let $I = (\zeta, \zeta')$, with $\zeta \leqslant 0 \leqslant \zeta'$. There are thus three possibilities: $0 \in I, \zeta = 0,$ and $\zeta' = 0$. Suppose that $0 \in I,$ and let us assume (temporarily) that $v(0) = 0$ and $k(0) = 1$. This yields $h(b) = g(b)$ for all $b \in I$. Equation 29 simplifies to

$$g(a + b) = v(a) + k(a)g(b) = v(b) + k(b)g(a). \tag{30}$$

Letting $a = 0,$ and $g(0) = \beta_1$, we obtain

$$v(b) = g(b) - k(b)\beta_1. \tag{31}$$

Replacing v in (30) by its expression in (31), we get

$$g(a + b) = g(a) - k(a)\beta_1 + k(a)g(b)$$
$$= g(a) + k(a)[g(b) - \beta_1].$$

Subtracting β_1 from each member and defining $f(a) = g(a) - \beta_1$, we obtain, finally,

$$f(a + b) = f(a) + k(a)f(b). \tag{32}$$

Notice that f is strictly increasing.

Case 1. k is a constant function. Thus, $k(a) = 1$ for all $a \in I$; (32) becomes

$$f(a + b) = f(a) + f(b).$$

From Theorem 3.2 we deduce that f is of the form $f(a) = \beta_0 a,$ for all $a \in I$ and some constant $\beta_0 > 0$. This implies that

$$g(a) = \beta_0 a + \beta_1 = h(a) \qquad \text{(by definition of } f\text{)}$$

$$v(a) = \beta_0 a + \beta_1 - \beta_1 = \beta_0 a \qquad \text{(by (31))}$$

$$k(a) = 1.$$

In general, $v(0) \neq 0$ and $k(0) \neq 1$. Say, for example, that $v(0) = \beta_2$ and $k(0) = \beta_3 > 0$. We obtain

$$h(a) = \beta_0 a + \beta_1 + \beta_2$$

$$v(a) = \beta_0 a + \beta_2$$

$$g(a) = (\beta_0 / \beta_3)a + (\beta_1 / \beta_3)$$

$$k(a) = \beta_3,$$

as asserted.

Case 2. k is not constant; we have $k(0) \neq k(\xi),$ for some $\xi \in I$. Then (32) gives $f(a + \xi) = f(a) + k(a)f(\xi) = f(\xi + a) = f(\xi) + k(\xi)f(a)$ yielding

$$f(a)[1 - k(\xi)] = f(\xi)[1 - k(a)].$$

Fixing ξ, and setting

$$\frac{f(\xi)}{1 - k(\xi)} = \beta_0,$$

$(k(\xi) \neq 1)$, this equation yields

$$f(a) = \beta_0[1 - k(a)], \tag{33}$$

for all $a \in I$. Notice that $\beta_0 \neq 0$ since f is strictly increasing. Thus, k is strictly increasing or strictly decreasing depending on whether $\beta_0 < 0$ or $\beta_0 > 0$. Replacing f in (32) by its expression in (33), dividing by β_0 and rearranging terms yields

$$k(a + b) = k(a)k(b).$$

If k is strictly increasing, we use 3.3, to yield

$$k(a) = e^{\lambda a} \tag{34}$$

for some $\lambda > 0$ and all $a \in I$. If k is strictly decreasing, $1/k$ is strictly increasing, and (34) also follows but with $\lambda < 0$. We obtain, then

$$f(a) = \beta_0(1 - e^{\lambda a}), \qquad \text{(by (33) and (34))}$$

$$g(a) = \beta_0(1 - e^{\lambda a}) + \beta_1 = h(a), \qquad \text{(by definition of } f)$$

$$v(a) = \beta_0(1 - e^{\lambda a}) + \beta_1 - e^{\lambda a}\beta_1, \qquad \text{(by (31))}$$

$$= (\beta_0 + \beta_1)(1 - e^{\lambda a}).$$

In general, $v(0) \neq 0$, $k(0) \neq 1$. If $v(0) = \beta_2$ and $k(0) = \beta_3 > 0$, we obtain the result of the theorem. The above argument goes through with only minor changes if h and g are assumed to be continuous. The discussion of the two remaining possibilities $I = (0,\zeta')$, $I = (\zeta,0)$, will be left to the reader (Exercise 9). ∎

Many useful results can be derived from this theorem by particularizing the functions of Equation 29. Consider, for example, the equation

$$r(\alpha s + \alpha' t) = \alpha r(s) + \alpha' r(t), \tag{35}$$

with $\alpha, \alpha' \neq 0$ two arbitrary constants, and r a real-valued, strictly increasing function. Assume (for a moment) that r is defined on $\mathbb{R}$. With $\alpha s = a$, $\alpha' t = b$, $\alpha r[(1/\alpha)a] = v(a)$, $\alpha' r[(1/\alpha')a] = g(a)$, and $h = r$, Equation 35 is equivalent to

$$h(a + b) = v(a) + g(b),$$

with h,g strictly increasing, holding for all real numbers a,b. Using Theorem 3.6, we obtain $v(a) = \beta_0 a + \beta_2 = \alpha r[(1/\alpha)a]$, $\beta_0 > 0$, for all $a \in \mathbb{R}$. That is $r(s) = \beta s + \gamma$, $\beta > 0$ for all $s \in \mathbb{R}$. Replacing r in (35) by its expression yields $\gamma = \alpha\gamma + \alpha'\gamma$. Thus, $\beta \neq 0$ implies that $\alpha + \alpha' = 1$. This result holds, in fact, even if r is only defined on an interval (ζ,ζ'), $\zeta \leqslant 0 \leqslant \zeta'$.

3.7. Theorem. *Let r be a real-valued, strictly monotonic (or continuous) function defined on an open interval I having 0 as a limit point. Let $\alpha, \alpha' \neq 0$ be two arbitrary* *constants, and suppose that (35) holds for all s, t, $(\alpha s + \alpha' t) \in I$. Then, for all $s \in I$, $r(s) = \beta s + \gamma$ for some constants β, γ with $\gamma \neq 0$ only if $\alpha + \alpha' = 1$.*

The proof of this theorem will be left to the reader (Exercise 10).

3.8. Remark.   Theorem 3.7 will be one of the key results in our discussion of Plateau's experiment in the next section. There are numerous other useful consequences of the theorems given so far in this section. It would be pointless to give a detailed derivation of all of these results here. The pattern of proof is more or less standard, and was illustrated in the two preceding proofs. Instead we will give a couple of tables providing a compact summary of the most frequently used results. The first table contains straightforward consequences of Theorem 3.7.

3.9. Table of results.   *Note.* The function f in the equations below is strictly increasing and, unless otherwise specified, is defined on an open interval (ζ, ζ'); $\alpha, \alpha' \neq 0$ are arbitrary constants.

Equations	Solutions
(i)	
$f(\alpha a + \alpha' b) = \alpha f(a) + \alpha' f(b)$; $\zeta \leqslant 0 \leqslant \zeta'$; (or $\alpha = \alpha' = 1$, f defined on $\mathbb{N}$).	$f(a) = \beta a + \gamma$; $\beta > 0$, γ, constants with $\gamma \neq 0$ only if $\alpha + \alpha' = 1$.
(ii)	
$f(\alpha a + \alpha' b) = f(a)^\alpha f(b)^{\alpha'}$; $f > 0$; $\zeta \leqslant 0 \leqslant \zeta'$; (or $\alpha = \alpha' = 1$, f defined on $\mathbb{N}$).	$f(a) = \gamma \exp(\beta a)$; β, $\gamma > 0$ constants, with $\gamma \neq 1$ only if $\alpha + \alpha' = 1$.
(iii)	
$f(a^\alpha b^{\alpha'}) = f(a)^\alpha f(b)^{\alpha'}$; $f > 0$, $0 < \zeta \leqslant 1 \leqslant \zeta'$; (or $\alpha = \alpha' = 1$, f defined on $\mathbb{N}$).	$f(a) = \gamma a^\beta$; β, $\gamma > 0$, constants, $\gamma \neq 1$ only if $\alpha + \alpha' = 1$.
(iv)	
$f(a^\alpha b^{\alpha'}) = \alpha f(a) + \alpha' f(b)$; $0 < \zeta \leqslant 1 \leqslant \zeta'$; (or $\alpha = \alpha' = 1$, f defined on $\mathbb{N}$).	$f(a) = \beta \ln a + \gamma$; $\beta > 0$, γ, constants, with $\gamma \neq 0$ only if $\alpha + \alpha' = 1$.

For example, line (iii) of the table contains the following result. Suppose that f is a real-valued, strictly increasing function. If f is defined on a positive, open interval (ζ, ζ'), with $\zeta \leqslant 1 \leqslant \zeta'$, and satisfying $f(a^\alpha b^{\alpha'}) = f(a)^\alpha f(b)^{\alpha'}$ for all a, b, $a^\alpha b^{\alpha'} \in (\zeta, \zeta')$, where $\alpha, \alpha' \neq 0$ are two constants, then f is of the form $f(a) = \gamma a^\beta, \gamma, \beta > 0$, with $\gamma \neq 1$ only if $\alpha + \alpha' = 1$. If f is defined on $\mathbb{N}$ and satisfies $f(ab) = f(a)f(b)$ for all positive integers a, b, then $f(a) = a^\beta$ for some constant $\beta > 0$.

I leave it to the reader to check these results (Exercise 11), which also hold, with appropriate specifications or changes of sign in the constants, if f is assumed to be strictly decreasing, continuous, or even semicontinuous. The table in 3.10 extends Theorem 3.6.

3.10. Table of results. The functions h, v, g, k in the following table are assumed to be real valued, defined on an open interval (ζ, ζ'), with h, g strictly increasing. The second column contains the solutions in the case where k is assumed to be a constant function. The third column contains the solutions in the case where k takes at least two distinct values. The proof of these results is left for the exercises (12, 13, and 14).

Equations	Solutions (k, constant)	Solutions (k, not constant)
i) $h(a + b) = v(a) + k(a)g(b)$ $\zeta \leqslant 0 \leqslant \zeta'$	$h(a) = \beta_0 a + \beta_1 + \beta_2$ $v(a) = \beta_0 a + \beta_2$ $g(a) = (\beta_0/\beta_3)a + (\beta_1/\beta_3)$ $k(a) = \beta_3$ $\beta_0, \beta_3 > 0$	$h(a) = \beta_0[1 - \exp(\lambda a)] + \beta_1 + \beta_2$ $v(a) = (\beta_0 + \beta_1)[1 - \exp(\lambda a)] + \beta_2$ $g(a) = (\beta_0/\beta_3)[1 - \exp(\lambda a)] + (\beta_1/\beta_3)$ $k(a) = \beta_3 \exp(\lambda a)$ $\beta_3 > 0, \beta_0 \lambda < 0$
ii) $h(a + b) = v(a)g(b)^{k(a)}$ $\zeta \leqslant 0 \leqslant \zeta'; h, v > 0$	$h(a) = \beta_1\beta_2 \exp(\beta_0 a)$ $v(a) = \beta_2 \exp(\beta_0 a)$ $g(a) = \beta_1^{(1/\beta_3)} \exp(a\beta_0/\beta_3)$ $k(a) = \beta_3$ $\beta_i > 0, 0 \leqslant i \leqslant 3$	$h(a) = \beta_1\beta_2 \exp\{\beta_0[1 - \exp(\lambda a)]\}$ $v(a) = \beta_2 \exp\{(\beta_0 + \ln \beta_1)[1 - \exp(\lambda a)]\}$ $g(a) = \beta_1^{(1/\beta_3)} \exp\{(\beta_0/\beta_3)[1 - \exp(\lambda a)]\}$ $k(a) = \beta_3 \exp(\lambda a)$ $\beta_i > 0, 1 \leqslant i \leqslant 3, \beta_0 \lambda < 0$
iii) $h(a + b) = v(a)k(a)^{g(b)}$ $\zeta \leqslant 0 \leqslant \zeta'; h, v > 0$	$h(a) = \beta_1\beta_2 \exp(\beta_0 a)$ $v(a) = \beta_2 \exp(\beta_0 a)$ $g(a) = (1/\ln \beta_3)(\beta_0 a + \ln \beta_1)$ $k(a) = \beta_3$ $\beta_i > 0, 0 \leqslant i \leqslant 2, \beta_3 > 1$	$h(a) = \beta_1\beta_2 \exp\{\beta_0[1 - \exp(\lambda a)]\}$ $v(a) = \beta_2 \exp\{(\beta_0 + \ln \beta_1)[1 - \exp(\lambda a)]\}$ $g(a) = \beta_3^{-1}\{\beta_0[1 - \exp(\lambda a)] + \beta_1\}$ $k(a) = \exp[\beta_3 \exp(\lambda a)]$ $\beta_i > 0, 1 \leqslant i \leqslant 3, \beta_0 \lambda < 0$
v) $h(ab) = v(a) + k(a)g(b)$ $0 < \zeta \leqslant 1 \leqslant \zeta'$	$h(a) = \beta_0 \ln a + \beta_1 + \beta_2$ $v(a) = \beta_0 \ln a + \beta_2$ $g(a) = (\beta_0/\beta_3) \ln a + (\beta_1/\beta_3)$ $k(a) = \beta_3$ $\beta_0, \beta_3 > 0$	$h(a) = \beta_0(1 - a^\lambda) + \beta_1 + \beta_2$ $v(a) = (\beta_0 + \beta_1)(1 - a^\lambda) + \beta_2$ $g(a) = (\beta_0/\beta_3)(1 - a^\lambda) + (\beta_1/\beta_3)$ $k(a) = \beta_3 a^\lambda$ $\beta_3 > 0, \beta_0 \lambda < 0$
) $h(ab) = v(a)g(b)^{k(a)}$ $0 < \zeta \leqslant 1 \leqslant \zeta'; h, v > 0$	$h(a) = \beta_1\beta_2 a^{\beta_0}$ $v(a) = \beta_2 a^{\beta_0}$ $g(a) = (\beta_1 a^{\beta_0})^{1/\beta_3}$ $k(a) = \beta_3$ $\beta_i > 0, 0 \leqslant i \leqslant 3$	$h(a) = \beta_1\beta_2 \exp[\beta_0(1 - a^\lambda)]$ $v(a) = \beta_2\beta_1^{(1 - a^\lambda)} \exp[\beta_0(1 - a^\lambda)]$ $g(a) = \{\beta_1 \exp[\beta_0(1 - a^\lambda)]\}^{1/\beta_3}$ $k(a) = \beta_3 a^\lambda$ $\beta_i > 0, 1 \leqslant i \leqslant 3; \beta_0 \lambda < 0$
) $h(ab) = v(a)k(a)^{g(b)}$ $0 < \zeta \leqslant 1 \leqslant \zeta'; h, v > 0$	$h(a) = \beta_1\beta_2 a^{\beta_0}$ $v(a) = \beta_2 a^{\beta_0}$ $g(a) = (1/\ln \beta_3)(\beta_0 \ln a + \ln \beta_1)$ $k(a) = \beta_3$ $\beta_i > 0, 0 \leqslant i \leqslant 3$	$h(a) = \beta_1\beta_2 \exp[\beta_0(1 - a^\lambda)]$ $v(a) = \beta_2\beta_1^{(1 - a^\lambda)} \exp[\beta_0(1 - a^\lambda)]$ $g(a) = \beta_3^{-1}[\beta_0(1 - a^\lambda) + \ln \beta_1)]$ $k(a) = \exp(\beta_3 a^\lambda)$ $\beta_i > 0, 1 \leqslant i \leqslant 3; \beta_0 \lambda < 0$

Many special cases of the results in these two tables will be of interest in later developments. These special cases are obtained by simple derivations, as exemplified below.

3.11. Examples. (a) Suppose $f > 0$ is a real-valued, strictly increasing function defined on an open interval (ζ,ζ'), with $0 < \zeta \leqslant 1 \leqslant \zeta'$, and satisfying $f(a/b) = f(a)/f(b)$ whenever $a, b, a/b \in (\zeta,\zeta')$. Then f is necessarily of the form $f(a) = a^\beta$, $\beta > 0$. Indeed, we use Table 3.9 (iii) with $\alpha = 1$, $\alpha' = -1$.

(b) Let h, v, g be three real-valued functions defined on an open interval (ζ,ζ'), $\zeta \leqslant 0 \leqslant \zeta'$ with h, g strictly increasing, $h,g > 0$, and satisfying $h(a + b) = v(a)g(b)$ whenever $a, b, a + b \in (\zeta,\zeta')$. Then, h, v, g have necessarily the forms: $h(a) = \beta_1\beta_2 \exp(\beta_0 a)$, $v(a) = \beta_2 \exp(\beta_0 a)$, $g(a) = \beta_1 \exp(\beta_0 a)$ for some constants $\beta_i > 0$, $0 \leqslant i \leqslant 2$. Indeed, $h,g > 0$ implies that $v > 0$. We then use Table 3.10(ii), with $k(a) = 1$.

(c) Notice that, in all six cases of Table 3.10 when k is a constant function, v,h are of the form $v = \alpha h + \beta$ for some constant $\alpha > 0$, β. This can be used as a quick check of the possibility (or impossibility) of some potential forms. For instance, there is no function g, defined, say on $(0,1)$, and satisfying $g(c - a) = \log c - a^3$ (Exercise 13).

Other examples are contained in the exercises. Simple consequences of this kind, from Tables 3.9 and 3.10, will be used freely in the future.

PLATEAU'S EXPERIMENT

In Example 3.1(a), we considered a function M of two variables, representing the value (on the lux scale) of the "midway" grays, and we assumed that the following relations were satisfied.

$$cM(a,b) = M(ca,cb), \tag{36}$$

(*the resulting gray is independent of the conditions of illumination*), and

$$u[M(a,b)] = \frac{u(a) + u(b)}{2} \tag{37}$$

(*the production of the midway gray can be represented by an arithmetical average, performed on some unspecified "sensation" scale*).

We claimed that under mild additional conditions, these two equations involved considerable restrictions on the possible form of the function u. In fact, there only two possibilities: either $u(a) = \alpha \log a + \beta$, or $u(a) = \alpha a^\beta + \gamma$, for two constants $\alpha > 0$, β (cf. Krantz, 1972). The results of 3.9 and 3.10 allow us to provide a short proof of these assertions.

Assume that u is strictly increasing, continuous, and defined on an open interval (ζ,ζ'), with $0 < \zeta \leqslant 1 \leqslant \zeta'$, (i.e., (ζ,ζ') is the part of the lux scale involved in the experiment, and we suppose that the unit is either a point or one of the boundary points of (ζ,ζ')). Thus, M maps $(\zeta,\zeta') \times (\zeta,\zeta')$ into (ζ,ζ'). We can suppose, without loss of generality, that the range of u contains 0. (If it does not, we define

a new function u_0, $u_0(a) = u(a) - u(a_0)$ and it is easy to see that u_0 satisfies (37).)
From (36) and (37) we derive

$$cu^{-1}\left[\frac{u(a) + u(b)}{2}\right] = u^{-1}\left[\frac{u(ca) + u(cb)}{2}\right]$$

Setting $u(a) = s$, $u(b) = t$ and applying u to both sides yields

$$u\left[cu^{-1}\left(\frac{s+t}{2}\right)\right] = \frac{u[cu^{-1}(s)] + u[cu^{-1}(t)]}{2}.$$

Fixing c, and defining $f_c(s) = u[cu^{-1}(s)]$, we obtain

$$f_c\left(\frac{s+t}{2}\right) = \frac{f_c(s) + f_c(t)}{2}.$$

Since $c > 0$, and u is strictly increasing and continuous, f_c is strictly increasing and defined on some open interval I, which contains 0 by a previous argument. We use Table 3.9(i) to assert

$$f_c(s) = \beta(c)s + \gamma(c)$$

for all $s \in I$. (The constants β, γ of 3.9(i) may depend on the value of c.) Since $f_c(s) = u[cu^{-1}(s)]$, this equation can be written with $u^{-1}(s) = a$,

$$u(ca) = \gamma(c) + u(a)\beta(c),$$

for all $a, c, ac \in (\zeta, \zeta')$. Using Table 3.10 (iv) we conclude that the following result holds.

3.12. Theorem.   *Let (ζ, ζ') be an open interval with $0 < \zeta \leqslant 1 \leqslant \zeta'$; let M be a function mapping $(\zeta, \zeta') \times (\zeta, \zeta')$ into (ζ, ζ'); let u be a real-valued, strictly increasing, continuous function on (ζ, ζ'). Suppose that both (36) and (37) hold. Then either*

$$u(a) = \alpha \log a + \beta,$$

for some constants $\alpha > 0, \beta$, or

$$u(a) = \alpha a^\beta + \gamma,$$

for some constants α, β, γ with $\alpha\beta > 0$.

This results is of great interest since *both* (36) and (37) can be investigated empirically. This is obvious for (36). In the case of (37), a set of axioms involving only the "observable" function M can be given that guarantees the existence of a function u satisfying this equation. These axioms, or at least some of them, can thus be tested empirically. This topic is discussed in Chapter 11. We must point out that there is arbitrariness in representing the "midway" operation by an arithmetical mean. A geometric mean would be equally plausible. (Incidentally, this arbitrariness will not be removed by the axioms of Chapter 11.) This remark is germane to an earlier observation regarding the arbitrariness of representing a physical concatenation by an arithmetic sum, rather than by a product (cf. 2.8). In any event, we emphasize the point in the following theorem, which is a straightforward consequence of the preceding result. The proof is left as an exercise.

3.13. Theorem.   *Let (ζ,ζ') and M be as in Theorem 3.12, and assume that* (36) *holds. Let $u > 0$ be a real valued, strictly increasing, continuous, function on (ζ,ζ') satisfying*

$$u[M(a,b)] = [u(a)u(b)]^{1/2} \tag{38}$$

for all $a,b \in (\zeta,\zeta')$. Then either

$$u(a) = \alpha a^\beta$$

for some constants $\alpha,\beta > 0$; or

$$u(a) = \alpha \exp(\gamma a^\beta)$$

for some constant α, β, γ, with $\gamma\beta > 0$.

The two preceding theorems suggest that (assuming that the data would support the assumptions) we would still have the choice between two "natural" representations, (37), (38), and four forms for the psychophysical scale u.

The choice may be made either by taking into account considerations of mathematical convenience, or possibly, by introducing additional data of a different type. We will encounter other instances of such a situation in the future.

*NORMAL DISTRIBUTION OF SENSORY VARIABLES

We justify here our claim in Example 3.1(c) regarding the normality of sensory variables under conditions of independence. We begin with a couple of preparatory theorems in which the solution of a given functional equation is a quadratic polynomial. These theorems are straightforward extensions of results contained in Feller (1966, pp. 77–80).

3.14. Theorem.   *Let f, g be two continuous functions, defined on an open interval containing 0. Suppose that*

$$f(x + y) + f(x - y) - 2f(x) = g(y)$$

whenever both members are defined; then necessarily

$$f(x) = \alpha x^2 + \beta x + \gamma,$$
$$g(x) = 2\alpha x^2,$$

for some constants α, β, γ.

In particular thus if g is a constant, then $g = 0$ and f is linear or constant.

3.15. Proof.   Let I be the common domain of f and g; then, $\delta, -\delta \in I$ for some $\delta > 0$. Define a function h on I by

$$h(x) = f(x) - \alpha x^2 - \beta x - \gamma,$$

with

$$\gamma = f(0), \qquad \beta = \frac{f(\delta) - f(-\delta)}{2\delta}, \qquad \alpha = \frac{f(\delta) + f(-\delta) - 2f(0)}{2\delta^2}.$$

It is easy to check that h satisfies

$$h(0) = h(\delta) = h(-\delta) = 0,$$

and

$$h(x + y) + h(x - y) - 2h(x) = k(y), \tag{39}$$

with $k(y) = g(y) - 2\alpha y^2$. The result follows if we can show that h vanishes on $[-\delta, \delta]$, since then, as a consequence of (39), k also vanishes on $[-\delta, \delta]$, and this implies that h vanishes everywhere on I. (For any $z \in I$, $h(z)$ can be written, using (39), as a linear combination of terms $h(x_i)$, $k(y_j)$, with $x_i, y_j \in [-\delta, \delta]$.) Let us show that $h(x) = 0$ if $-\delta \leqslant x \leqslant \delta$. The image of $[-\delta, \delta]$ by the continuous function h is a closed interval, say $[s, t]$. Suppose that $t > 0$. The set $W^+ = \{x | -\delta \leqslant x \leqslant \delta, h(x) = t\}$ is a compact subset of $[-\delta, \delta]$; let x_0 be a point of its boundary. Then $x_0 \in W^+ \cap (-\delta, \delta)$ (since $h(-\delta) = h(\delta) = 0$), and there exists $y > 0$ such that $y, (x_0 + y), (x_0 - y) \in [-\delta, \delta]$ and

$$h(x_0 + y) + h(x_0 - y) - 2h(x_0) = k(y) < 0, \tag{40}$$

since at least one of $x_0 + y$, $x_0 - y$ is not in W^+. If $s < 0$, a symmetrical argument, involving the set $W^- = \{x | -\delta \leqslant x \leqslant \delta, h(x) = s\}$ yields $k(y) > 0$, contradicting (40). Thus, $h(0) = 0 \leqslant h(x)$ whenever $-\delta \leqslant x \leqslant \delta$. Setting $x = 0$ in (39), we obtain

$$h(y) + h(-y) - 2h(0) = k(y) \geqslant 0,$$

again a contradiction. We conclude that $t = 0$ and by symmetry, $s = 0$. Thus, $h(x) = 0$ for all $x \in [-\delta, \delta]$. ∎

3.16. Theorem. *Let f_i, h_i $(i = 1,2)$ be continuous functions defined on an open interval containing 0; let $\zeta_{ij} \neq 0$ $(i = 1,2; j = 1,2)$ be constants satisfying*

$$\zeta_{11}\zeta_{22} - \zeta_{12}\zeta_{21} \neq 0. \tag{41}$$

Suppose that

$$f_1(\zeta_{11}x + \zeta_{12}y) + f_2(\zeta_{21}x + \zeta_{22}y) = h_1(x) + h_2(y), \tag{42}$$

whenever both members are defined. Then, there are constants α_i, β_i, γ_i such that

$$f_i(x) = \alpha_i x^2 + \beta_i x + \gamma_i \ (i = 1,2)$$

with

$$\alpha_1\zeta_{11}\zeta_{12} + \alpha_2\zeta_{21}\zeta_{22} = 0. \tag{43}$$

Notice that $\alpha_1 = 0$ iff $\alpha_2 = 0$, by (43). This means that f_1 in (42) is a polynomial of the second degree if and only if f_2 also is. If the f_i were assumed to be differentiable, the following argument could be used. Differentiating in (42) successively with respect to x,y, yields

$$\zeta_{11}\zeta_{12}f_1''(\zeta_{11}x + \zeta_{12}y) + \zeta_{21}\zeta_{22}f_2''(\zeta_{21}x + \zeta_{22}y) = 0. \tag{44}$$

We can vary $\zeta_{11}x + \zeta_{12}y$ in this equation in such a way that $\zeta_{21}x + \zeta_{22}y$ remains constant (using (41)). Thus, (44) implies that f_1'' is constant; in other words, f_1 is a polynomial of second degree or lower. The argument used in the following proof is similar, the derivatives being replaced by differences.

Proof.   Let I be the domain of the functions f_i, h_i. We define a difference operator on functions v of two variables by

$$\Delta_{z,w}v(x,y) = v(x + z, y + w) - v(x + z, y - w) - v(x - z, y + w)$$
$$+ v(x - z, y - w).$$

From (42), it can be checked by a simple computation that

$$\Delta_{z,w}f_1(\zeta_{11}x + \zeta_{12}v) + \Delta_{z,w}f_2(\zeta_{21}x + \zeta_{22}y) = 0. \tag{45}$$

This equation (which replaces (44) in the informal argument using derivatives) holds whenever the terms are defined, that is, whenever all the quantities x, y, $\zeta_{11}x + \zeta_{12}y$, $\zeta_{11}(x + z) + \zeta_{12}(y + w)$, etc. are members of I. No special difficulty arises here since I is an open interval containing 0; thus, the Δf_i are defined if $|x|, |y|, |z|$, and $|w|$ are small enough. As a consequence of (41), we can vary $\zeta_{11}x + \zeta_{12}y$ in (45) while $\zeta_{21}x + \zeta_{22}y$ remains constant, and vice versa. This implies that $\Delta_{z,w}f_i(\zeta_{i1}x + \zeta_{i2}y)$ is a constant (which may, of course, depend on z,w). Writing $t = \zeta_{i1}z + \zeta_{i2}w$, $s = \zeta_{i1}x + \zeta_{i2}y$, and choosing z,w satisfying $\zeta_{i1}z - \zeta_{i2}w = 0$, we obtain

$$f_i(s + t) + f_i(s - t) - 2f_i(s) = g_i(t),$$

for some continuous function g_i. From theorem 4.14, we deduce that there are constants α_i, β_i, γ_i such that

$$f_i(x) = \alpha_i x^2 + \beta_i x + \gamma_i. \qquad (i = 1,2)$$

Replacing the f_i's in (42) by their expressions, we see that each of the h_i's is differentiable. Taking derivatives with respect to x,y (as in the informal argument) yields (44), which reduces, in fact, to (43). ∎

We use this theorem to prove the following generalization of Example 3.1(c).

3.17. Theorem.   *Let* $\mathbf{X}_a, \mathbf{X}_b$ *be two random variables having strictly positive, continuous densities; let* $\zeta_{ij} \neq 0$ $(i = 1,2; j = 1,2)$ *be constants satisfying* (41); *let* G *be a strictly increasing function. Suppose that* $\mathbf{X}_a, \mathbf{X}_b$ *are independent, and that* $G(\zeta_{11}\mathbf{X}_a + \zeta_{12}\mathbf{X}_b)$, $G(\zeta_{21}\mathbf{X}_a + \zeta_{22}\mathbf{X}_b)$ *are also independent. Then* $\mathbf{X}_a, \mathbf{X}_b$ *are normally distributed.*

The assumptions of this theorem can be weakened. For instance, the condition that $\mathbf{X}_a, \mathbf{X}_b$ have strictly positive, continuous densities can be dropped (Feller, 1966, p. 78; Skitlovič, 1954.)

3.18. Proof. Let v be the joint density of the two random variables $\mathbf{Z}_1 = \zeta_{11}\mathbf{X}_a + \zeta_{12}\mathbf{X}_b$, $\mathbf{Z}_2 = \zeta_{21}\mathbf{X}_a + \zeta_{22}\mathbf{X}_b$, and let w be the joint density of $\mathbf{X}_a,\mathbf{X}_b$. The transformation $(x,y) \mapsto (\zeta_{11}x + \zeta_{12}y, \zeta_{21}x + \zeta_{22}y)$ is a 1 to 1 (linear) mapping of the plane onto itself. Consequently, any event A in the space of $(\mathbf{X}_a,\mathbf{X}_b)$ is mapped onto an event A' in the space of $(\mathbf{Z}_1,\mathbf{Z}_2)$, and the probabilities of A,A' in their respective probability spaces are identical. In terms of densities, this means that

$$v(\zeta_{11}x + \zeta_{12}y, \zeta_{21}x + \zeta_{22}y) = w(x,y). \tag{46}$$

We denote the marginal densities of $(\mathbf{X}_a,\mathbf{X}_b)$ by w_1,w_2. Since $\mathbf{X}_a,\mathbf{X}_b$ are independent, we have $w_1(x)w_2(y) = w(x,y)$. Notice that since G is strictly increasing, $\mathbf{Z}_1$ and $\mathbf{Z}_2$ are also independent. Denoting by v_1,v_2 their respective densities, we rewrite (46) as

$$v_1(\zeta_{11}x + \zeta_{12}y)v_2(\zeta_{21}x + \zeta_{22}y) = w_1(x)w_2(y).$$

Since $w_1,w_2 > 0$, we can take logarithms on both sides of this equation, yielding

$$f_1(\zeta_{11}x + \zeta_{12}y) + f_2(\zeta_{21}x + \zeta_{22}y) = h_1(x) + h_2(y),$$

with $f_i = \ln v_i$, $h_i = \ln w_i (i = 1,2)$. Since f_i is the density of a sum of two continuous random variables, $f_i = \ln v_i$ is continuous. All the conditions of Theorem 3.16 are then satisfied. This means that f_i, and thus h_i, must be quadratic functions. We conclude that for some constants α_i, β_i, γ_i and all real numbers x

$$w_i(x) = \exp(\alpha_i x^2 + \beta_i x + \gamma_i) \qquad (i = 1,2.)$$

The result follows by showing that only normal random variables have densities with such a form (Exercise 22). ∎

A FUNCTIONAL INEQUALITY

Inequalities are sometimes very revealing regarding the shape of some unknown functions. An example is given in this section, which deals with the following generalization of the basic Cauchy Equation 15:

$$f(a + b) \leqslant f(a) + f(b). \tag{47}$$

Under continuity or monotonicity assumptions, the Cauchy Equation 15 gave the solution,

$$f(a) = \beta a,$$

with β, a constant. In the case of (47) essentially the same solution is obtained asymptotically, in the sense that

$$\lim_{a \to \infty} \frac{f(a)}{a} = \beta.$$

This material will be useful, particularly in our discussion of the so-called Weber's inequality, in Chapter 8 (cf. Example 3.1(f)).

3.19. Theorem. (Polya & Szego, 1972.) *Let f be a real-valued, strictly increasing function defined on* $\mathbb{N}$ *or* $\mathbb{R}^+$, *and satisfying*

$$f(a + b) \leqslant f(a) + f(b);$$

then

$$\lim_{a \to \infty} \frac{f(a)}{a} = \beta \geqslant 0, \qquad (48)$$

where

$$\beta = \mathrm{Inf}\left\{ \frac{f(a)}{a} \,\middle|\, a \in \mathcal{D}(f) \right\}. \qquad (49)$$

For example, with $f(a) = a^{1/2}$, we have

$$(a + b)^{1/2} \leqslant a^{1/2} + b^{1/2},$$

and

$$\lim_{a \to \infty} \frac{a^{1/2}}{a} = 0.$$

Proof. We consider first the case $\mathcal{D}(f) = \mathbb{N}$. Let β be defined by (49). Notice that β is nonnegative if the equality in (48) holds, since

$$\frac{f(1)}{n} \leqslant \frac{f(n)}{n}.$$

Take any $\varepsilon > 0$. Then

$$\beta \leqslant \frac{f(m)}{m} < \beta + \varepsilon$$

for some $m \in \mathbb{N}$. Any $n \in \mathbb{N}$ can then be written $n = km + p$, with $k \in \mathbb{N} \cup \{0\}$, $p \in \mathbb{N}, 1 \leqslant p \leqslant m - 1$. We have

$$f(n) = f(km + p) \leqslant kf(m) + f(p)$$

yielding, successively,

$$\beta = \frac{f(n)}{n}$$

$$\leqslant \frac{kf(m) + f(p)}{km + p}$$

$$= \frac{f(m)}{m} \cdot \frac{mk}{mk + p} + \frac{f(p)}{n}$$

$$< (\beta + \varepsilon) \cdot \frac{mk}{mk + 1} + \frac{f(m - 1)}{n}.$$

Thus, $f(n)/n \leqslant \beta + \varepsilon$ for n sufficiently large, and we conclude that (48) holds. The case $\mathscr{D}(f) = \mathbb{R}^+$ follows immediately, since for $a \geqslant 1$,

$$\frac{f(\langle a \rangle)}{\langle a \rangle + 1} \leqslant \frac{f(a)}{a} \leqslant \frac{f(\langle a \rangle + 1)}{\langle a \rangle}$$

where $\langle a \rangle$ is the largest integer contained in a, and clearly

$$\lim_{a \to \infty} \frac{f(\langle a \rangle)}{\langle a \rangle + 1} = \lim_{a \to \infty} \frac{f(\langle a \rangle + 1)}{\langle a \rangle}. \quad \blacksquare$$

With the exception of our discussion of Plateau's experiment, all the functional equations encountered so far involve functions of one variable in various combinations. The next section is devoted to a simple, but very useful, result regarding a function of two variables.

SINCOV EQUATIONS

Suppose that we have a real valued function θ of two variables x,y. Under which conditions can θ be decomposed according to the equation

$$\theta(x,y) = g(x) - g(y) \tag{50}$$

for some function g? Such a problem arises frequently in psychophysics in a case where θ is a "data" function; that is, θ is determined—or can be estimated— empirically. The question then is whether this data can be "explained" by the difference $g(x) - g(y)$ of the values of x and y on some psychophysical scale g. A well-known example is the Bradley-Terry-Luce model (also called "strict utility model") where (50) takes the form

$$\ln \frac{P_{x,y}}{1 - P_{x,y}} = g(x) - g(y).$$

(Luce, 1959; Suppes and Zinnes, 1963). In this equation, $P_{x,y}$ is the probability that the subject chooses x when presented with the ordered pair of alternatives (x,y).[4] The Bradley-Terry-Luce model will be discussed in detail in Chapter 5 (see, however, Example 3.25). The inclusion at this point of a discussion of (50) from the viewpoint of functional equations has a particular purpose. The results are specifically needed in Chapter 4, where we discuss Fechner's psychophysics. A convenient language will be introduced for the discussion of Equation 50. This language, and in general, the results of this section, will be used in the future only in the proof of theorems. This material can thus be skipped at first reading without much loss of continuity. We begin with a couple of definitions.

3.20. Definition. Let Y be a set, $B \subset Y \times Y$ and θ a function mapping B into the reals. If xBy, we say that x is *linked* to y. A finite sequence, $x_1, x_2, \ldots, x_n \in Y$, is called a *path (of length $n - 1$) connecting x_1 to x_n* iff $x_i B x_{i+1}$ for $1 \leqslant i \leqslant n - 1$; if

---

4. Frequently, this condition on the probabilities is written under the more familiar equivalent form, $P_{x,y} = v(x)[v(x) + v(y)]^{-1}$.

$x_1 = x_n$, the path is called *cyclic*. The sum $\sum_{i=1}^{n-1} \theta(x_i, x_{i+1})$ is called the *value* (or θ *value*) of the path. With Y, B, and θ as above, the triple (Y, B, θ) is called a *connected system of valued paths* iff for all $x, y, z \in Y$:

1. xBx (B is reflexive).
2. If $\theta(x,y) \leqslant 0 \leqslant \theta(y,z)$ or $\theta(y,z) \leqslant 0 \leqslant \theta(x,y)$, then zBx.
3. There is a path connecting every two points.

A connected system of valued paths is called a *Sincov system* iff

4. Every cyclic path has value zero.

A connected system of valued paths (Y, B, θ) is called *complete* iff $B = Y \times Y$. In such case, Conditions 1 to 3 are automatically satisfied and Condition 4 is equivalent to the condition: if xBy, yBz, and xBz, then

$$\theta(x,z) = \theta(x,y) + \theta(y,z). \tag{51}$$

Indeed, (51) implies $\theta(x,x) + \theta(x,x) = \theta(x,x)$, yielding $\theta(x,x) = 0$. Hence, the value of any cyclic path $\{x_i \mid 1 \leqslant i \leqslant n\}$ is $\sum_{i-1}^{n-1} \theta(x_i, x_{i+1}) = \theta(x_1, x_1) = 0$. Conversely, Condition 4 implies that

$$\theta(x,y) + \theta(y,z) + \theta(z,x) = 0$$

and

$$\theta(x,z) + \theta(z,x) = 0,$$

which together imply (51). Equation 51 was investigated by Sincov (1903a, 1903b; Aczél, 1966, p. 223). The next theorem generalizes a well-known result. Comments on the axioms follow the theorem.

3.21. Theorem.   *Suppose that (Y, B, θ) is a Sincov system. Then there exists a function g mapping Y into the reals such that whenever xBy,*

$$\theta(x,y) = g(x) - g(y).$$

Moreover, if h is another function satisfying these conditions, then $h = g + \beta$ for some constant β.

Clearly, Axiom 4 is necessary for the existence of a function g satisfying (50). Axiom 3 is necessary for the uniqueness of g. For instance, take $Y = \{x, y\}$, $B = \{(x,x), (y,y)\}$, $\theta(x,x) = \theta(y,y) = 0$. Then, clearly Axioms 1, 2, and 4 are satisfied; Axiom 3 fails, and Equation 50 holds for *any* real-valued function g on Y. In particular, with $g(x) = h(x) = 0$, $g(y) = 1$, $h(y) = 2$, there is no β such that $h = g + \beta$. The remaining Axioms 1 and 2 are not necessary. These axioms specify B as a subset of $Y \times Y$. If we assume that (Y, B, θ) is complete, the situation is very simple. In fact, Theorem 3.21 becomes almost trivial. This, however, will frequently be unrealistic from an empirical standpoint. Axioms 1 and 2 ensure that B contains all the pairs in $Y \times Y$, except possibly those pairs (x,y) such that the absolute value of the difference $g(x) - g(y)$ is large. From this viewpoint, Axiom 1 is clear. Axiom 2 states, intuitively, that if x and z are on the same side of some y that is linked to both of them, then they are also linked.

Suppose that (Y,B,θ) is a connected system of valued paths in which every cyclic path of length $\leqslant 3$ has value zero. (Thus, $\theta(x,x) = 0$ for all $x \in Y$.) If xBy, then either $\theta(x,y) \leqslant 0 = \theta(y,y)$, or $\theta(y,y) = 0 < \theta(x,y)$, and yBx follows from Axiom 2. Thus, B is symmetric with $\theta(x,y) = -\theta(y,x)$ whenever xBy, since $\theta(x,y) + \theta(y,x) + \theta(x,x) = 0$. With these facts in mind we turn to the proof of the theorem.

Proof. Let (Y,B,θ) be a Sincov system and let us assume that it is complete. Fix $y_0 \in Y$ and define a function g on Y by $g(x) = \theta(x,y_0)$. Then for all $x,y \in Y$, $\theta(x,y) = \theta(x,y_0) + \theta(y_0,y) = \theta(x,y_0) - \theta(y,y_0) = g(x) - g(y)$. If h is another function on Y such that $\theta(x,y) = h(x) - h(y)$, with $h(y_0) = \beta$, then for all $x \in Y$, $h(x) = \theta(x,y_0) + h(y_0) = g(x) + \beta$.

Assume, therefore, that (Y,B,θ) is not complete. We define a function $\bar{\theta}$ on $Y \times Y$ by

$$\bar{\theta}(x,y) = \sum_{i=1}^{n-1} \theta(x_i,x_{i+1}),$$

where $\{x_i | 1 \leqslant i < n\}$ is a path connecting x and y. The function $\bar{\theta}$ is a well-defined extension of θ to $Y \times Y$. Indeed, suppose that for some $x,y \in Y$, $\{x_i | 1 \leqslant i \leqslant n\}$, $\{x'_j | 1 \leqslant j \leqslant m\}$ are two paths connecting x and y with $\sum_{i=1}^{n-1} \theta(x_i,x_{i+1}) \neq \sum_{j=1}^{m-1} \theta(x'_j,x'_{j+1})$. This implies that

$$\sum_{i=1}^{n-1} \theta(x_i,x_{i+1}) + \sum_{j=1}^{m-1} \theta(x'_{j+1},x'_j) \neq 0$$

contradicting Axiom 4. (Since $x_1 = x = x'_1$, and $x_n = y = x'_{m'}$, we have a cyclic path with a value different from zero.) Moreover, the function $\bar{\theta}$ clearly satisfies Axiom 4. Thus, $(Y, Y \times Y, \bar{\theta})$ is a complete Sincov system and the function g can be constructed by the procedure used above. This yields, if xBy, $\theta(x,y) = \bar{\theta}(x,y) = g(x) - g(y)$. The argument for uniqueness applies here without change. ■

In the above discussion the question is implicitly raised whether Theorem 3.21 still holds if Axiom 4 is replaced by the weaker condition: every cyclic path of length $\leqslant 3$ has value zero. The answer is no, as shown by the following example.

$$Y = \{x_1,x_2,x_3,x_4\};$$

$$x_i B x_j \quad \text{iff} \quad \begin{cases} j - 1 \leqslant i \leqslant j + 1 \\ \qquad \text{or} \\ i = j \pm 3; \end{cases}$$

θ, a function defined on B by

$$\theta(x_i,x_j) = \begin{cases} 0 \text{ if } i = j \\ 1 \text{ if } i = j - 1 \text{ or } i = j + 3 \\ -1 \text{ if } i = j + 1 \text{ or } i = j - 3. \end{cases}$$

It is easy to check that (Y,B,θ) is a connected system of valued paths in which every cyclic path of length $\leqslant 3$ has value zero. Clearly however, no function g can exist satisfying (50). In particular, since $\sum_{i=1}^{3} \theta(x_i,x_{i+1}) + \theta(x_4,x_1) = 4$, we have a cyclic path of length 4 with a value different from zero. The situation is clarified by Theorem 3.23, which is suggested by the above example. We state a preliminary definition.

3.22. Definition. In a connected system of valued paths (Y,B,θ), a path $x_1,x_2,\ldots,x_n$ is called *directional* iff either $\theta(x_i,x_{i+1}) \geqslant 0$ for $1 \leqslant i \leqslant n - 1$, or $\theta(x_i,x_{i+1}) \leqslant 0$, for $1 \leqslant i \leqslant n - 1$.

3.23. Theorem. *In a connected system of valued paths the following conditions are equivalent:*

   (i) *Every cyclic path has value zero.*
   (ii) *Every cyclic path of length $\leqslant 3$ has value zero.*
   Moreover, every two points in a directional cyclic path are linked.

Condition (ii) effectively rules out the counterexample above since x_1, x_2, x_3, x_4, x_1 constitute a directional cyclic path. Thus, for example $\theta(x_1,x_3)$ is defined and equal to $\theta(x_1,x_2) + (x_2,x_3) = 2$. Thus, $-1 = \theta(x_1,x_4) = \theta(x_1,x_3) + \theta(x_3,x_4) = 3$, a contradiction.

Proof. Suppose that (Y,B,θ) is a Sincov system and let $\{x_i | 1 \leqslant i \leqslant n\}$ be a directional cyclic path. Then clearly $\theta(x_i,x_{i+1}) = 0$ for $1 \leqslant i \leqslant n - 1$. In particular, $\theta(x_{i-1},x_i) = 0 = \theta(x_i,x_{i+1})$, implying $x_{i-1}Bx_{i+1}$, by Axiom 2 of a connected system of valued paths. Pursuing this argument we conclude that, x_iBx_j for any two points x_i,x_j in the path.

Suppose that (Y,B,θ) is a connected system of valued paths satisfying condition (ii) of the theorem, and let $\{x_i | 1 \leqslant i \leqslant n\}$ be any cyclic path. If $\theta(x_{j-1},x_j) \leqslant 0 \leqslant \theta(x_j,x_{j+1})$ for some index j, then $x_{j-1}Bx_{j+1}$ by Axiom 2 and the symmetry of B. Thus, the term x_j can be deleted. In fact, since $\theta(x_{j-1},x_{j+1}) = \theta(x_{j-1},x_j) + \theta(x_j,x_{j+1})$ the value of the cyclic path after deletion of x_j remains unchanged. The same argument is applied if $\theta(x_j,x_{j+1}) \leqslant 0 \leqslant \theta(x_{j-1},x_j)$. Clearly, this deletion process can be pursued until a directional cyclic path is obtained the value of which is the same as the original path.
Let us denote $\{x'_k | 1 \leqslant k \leqslant m\}$ this directional path. Thus, $\sum_{i=1}^{n-1} \theta(x_i,x_{i+1}) = \sum_{k=1}^{m-1} \theta(x'_k,x'_{k+1})$. Since all the points of the directional cyclic path are linked, we have successively

$$\theta(x'_1,x'_2) + \theta(x'_2,x'_3) + \cdots + \theta(x'_{k-1},x'_1)$$
$$= \theta(x'_1,x'_3) + \cdots + \theta(x'_{k-1},x'_1)$$
$$= \theta(x'_1,x'_1) = 0 \quad \blacksquare$$

3.24. Remark. Observe that in a Sincov system there is a directional path connecting every two points. This results from a minor modification of the argument used in the above proof with regard to the elimination of the x_i's.

3.25. Example. (The Bradley-Terry-Luce model.) Theorem 3.23 readily suggests an axiom system for the Bradley-Terry-Luce model mentioned at the beginning of this section. Let Y be a set and P a function mapping a subset $C \subset Y \times Y$ into the open interval $(0,1)$. Thus, $P_{x,y}$ is to be interpreted as the probability that the subject chooses x when presented with the ordered pair of alternatives (x,y). Suppose that the triple (Y,C,P) satisfies the following conditions. For all $m \in \mathbb{N}$ and $x,y,z,y_1,y_2,\ldots,y_m \in Y$:

(i) xCx.

(ii) If $P_{x,y} \leqslant \frac{1}{2} \leqslant P_{z,x}$ or $P_{y,x} \leqslant \frac{1}{2} \leqslant P_{x,z}$, then zCy.

(iii) There exists $n \in \mathbb{N}$ and $x_1,x_2,\ldots,x_n \in Y$ such that $x_1 = x$, $x_n = y$ and $x_i C x_{i+1}$ for $1 \leqslant i \leqslant n - 1$.

(iv) If $P_{y_i,y_{i+1}} \leqslant \frac{1}{2}$ for $1 \leqslant i \leqslant m - 1$, then $P_{y_1,y_m} = \frac{1}{2}$ implies that $P_{y_i,y_{i+1}} = \frac{1}{2}$ for $1 \leqslant i \leqslant m - 1$.

(v) $P_{x,y} + P_{y,x} = 1$, whenever xCy and yCx.

In the terminology of Exercise 27 in Chapter 1, these five axioms define a *probabilistic low order*.

Moreover, suppose that whenever the relevant probabilities are defined, we have:

(vi) $\dfrac{P_{x,y}}{P_{y,x}} \cdot \dfrac{P_{y,z}}{P_{z,y}} \cdot \dfrac{P_{z,x}}{P_{x,z}} = 1$.

It follows easily from Theorems 4.21 and 4.23 that, under Conditions (i) to (vi), there exists a function v satisfying

$$P_{x,y} = \frac{v(x)}{v(x) + v(y)}$$

(Exercise 19). This example points out a connection between Sincov systems and probabilistic low orders and is suggestive of the approach taken in Chapter 4 for a much more difficult case.

ADDITIVE SYSTEMS

In our discussion of extensive measurement in Chapter 2, we ask: When can a concatenation be represented by the addition of arithmetic? The problem discussed below is similar. We consider a real valued function M of two real arguments, and we ask: When does there exist a function f satisfying

$$f[M(a,b)] = f(a) + f(b)?$$

(Compare with Theorem 2.7 (ii).) Our answer in Theorem 3.27 is one of the key results of this book. Many of our later developments will be based on the results of this chapter, particularly via Theorem 3.27. The proof of this theorem, which is relegated to the last section of this chapter, is rather long and it may be advisable to skip it at first reading.

Let h be a strictly increasing, continuous function, mapping an open interval $(0,\zeta)$ onto an interval I. Define a function M

$$M(a,b) = h[h^{-1}(a) + h^{-1}(b)].\tag{52}$$

Thus, M maps the set

$$B = \{(a,b) \in I \times I \mid 0 < h^{-1}(a) + h^{-1}(b) < \zeta\}$$

into I. Unless h is the identity function on $(0,\zeta)$, M is not the usual addition of arithmetic, that is, we do not have $M(a,b) = a + b$. In all essential respects, however, M behaves very much like an addition. For example, it is associative, in the sense that, for any a, b, c such that both members are defined, we have

$$M[a, M(b,c)] = M[M(a,b), c].\tag{53}$$

(The reader should check this. This particular way of expressing associativity should not be puzzling. Indeed, defining a binary operation $(a,b) \mapsto a \nabla b = M(a,b)$, we see that (ii) is equivalent to the more traditional $a \nabla (b \nabla c) = (a \nabla b) \nabla c$.)

Since the addition of arithmetic is a convenient operation, it is often of interest for practical reasons to reverse the above construction and to transform a given function M into an addition. When will this be possible? One answer is contained in our next definition.

3.26. Definition.   Let I be a real interval; Let B be a nonempty subset of $I \times I$, (we write aBb for $(a,b) \in B$); let M be a mapping of B into I. We say that (I,B,M) is an *additive system* iff for all a, b, c, a', $b' \in I$,

1. (Associativity)

   $$[aBb \text{ and } M(a,b)Bc] \qquad \text{iff} \qquad [bBc \text{ and } aBM(b,c)],$$

   and when both conditions hold, then

   $$M[a, M(b,c)] = M[M(a,b), c];$$

2. M is strictly increasing in both arguments.
3. If $a \leqslant a'$, $b \leqslant b'$ and $a'Bb'$, then aBb.
4. $a < M(a,b)$.
5. If $c < a$, then there exists $c' \in I$ such that $M(c,c') = a$.

Thus, the notation aBb is an abbreviation to state that the function M is defined at the point $(a,b) \in B$. It is easy to check that all the axioms are satisfied if M is the natural addition ($M(a,b) = a + b$). Since B is not empty, we must have $a < M(a,b)$ for some $a,b \in I$, with also $M(a,b) \in I$; thus I is not a degenerate interval. Notice that if (I,B,M) is an additive system, then another one can obtained simply by taking an arbitrary strictly increasing, continuous mapping f of I into the reals. Indeed, with

$$B_f = \{(s,t) \mid f^{-1}(s)Bf^{-1}(t)\},$$
$$M_f(s,t) = f\{M[f^{-1}(s), f^{-1}(t)]\}$$

it is easy to show that $(f(I), B_f, M_f)$ is an additive system (Exercise 23). Theorem 3.27 states that there is at least one such f such that $M_f(s,t) = s + t$, thus transforming M into an addition.

3.27. Theorem. *Let (I, B, M) be an additive system. Then, there exists a real-valued, strictly increasing function f on I, such that whenever aBb, then $f[M(a,b)] = f(a) + f(b)$. If g is another function satisfying these conditions, then $g = \alpha f$ for some constant $\alpha > 0$. Moreover, the function f is continuous with $f > 0$ and $\inf f(I) = 0$.*

(Thus, $f(I)$ is of the form $(0, \zeta)$ or $(0, \zeta]$ for some real number ζ.) The proof of this theorem is based on Theorems 2.7 and 2.17. Using the axioms of an additive system, we construct a set X of strings of the interval I, and a weak order $\precsim$ on X, such that $(I, X, \precsim)$ is an extensive system. The existence and uniqueness of the function f follows then from an application of Theorem 2.7. Other properties of f are derived from Theorem 2.17. Considering this pattern of proof, a comparison of the axioms of Definition 2.26 with those of Definition 2.6 is in order. Associativity was not needed in Definition 2.6 since the notion of a string involves an implicit associative operation. Axioms 2 and 3 of an additive system together correspond to Axiom 3 of an extensive system. Axioms 4 and 5 are mere translations, respectively, of Axioms 4 and 5 in Definition 2.6. No Archimedean axiom is required mainly because we are within the real number system: the Archimedean property in Axiom 6 of Definition 2.6 can be derived from properties of real numbers.

The last section of this chapter is devoted to the proof of this and of an earlier, related result.

*TWO PROOFS

3.28. Proof of Theorem 3.27. Let us first prove the symmetrical counterpart of Axiom 4.

Lemma 1. *If aBb, then $b < M(a,b)$.*

Proof. Suppose that $M(a,b) \leqslant b$. Successively using Axioms 3, 2, Associativity, 4, and 2, again we obtain successively $M(a,b) \geqslant M[a, M(a,b)] = M[M(a,a), b] > M(a,b)$, a contradiction. ∎

Next we construct an appropriate extensive system. We define a set X of strings of I and a function v mapping X into I recursively as follows.

(i) $I \subset X$ and $v(x) = x$ iff $x \in I$.
(ii) If $x, y \in X$, and $v(x)$, $v(y)$ are defined, then $xy \in X$ iff $v(x)Bv(y)$ with $v(xy) = M[v(x), v(y)]$; otherwise $xy \notin X$ and $v(xy)$ is not defined. (*Warning.* In this paragraph the juxtaposition $a_1 a_2 \cdots a_n$ of real numbers $a_1, a_2, \ldots, a_n \in I$ may denote a string of I or the ordinary multiplication. The context will always eliminate ambiguities.)

Let us show that X and v are well defined. Suppose that four strings x, y, x', y' are such that $xy = x'y'$, and $v(x), v(y)$ are defined with $v(x)Bv(y)$. We must prove that $v(x'), v(y')$ are also define with $v(x')Bv(y')$ and

$$M[v(x), v(y)] = M[v(x'), v(y')].$$

We proceed by induction on the number of terms of the strings. Let $X_n, (n \in \mathbb{N})$ be the subset of X containing the strings of length n or less; that is, $x \in X_n$ means that $x = a_1 a_2 \cdots a_m$ for some $m \in \mathbb{N}$, $m \leqslant n$ and some $a_1, a_2, \ldots, a_m \in I$. For $n = 1, X_1 = I$, and v is well defined on I, since $v(x) = x$ if $x \in I$. For $n = 2$, there is no problem either since in that case $xy = x'y'$ only if $x = x', y = y'$. Suppose that for some $n \geqslant 2$ and all positive integers $m \leqslant n$, X_m is well defined and v is well defined on X_m. Consider the string $xy = x'y'$ of length $n + 1$. If $x \neq x'$, we have two cases: (i) $x = x'z$ for some string z, thus $y' = zy$; (ii) $y = zy'$ for some string z, thus $x' = xz$. We prove (i) and leave (ii) to the reader. Successively,

$$
\begin{aligned}
M[v(x'z), v(y)] &= M\{M[v(x'), v(z)], v(y)\} &&\text{(by hypothesis)} \\
&= M\{v(x'), M[v(z), v(y)]\} &&\text{(by associativity)} \\
&= M[v(x'), v(zy)] &&\text{(by hypothesis)} \\
&= M[v(x'), v(y')]. &&\text{(by hypothesis)}
\end{aligned}
$$

By induction, this proves that X and v are well defined. Notice that, since B is nonempty, X is operant. We define a binary relation $\precsim$ on X as follows: $x, y \in X$, $x \precsim y$ iff $v(x) \leqslant v(y)$.

Lemma 2. $(I, X, \precsim)$ *is an extensive system.*

Proof.   We show that Axioms 1 to 6 of Definition 2.6 are satisfied.
1. True by definition of X.
2. Follows immediately from the definition of $\precsim$.
3. Suppose that $x' \precsim x$, $y' \precsim y$ and $xy \in X$. Then $v(x') \leqslant v(x), v(y') \leqslant v(y)$, with $v(x)Bv(y)$. Using Axiom 3, we conclude that $v(x')Bv(y')$. Observe that we also have $v(x)Bv(y')$. Since M is strictly increasing in both arguments, we have $M[v(x'), v(y')] \leqslant M[v(x), v(y')] \leqslant M[v(x), v(y)]$. Thus, $x'y' \precsim xy$.
4–5. Immediate consequences of the definition of v and of Axioms 4 and 5, respectively.
6. Suppose that $v(n * x) < v(y)$ for some $x, y \in X$ and all $n \in \mathbb{N}$. We write $z_n = v(n * x)$; thus, in particular $z_1 = v(x)$. Since $n * x \prec (n + 1) * x$ by 4 above, (z_n) is a strictly increasing sequence of real numbers bounded above by $v(y)$. This sequence converges to some $\bar{z} \in I$. Since $z_1 < \bar{z}$, we have, by Axiom 5, some $b \in I$ satisfying $M(z_1, b) = \bar{z}$, with $b < M(z_1, b)$ by Lemma 1. We have thus, $b < z_m \leqslant \bar{z}$ for some term z_m in the sequence. Successively, $\bar{z} \geqslant z_{m+1} = M(z_m, z_1) = M(z_1, z_m) > M(z_1, b) = \bar{z}$.

This contradiction establishes the result. ■

Let $\{X',X''\}$ be a cut of $(X,\precsim)$ (Definition 2.16). Thus, $v(x') \leqslant v(x'')$ for all $x' \in X', x'' \in X''$. We have $I = v(X') \cup v(X'')$ where both $v(X'), v(X'')$ are real intervals with $v(X') \cap v(X'') = \emptyset$. Define $\gamma = \sup v(X')$. Then $v(x') \leqslant v(\gamma) \leqslant v(x'')$ implying that $x' \precsim \gamma \precsim x''$, for all $x' \in X'$, $x'' \in X''$. In other words, γ is a separating point of the cut $\{X',X''\}$. Moreover, if x is another separating point of the same cut, we have necessarily $v(x) = \gamma$, $x \sim \gamma$. Thus, all cuts of $(X,\precsim)$ have separating points and if x,y are separating points of the same cut, then $x \sim y$. That is, $(I,X,\precsim)$ is Dedekind complete. Using Lemma 2, Theorem 2.7, and Theorem 2.17, we conclude the following. There exists a mapping ℓ of X into the positive reals such that for all $x,y \in X$

(i) $\ell(x) \leqslant \ell(y)$ iff $x \precsim y$.

(ii) If $xy \in X$, $\ell(xy) = \ell(x) + \ell(y)$.

(iii) If k is another mapping satisfying the above conditions, then $k = \alpha\ell$ for some constant $\alpha > 0$;

(iv) $\ell(X)$ is a real, positive interval having zero as a limit point. Notice also that since $v[v(x)] = v(x)$, we have $v(x) \sim x$, for all $x \in X$. Thus, $\ell[v(x)] = \ell(x)$ implying that $\ell(X) = \ell(I)$. We have, for all $a,b \in I$ such that aBb, successively,

$$\ell[M(a,b)] = \ell\{M[v(a),v(b)]\}$$
$$= \ell[v(ab)]$$
$$= \ell(ab)$$
$$= \ell(a) + \ell(b).$$

Let f be the restriction of ℓ to the interval I. Then, clearly f is strictly increasing, with $f[M(a,b)] = f(a) + f(b)$ if aBb. Suppose that g is some other function on I satisfying these properties. Let $\bar{g}$ be the extension of g to X, defined by $g(x) = g[v(x)]$. We must have $\bar{g} = \alpha\ell$ for some constant $\alpha > 0$. Indeed, if $x,y \in X$, then $\bar{g}(x) \leqslant \bar{g}(y)$ iff $g[v(x)] \leqslant g[v(y)]$ iff $v(x) \leqslant v(y)$ iff $x \precsim y$; and also if $xy \in X$, then $\bar{g}(xy) = g[v(xy)] = g\{M[v(x),v(y)]\} = g[v(x)] + g[v(y)] = \bar{g}(x) + \bar{g}(y)$.

Thus, $\bar{g}$ satisfies properties (i) and (ii) above and property (iii) applies. We conclude that, for any $a \in I$, $g(a) = \bar{g}(a) = \alpha\ell(a) = \alpha f(a)$, as required. Finally, since $f(I)$ is a real positive interval, f is continuous and $\ell > 0$ implies that $f > 0$; however, $\inf f(I) = \inf \ell(X) = 0$. This completes the proof of the theorem. ∎

3.29. Remark. Under the conditions of Theorem 3.27, there also exists a mapping g of I into the reals, strictly increasing, continuous, such that: $g > 1$; $\inf g(I) = 1$; if aBb, then $g[M(a,b)] = g(a)g(b)$; and if v is another function satisfying these conditions, then $v = g^{\alpha}$ for some $\alpha > 0$. Indeed, it suffices to define $g = \exp \circ f$.

3.30. Proof of Theorem 3.2. Suppose that f is a real-valued function, defined on an open interval I having 0 as a limit point, and satisfying

$$f(a + b) = f(a) + f(b). \tag{54}$$

We must show that if f is continuous or strictly monotonic, then

$$f(a) = \beta a$$

for some constant β and all $a \in I$.

Case 1. Assume that f is continuous. We already proved the subcase $I = \mathbb{R}^+$. In fact, the argument used there applies without change to the more general subcase, $I = (0,\zeta)$. In the subcase $I = (\zeta,0), \zeta < 0$, we define a function f_0 on $(0,-\zeta)$ by $f_0(a) = -f(-a)$. Then, clearly, f_0 is strictly increasing on $(0,-\zeta)$, and satisfies (54) for all a, b, $(a + b) \in (0,-\zeta)$. Using the above argument, we obtain $f_0(a) = \beta a, \beta > 0$. Thus, for all $a \in (\zeta,0), f(a) = -f_0(-a) = -\beta(-a) = \beta a$. Finally, we have the case $I = (\zeta,\zeta'), \zeta < 0 < \zeta'$. Taking the restriction of the function f to the set $\{a \in I \,|\, a > 0\}$, and using the argument in the first part of this proof, we know that for some constant $\beta > 0$, $f(a) = \beta a$ for all $a \in I, a > 0$. Observing that $f(0 + 0) = f(0) + f(0)$, we obtain that $f(0) = 0 = \beta \cdot 0$. For $a \in I, a < 0$, we consider two possibilities: if $-a \in I$, then $f(a - a) = f(a) + f(-a) = f(a) + \beta(-a) = 0$, yielding $f(a) = a\beta$; if $-a \notin I$, we find $b \in I$ such that $-b \in I$ and $a = nb$, for some $n \in \mathbb{N}$. Successively, $f(a) = f(nb) = nf(b) = n\beta b = \beta a$.

Case 2. Assume that f is strictly monotonic, say increasing. It suffices to prove the case $I = (0,\zeta)$. Let f^{-1} be the inverse of f. We define a function M, mapping the set $B = \{(a,b) \in I \times I \,|\, a + b \in I\}$ into I by

$$M(a,b) = f^{-1}[f(a) + f(b)]. \tag{55}$$

It is easy to see that since $M(a,b) = a + b, (I,B,M)$ is an additive system. (I leave it to the reader to verify, in detail, that the conditions of Definition 3.26 are indeed satisfied.) Consequently, if f_1 and f_2 are two strictly increasing functions satisfying (55), we must have $f_1 = \beta f_2$ for some constant $\beta > 0$ (Theorem 3.27). Since the identity on I is such a function, f is of the form $f(a) = \beta a, \beta > 0$. ∎

Remark. It is worth pointing out that the key argument in the proof of Case 2 relies on the uniqueness part of Theorem 3.27.

EXERCISES

1. In Example 3.1(a), replace (2) by the more general

$$u[M(a,b)] = \xi u(a) + (1 - \xi) u(b) \tag{*}$$

   (i) Can you distinguish empirically between (*) and Equation 2? (Remember that only M is known.)
   (ii) Find some interesting empirical property on M satisfied by (*).
   (iii) Is (*) compatible with (1) together with either of the two scales, $u(a) = \alpha a^\beta + \gamma, u(a) = \alpha \log a + \beta$? Can you prove Theorem 3.12 in this more general case? What can you say about the still more general case

$$u[M(a,b)] = \xi u(a) + \theta u(b) + \mu?$$

(Cf. Krantz et al., 1971; Pflanzagl, 1968.)

2. Let I be an open interval having 0 as a limit point; let r be a real-valued function on I, strictly increasing, satisfying $r(s + t) = r(s)r(t)$. Prove that, necessarily, $r(s) = \exp \beta s$ for some constant $\beta > 0$ and all $s \in I$ (cf. 3.3).

3. Prove Theorem 3.4.

4. Example 3.1(e)—a memoryless phenomenon. Let $\mathbf{T}$ be a random variable with a mass concentrated on the set of positive real numbers; let g be a real-valued, strictly decreasing function. Suppose that $\mathbb{P}\{\mathbf{T} > t + s | \mathbf{T} > t\} = g(s)\}$ for all $s,t > 0$. Prove that $\mathbf{T}$ is exponentially distributed: $\mathbb{P}\{(\mathbf{T} \leqslant t) = 1 - e^{-\alpha t}\}$, $\alpha > 0$.

5. Check that Theorem 3.2 still holds if f is only assumed to be continuous at one point.

*6. Example 3.1(d)—rating the number of excitations. Use the results of the preceding exercise to solve the following problem. For any real numbers t, τ with $0 \leqslant \tau < t$, let $\mathbf{L}(\tau,t)$ be a random variable with a mass concentrated on the set $\mathbb{N}_0$ of nonnegative integers; let G be a real-valued, strictly increasing function on $\mathbb{N}_0$; define a new random variable $\mathbf{R}(\tau,t) = G[\mathbf{L}(\tau,t)]$. Suppose that (a) whenever $0 \leqslant \tau < t \leqslant \tau' < t'$, the random variables $\mathbf{R}(\tau,t), \mathbf{R}(\tau',t')$ are independent; (b) whenever $0 \leqslant \tau < t$ and $r \in G(\mathbb{N}_0)$ the probability that $\mathbf{R}(\tau,t)$ equals r only depends on $t - \tau$ (and of course, r). For simplicity, define for any real numbers τ, t with $0 \leqslant \tau < t$ and any nonnegative integer $k, v_k(t - \tau) = \mathbb{P}\{(\mathbf{L}(\tau,t) = k)\}$. Prove successively (i) $v_0(s + t) = v_0(s)v_0(t)$; (ii) $v_0(t) = e^{-\lambda t}$; (iii) $v_n(t + s) = \sum_{k=0}^{n} v_k(t)v_{n-k}(s)$; (iv) $v_1(t) = \alpha_1 t e^{-\lambda t}$; (v) $v_2(t) = e^{-\lambda t}\left[\frac{(\alpha_1 t)^2}{2} + \alpha_2 t\right]$. (vi) Compute $v_3(t)$ (cf. Aczél, 1966, pp. 111–114).

7. *(Continuation.)* Prove by induction that

$$v_n(t) = e^{-\lambda t} \sum_{r_1 + 2r_2 + \cdots + nr_n = n} \prod_{i=1}^{n} \frac{(\alpha_i t)^{r_i}}{r_i'} \qquad (n = 0,1,2,\ldots)$$

(iv), (v), and (vi) are three particular cases of this expression, which defines a homogeneous compound Poisson distribution.

8. Find (construct) a nonlinear continuous function f, defined on the open interval (ζ,ζ') with $0 < \zeta$, and satisfying $f(a + b) = f(a) + f(b)$.

*9. Complete the proof of Theorem 3.6 in the case where 0 is a limit point (but not necessarily a point) of the domain I of the functions h,v,k,b.

*10. Prove Theorem 3.7.

11. The proof of a result stated in Table 3.9(i) was requested in the preceding exercise. Assuming this result, derive the other results of Table 3.9.

12. The result in Table 3.10(i) is, in fact, Theorem 3.6. Assuming this result, check the other results in this table in two phases. (a) Check whether the solution in the last two columns satisfies the corresponding functional equation in the first column. (b) Provide a (short) proof of each result.

13. Prove that there is no function g defined on $(0,1)$ and satisfying $g(a - b) = \log a - b^3$. Prove that the functional equation $(a + b)^3 = h^{-1}[h(a) + g(b)]$ has no strictly increasing solution h,g. (The functions h,g are mapping $(0,1)$ into the reals.)

14. Let h, v, g be three real-valued functions defined on an open interval (ζ,ζ'), with $0 < \zeta \leqslant 1 \leqslant \zeta'$ and g strictly increasing. Find the only possible forms of

these functions if we assume that $h(ab) = v(a) + g(b)$ holds. Prove your result. Answer a similar question for the functional equation $h(ab) = v(a)g(b)$.

15. Example 3.1(b)—sound localization. Let I be a positive, open interval, having 1 as a limit point; let M be a real-valued function defined on $I \times I$; let ℓ, r be two real-valued strictly increasing functions defined on I. Suppose that $M(a,b) = M(ca,cb)$ and $M(a,b) = F[\ell(a) - r(b)]$, for some strictly monotonic function F, whenever a, b, ca, $cb \in I$. Prove that necessarily, $\ell(a) = \alpha \log a + \beta$, $r(a) = \alpha \log a + \beta'$ for some constant $\alpha > 0, \beta, \beta'$.

16. Modify the preceding exercise in the case $M(a,b)$ is assumed to depend on the ratio $\ell(a)/r(b)$.

17. Let $\mathbf{X}_a, \mathbf{X}_b$ be two independent, normally distributed, random variables with equal variances; let G be a real-valued, strictly increasing function defined on the reals; define two new random variables $\mathbf{Z}_1 = G(2\mathbf{X}_a - \mathbf{X}_b)$, $\mathbf{Z}_2 = G[(1/3)\mathbf{X}_a + (2/3)\mathbf{X}_b]$. Prove that $\mathbf{Z}_1$ and $\mathbf{Z}_2$ are independent.

18. Prove Theorem 3.13.

19. Example 3.25. Let Y be a set and P a function mapping some set $B \subset Y \times Y$ into the open interval $(0,1)$. Suppose that the triple (Y,B,P) satisfies Conditions (i) to (vi) of 3.25. Prove that there exists a function v on y, satisfying $P_{x,y} = v(x)[v(x) + v(y)]^{-1}$ whenever xBy.

20. (*Continuation.*) Prove that if v' is another function satisfying the condition, then necessarily $v' = \alpha v$ for some constant v. (See Suppes & Zinnes, 1963.)

21. Let h, v, g, k be four real-valued functions, defined on the interval $(0,200)$, satisfying $h(ab) = v(a)g(b)^{k(a)}$, with h,g strictly increasing, and $h,v > 0$. Suppose that $v(1) = g(1) = k(1) = k(2) = 1$, $h(2) = 2$. Compute $v(10)$.

22. Suppose that w is the density of some real random variable X, with $w(x) = \exp(\alpha x^2 + \beta x + \gamma)$ for some constants α, β, and γ and all real numbers x. Prove that X is normally distributed.

23. Let (I,B,M) be an additive system; let f be a real-valued, strictly increasing, continuous function on I; define $B_f = \{(s,t)\} | f^{-1}(s)Bf^{-1}(t)\}$, $M_f(s,t) = f\{M[f^{-1}(s), f^{-1}(t)]\}$. Prove that $(f(I), B_f, M_f)$ is an additive system.

24. Let G be a real-valued function of two real variables, strictly increasing in the first variable. Suppose that $G(s,t) = G(s',t')$ iff $G(\alpha s,t) = G(\alpha s',t')$, for all s, s', t, t', $\alpha \in \mathbb{R}$. Prove that, necessarily, there are functions F, h such that $G(s,t) = F[sh(t)]$ (cf. Burt & Sperling, 1981).

25. Let (Y,B,P) be a probabilistic low order, in the sense of Exercise 27 in Chapter 1. Find necessary and sufficient conditions for the so-called Thurstone model, Case 5 to hold, namely

$$P_{x,y} = \frac{1}{\sqrt{2\pi}} \int_{-\infty}^{u(x)-u(y)} e^{-z^2/2} \, dz,$$

for some strictly increasing, continuous function u. Generalize this result for an arbitrary, continuous distribution function.

II
THEORY

4

Fechner's Psychophysics

...Indeed, we will demonstrate that in principle our psychic measurement will amount to the same as physical measurement, the summation of so-and-so many multiples of an equal unit.

It would be quite in vain to try the engage in such a summation directly. Sensation does not divide into equal inches or degrees by itself, units that we can count and summate. Let us keep in mind, however, that the same problem arises for physical magnitudes. After all, do we count periods of time directly in terms of time, when measuring time, or spatial units directly in terms of space, when we measure space? Do we not rather employ an independent yardstick, a measuring rod, which for time does not consist of pure time, nor for space of pure space and for matter of pure matter alone? Measuring any of these three quantities demands something else as well. Why should the case not be the same in the mental or psychological sphere?

G. T. Fechner, *Elements of Psychophysics*[1]

GUSTAV THEODOR FECHNER, THE PSYCHOPHYSICIST

A professor of physics until the age of 39, Fechner resigned his chair at the University of Leipzig in 1840, as a result of a long illness. After his recovery, his lifelong, but casual, interest for philosophy and psychology became systematic (Boring, 1950, pp. 275–283). He set out to apply the procedures of extensive measurement to the quantification of sensory events, thereby creating a field that he christened "psychophysics."

In this chapter, Fechner's psychophysical scheme is described as Fechner himself might have presented it, were he alive today. As evidenced by his massive and diverse output as a physicist, Fechner was a very sophisticated scientist. It is only reasonable to suppose that a modern Fechner would be well in command of the relevant literature—in particular, obviously, concerning measurement theory. Such updating is rarely done in standard textbooks covering this field, in which Fechner's methods are typically described as if little or no theoretical progress had been made since the publication of *Elemente der Psychophysik*, in 1860.[2] This is unfortunate, since a serious analysis of the foundations of

1. D. H. Howes and E. C. Boring, Eds. Translated by H. E. Adler. Holt, Rinehart and Winston, Inc., Henry Holt Editions in Psychology, 1966, p. 47. (Originally published as *Elemente der Psychophysik*, 1860.)

2. Fechner's ideas are then open to easy, but rather superficial, objections. By way of comparison, think of an introduction to the theory of evolution solely based on Darwin's text, and how vulnerable it would be to modern standards.

Fechner's psychophysics is essential to a good understanding of the theoretical basis of current methodological practice.

As an introduction, we describe an algorithm for the construction of a psychophysical scale in Fechner's style. Our discussion stresses the analogy between such an algorithm and those used in Chapter 2 to measure length.

CONSTRUCTION OF A FECHNERIAN SCALE

4.1. Method.   Suppose that $a, b, c, \ldots$ are numbers representing, in conventional units, the values of some physical magnitude such as mass (or sound pressure, luminance, etc.). For simplicity, we refer to $a, b, c, \ldots$, as stimuli. Let $P_{a,b}$ be the probability that a subject, presented with the pair (a,b) of stimuli in some experimental paradigm, judges a at least as heavy (loud, bright, etc.) as b. For the time being, consider only the data obtained for pairs (a,b) such that $a \geqslant b$. Assume that each stimulus is mapped to a point of some unknown psychophysical scale. Assume also that this mapping preserves the physical order of the stimuli (i.e., $b < a$ iff the scale value of a exceeds that of b) and that $P_{a,b}$ is strictly increasing with the distance between the points representing a and b. The following illustrative device is helpful: identify a and b in the pair (a,b) as names given to the two end points of a "rod" positioned horizontally; a is the name of the right end point and b that of the left end point. In fact, to stress the analogy with extensive measurement, we refer to the pairs (a,b) in this section as "rods." Thus, $P_{a,b}$ increases strictly monotonically with the "length" of the "rod" (a,b). We write

$$
\begin{aligned}
(a,b) &\prec (c,d) &&\text{iff} && P_{a,b} < P_{c,d} \\
(a,b) &\sim (c,d) &&\text{iff} && P_{a,b} = P_{c,d} \\
(a,b) &\precsim (c,d) &&\text{iff} && P_{a,b} \leqslant P_{c,d}.
\end{aligned}
$$

Figure 4.1 summarizes the situation.

Clearly, $\precsim$ is a weak order (Definition 1.14). The rod analogy suggests a concatenation procedure. For example, (a,b) concatenated with (b,c) should have a length equal to that of (a,c). That is,

$$(a,b)(b,c) \sim (a,c).$$

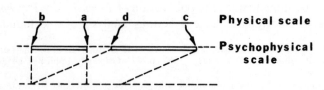

FIGURE 4.1. The pairs $(a,b),(c,d)$ as "rods"; $(a,b) \prec (c,d)$. The length of the rods is assumed to be measured on the psychophysical scale.

Thus, comparing $(a,b)(b,c)$ with (d,e) is made possible by comparing (a,c) with (d,e). For example, if $(a,c) \precsim (d,e)$, one concludes that

$$(a,b)(b,c) \precsim (d,e).$$

This, of course, is a special case. Generally, two rods to be concatenated need not have a common end point. A discussion of the more general situation, although quite straightforward, would involve us in premature developments and we postpone it.[3]

We have thus a set of "rods," a comparison procedure, and a concatenation procedure. Let us proceed to construct a scale measuring the "length" of the "rods" (keeping in mind that the "length" of (a,b) is the distance between the stimuli a,b on some psychophysical scale). Suppose that we decide to use Method 2.2 to measure the "length" of some "rod" (a,a'). We pick some "rod" (b_0,b_1) as a unit, together with any number of exact copies of that "rod,"

$$(b_0,b_1) \sim (b_1,b_2) \sim \cdots \sim (b_i,b_{i+1}) \sim \cdots,$$

with

$$b_0 \geqslant b_1 \geqslant b_2 \geqslant \cdots \geqslant b_i \geqslant b_{i+1} \geqslant \cdots$$

We have thus, by definition of the concatenation,

$$(b_0,b_1)(b_1,b_2)\cdots(b_{i-1},b_i) \sim (b_0,b_i), \qquad i = 1,2,\ldots$$

The length n will be assigned to (a,a') (n being some positive integer), if

$$(b_0,b_n) \precsim (a,a') \prec (b_0,b_{n+1});$$

that is, if correspondingly, the probabilities satisfy the inequalities

$$P_{b_0,b_n} \leqslant P_{a,a'} < P_{b_0,b_{n+1}}. \tag{1}$$

The number n is thus a measure of the "length" of the "rod" (a,a'), that is, of the distance between a and a' on the psychophysical scale. Let us apply this idea in an example. Suppose that the probabilities for all the pairs of stimuli in a set $\{b_0,b_1,b_2,b_3,b_4\}$ are given by the following matrix in which $P_{b_0,b_1} = .75$, $P_{b_0,b_2} = .80$, etc.

	b_0	b_1	b_2	b_3	b_4
b_0	.5				
b_1	.75	.5			
b_2	.80	.75	.5		
b_3	.90	.80	.75	.5	
b_4	.95	.90	.80	.75	.5

$$(2)$$

3. Such discussion is actually embedded in the details of the proof of Theorem 4.13 (see 4.17).

If we take (b_0,b_1) as a unit, this method leads us to assign the values in the matrix below, as measuring the distance between the points:

	b_0	b_1	b_2	b_3	b_4
b_0	0				
b_1	1	0			
b_2	2	1	0		
b_3	3	2	1	0	
b_4	4	3	2	1	0

$$(3)$$

I leave it to the reader to verify this in detail.[4] The five stimuli can thus be represented as points on a straight line, the distance between b_i and b_{i+1} being constant, equal to 1. Except for unessential (and tedious) details, this is Fechner's fundamental idea.

4.2. Remarks.   (1) In our deliberate emphasis of the relation between Fechner's scaling method and extensive measurement, we were led, for simplicity's sake, to make a somewhat unrealistic assumption. We supposed that any "rod" (a,a') could be "squeezed" between two rods (b_0,b_n) and (b_0,b_{n+1}) in the sense of Equation 1. In practice, however, if a and a' are far enough apart, the probability $P_{a,a'}$ will be equal to 1 (or 0, if $a < a'$) and will be unaffected by small changes of the values of a and a'. This means, of course, that Formula (1) cannot hold. A minor modification of the algorithm takes care of this difficulty, without altering the spirit of the method. We assign the number n to (a,a') (say, with $a' < a$) if there exists a sequence $b_0,b_1,\ldots,b_{n+1}$ such that

(i) $a = b_0 > b_1 > \cdots b_n \geqslant a' > b_{n+1}$.
(ii) $P_{b_i,b_{i+1}} = .75$ for $0 \leqslant i \leqslant n$.

(2) The distance $b_i - b_{i+1}$ is often referred to as a "just-noticeable-difference" or "Jnd." Unfortunately, this term is used for a variety of closely related, but different, indices. To eliminate confusion, we reserve the term for one particular such index, which is defined in Chapter 8.

(3) The Fechnerian method of scale construction described in 4.1 is an adaptation of the algorithm for the measurement of the length of rods discussed earlier (cf. First Method 2.2). We have seen that such an algorithm lacks precision. In fact, it can be shown that a full psychophysical scale—one that would assign a scale value to each stimulus—could not be constructed using this method. A more sophisticated algorithm must be used, similar to the Third Method described in 2.4. This point was made by Luce and Edwards (1958).

(4) Even assuming that an appropriate refinement of the algorithm is used, there is no guarantee that the method will work. The analogy of this method with

---

4. The values 0 to 3 follow from a straightforward application of the criterion represented by (1). The value 4 would require a refinement of this criterion (Exercise 1).

that used in extensive measurement indicates that some axioms are implicitly assumed. This analogy even suggests which axioms might be involved. For example, one of the axioms of extensive measurement is Axiom 3 of Definition 2.6. That is, in an extensive system $(A, X, \precsim)$,

if $x' \precsim x$, $y' \precsim y$ and $xy \in X$ then $x'y' \in X$ and $x'y' \precsim xy$.

This axiom has a natural translation in the notations of this chapter. Indeed, identifying

x with the "rod" (a,b),

x' with the "rod" (a',b'),

y with the "rod" (b,c),

y' with the "rod" (b',c'),

suggests the following condition:

if $P_{a',b'} \leqslant P_{a,b}$ and $P_{b',c'} \leqslant P_{b,c}$, then $P_{a',c'} \leqslant P_{a,c'}$

provided that the last two probabilities are defined (see Figure 4.2). We will see that versions of this condition—to which the name bicancellation will be attached—will play a major role in the axiomatization of Fechner's methods.

This condition sets constraints on the results of an experiment intended to provide the basic data for the construction of a Fechnerian scale. A priori, there is no reason to believe that this condition would be satisfied experimentally, for a given psychophysical continuum. To my knowledge, no direct test of this axiom has ever been made. As can be shown easily, Weber's law—a strong form of it, that is—implies it (cf. Exercise 2). (Weber's law is discussed in Chapter 8.) Weber's law itself however is not always satisfied experimentally, and in any event is not necessary for the method to be applicable. (Fechner was well aware of this fact; cf. Fechner, 1966, pp. 54–55.) More generally, two questions are raised here. (1) Which axioms are involved in Fechner's method of scale construction? (2) Are these axioms satisfied experimentally?

(5) Important errors of measurement will unavoidably result from any method that is based on successive concatenation of rods, possibly a large number of times. The method described in 4.1 for example, involves, as a first step, fixing (b_0, b_1) as a "unit." Second, b_2 is estimated such that (approximately) $P_{b_1, b_2} = P_{b_0, b_1}$. Next, b_3 is estimated such that (approximately) $P_{b_0, b_1} = P_{b_2, b_3}$, and so on. Any error made on the estimation of the location of b_2 will affect

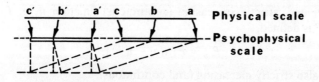

FIGURE 4.2. Axiom 3, Definition 2.6, adapted to Fechner's psychophysical situation: bicancellation and the "rod" analogy.

the estimated location of b_3. In general, the location of b_n will be affected by the accumulated errors made in the location of $b_2, b_3, \ldots, b_{n-1}$. Fechner realized this difficulty, which he bypassed by solving a functional equation: he did not actually construct the psychophysical scale, but simply derived its mathematical form under the constraints imposed by Weber's law. We will address these issues later.

(6) Finally, the status of the Fechnerian scale obtained by this method is ambiguous. Exactly what problems are we solving by such construction? Why would this particular scale be of central importance in psychophysical theory? Fechner's viewpoint seems to have been that such a scale is adequate as a measure of the magnitude of the sensation evoked by the stimulus. As is well known, this position has been sternly criticized, in particular by a contemporary school of psychophysics which originated with S. S. Stevens (1957). (See also Marks, 1974, and many references in that book. We return to this question in Chapter 13.)

In the discussion of such issues, it is important to distinguish clearly between the factual ones (mathematical or empirical) and the philosophical or semantic ones. In this chapter we are mainly concerned with the mathematical aspects, a suitable framework for which is offered by what is called, in the modern literature, *Fechner's problem* (Falmagne, 1971, 1974; Krantz, 1971, 1972a, 1972b; Levine, 1971, 1972; Luce, 1959; Luce & Edwards, 1958; Luce & Galanter, 1963). Reference notes can be found at the end of the chapter.

FECHNER'S PROBLEM

4.3. Notation.   We assume that the physical variable under consideration takes its values in some real, open interval I. (We recall that a real interval is called *closed* (respectively, *open*) when it contains (respectively, does not contain) its end points.) Thus, in a weightlifting experiment, I might contain all weights between say, 0 and 500 g. Since the probabilities $P_{a,b}$ are defined for pairs (a,b) of stimuli, P can be regarded as a function of two variables, taking its values in the open interval $(0,1)$. Let C be the domain of the function P that is the set of all pairs (a,b) for which $P_{a,b}$ is defined. For reasons that will be made clear in a moment, we do not assume that P is necessarily defined for *all* pairs (a,b) of stimuli. In other words, we do not assume that we have necessarily $C = I \times I$. From a mathematical standpoint, the problem implicitly proposed by Fechner can be stated as follows.

4.4. Problem.   Let I be a real, open interval; let C be a subset of $I \times I$; let P be a mapping of C into the open interval $(0,1)$. Find an algorithm for the construction of a real-valued, strictly increasing (continuous) function u on I, such that whenever P is defined,

$$P_{a,b} = F[u(a) - u(b)], \tag{4}$$

where F is also strictly increasing (and continuous).

Thus, in the "rod" analogy used in 4.1, $u(a) - u(b)$ is the length of the rod (a,b) (when $b \leqslant a$). Note that in Problem 4.4, however, we do *not* assume that $P_{a,b}$ is defined only if $b \leqslant a$. Under a slightly different form, this problem was proposed by Luce and Galanter (1963) under the name *Fechner's problem*. That problem immediately suggests the following.

4.5. Representation problem.   Let I, C, and P be as in Problem 4.1. Under which conditions on (I, C, P) does Problem 4.4 have a solution?

The answer would be a list of axioms on (I, C, P) ensuring the existence of a pair (u, F) of functions satisfying (4).

4.6. Remarks.   (1) With suitable refinements (cf. 4.2.(1) and 4.2.(3)), Fechner's scaling algorithm provides a solution to Problem 4.4. This method, however, is applicable only if (I, C, P) satisfies all the axioms in a list constituting a solution to the Representation Problem. There is more than one such solution. For example, in the framework of appropriate side conditions, Weber's law itself is a solution to the Representation Problem. This solution, however, is only a particular case and there are many more.

(2) There is, obviously, a degree of arbitrariness in the choice of Equation 4 to represent the subject's ability to discriminate between adjacent stimuli. In particular, if Equation 4 holds, then

$$P_{a,b} = H[g(a)/g(b)] \tag{5}$$

also holds with $g(a) = e^{u(a)}, H(s) = F(\ln s)$. Instead of differences, we could thus equally well represent pairs of stimuli by ratios. Clearly, (4) and (5) are equivalent, in the sense that they impose identical constraints on the choice probabilities. In the sequel, we occasionally adopt (5) rather than (4) whenever it is convenient.

(3) The errors of estimation inherent in Fechner's method of scale construction are so severe as to rule out such construction as impractical. One may thus wonder whether the Representation Problem is worth investigating. Actually, Fechner's algorithm can be improved. More important, it must be realized that the axioms of a solution to the Representation Problem constitute a genuine psychophysical theory. If these axioms are found to hold experimentally, this is important whether or not a practical method is available to construct the scale.

(4) Equation 4 is sometimes objected to on the grounds that it is too abstract and offers little intuition regarding the mechanisms responsible for the subject's choices. The fundamental importance of Equation 4 in psychophysical theory, however, is that it characterizes a large family of models, some which postulate compelling, explicit choice mechanisms. Several examples of such models are discussed in Chapter 5.

PSYCHOPHYSICAL DISCRIMINATION SYSTEMS

In view of the central importance of the Representation Problem for Fechnerian scaling, two complete solutions will be given. We proceed by first stating a number of background conditions on the choice probabilities. Some of the conditions 1 to 4 gathered in Definition 4.7 may be puzzling at first reading, in part perhaps since the mathematical symbolism may be unfamiliar. To facilitate the reader's approach to these notions, each condition is followed by a paraphrase in parentheses. Some reflection will certainly convince the reader that, in each case, the condition is reasonable from an empirical viewpoint (see the comments following Definition 4.7). The set C in the definition is the set of all pairs (a,b) of stimuli that could be presented to the subject. Note that this set is much larger than the set of pairs actually used in an experiment. This last set is a finite subset of C. We do not assume that all pairs of stimuli could be used, even in an idealized experiment. The reason for this is that some pairs (a,b) of stimuli are uninformative, since the corresponding discrimination probability is 0 or 1 and is unaffected by small changes of the values of a,b. Accordingly, we require the function P to be strictly monotonic in both variables (see Axioms 3 and 4 below).

4.7. Definition.   Let I be a real, open interval; let C be an open[5] subset of $I \times I$. When a pair (a,b) of stimuli belong to the set C, we sometimes say that a is *comparable* to b. Since C is a binary relation, we denote this fact by aCb. Let $(a,b) \mapsto P_{a,b}$ be a function mapping C into the open interval $(0,1)$. Then (I,C,P) is a (*psychophysical*) *discrimination system* iff for all stimuli $a,b \in I$:

1. aCa (every pair (a,a) can be presented to the subject for discrimination).
2. aCb implies bCa (if a is comparable to b, then b is comparable to a).
3. P is strictly increasing in the first variable, strictly decreasing in the second variable, and continuous in both (for every fixed $b \in I$, the two functions p_b and q_b of one variable, defined by $p_b(a) = P_{a,b}$ and $q_b(a) = P_{b,a}$, are continuous; moreover, $a < a'$ iff $p_b(a) < p_b(a')$ iff $q_b(a') < q_b(a)$).
4. The sets $\{c \in I \,|\, cCb\}$ and $\{c \in I \,|\, bCc\}$ are real, open intervals (for every fixed $b \in I$, the domains of the functions p_b and q_b are real, open intervals).

In the sequel, the adjective *psychophysical* will be dropped for simplicity.

Axioms 1 and 2 are quite natural. The function p_b, introduced in the paraphrase of Axiom 3, is the so-called "psychometric function with standard stimulus b," a familiar and important concept in psychophysical practice, which is discussed in detail in Chapters 6 and 7. In terms of this concept, Axioms 3 and 4 imply that any psychometric function is strictly increasing and continuous, and is defined on an open interval. Similar conclusions hold for the functions q_b.

It can be derived from the assumptions defining a discrimination system, that any two stimuli (no matter how distant) can be "linked" by a sequence of pairwise successively comparable stimuli. This is a crucial property. The psychometric functions provide sensitive, local information concerning the discriminability of stimuli. The construction of the scale u of Equation 4 requires that such local information can be pieced together through the entire sensory continuum,

---

5. We recall that a subset $S \subset \mathbb{R}^2$ is called *open* iff for every point $s \in S$ there is an open circle $\{t \in \mathbb{R}^2 \,|\, d(s,t) < r\} \subset S$, with center s and radius r, where d is the Euclidean distance.

especially if reasonable uniqueness properties are desirable (cf. Theorem 4.13). Theorem 4.8 specifies this linkage.

4.8. Theorem. *Let* (I,C,P) *be a discrimination system. For any* $a,b \in I$ *there exists a positive integer n and a sequence* $a_1,a_2,\ldots,a_n \in I$ *such that* $a_1 = a$, $a_n = b$, *and* $a_i C a_{i+1}$ *for* $1 \leqslant i \leqslant n - 1$.

We will postpone the proof of this result (see 4.14). The following condition is widely used.

4.9. Definition. A discrimination system (I,C,P) is called *balanced* iff

$$P_{a,b} + P_{b,a} = 1$$

whenever both aCb and bCa.

In some cases, the balance condition will hold by virtue of the paradigm or of the mode of data collection. An example is a brightness discrimination experiment (such as Cornsweet & Pinsker, 1965) where the position of two patches of light is varied randomly, over trials, from above to below a fixation point, and the data are pooled over position. In other cases, however, such averaging is not legitimate and may mask an important phenomenon. For instance, the order of the stimuli in the notation (a,b) may symbolize the fact that stimulus a is presented first, followed by stimulus b. The balance condition states, in effect, that the order of presentation has no effect on the result of a comparison. This may not be true, for example, for auditory stimuli presented successively. This case is considered in Chapter 6 where a more general theory is discussed.

Notice that, taken by themselves, the axioms of a balanced psychophysical discrimination system are not sufficient to ensure that Equation 4

$$P_{a,b} = F[u(a) - u(b)]$$

holds for some strictly increasing, continuous functions u,F. Indeed, suppose that

$$P_{a,b} = \Phi\left[\frac{a - b}{(a + b)^{1/2}}\right] \tag{6}$$

for all positive real numbers a,b. (As customary, we denote by Φ the distribution function of a standard, normal random variable.) It is easy to check that, as defined by (6), the probabilities $P_{a,b}$ satisfy all the conditions of a balanced psychophysical discrimination system. (This verification is left to the reader.)

This model, however, is incompatible with Equation 4. The reason for this is that the (functional) equation

$$P_{a,b} = \Phi\left[\frac{a - b}{(a + b)^{1/2}}\right] = F[u(a) - u(b)]$$

has no solution for the functions u,F. (That is, there are no functions u,F "solving" this equation; cf. Iverson, 1979; see also Exercise 3.) Thus, additional conditions on the choice probabilities are needed if Equation 4 is to hold. Two such conditions are introduced in Definition 4.10.

SOME NECESSARY CONDITIONS

4.10. Definition.   A discrimination system (I,C,P) is called *Fechnerian* iff the equation $P_{a,b} = F[u(a) - u(b)]$ holds for some strictly increasing continuous functions u, F. In such case, the pair (u, F) of functions will be called a *Fechnerian representation* of (I,C,P).

We say that (I,C,P) satisfies the *bicancellation condition* iff

$$\text{whenever} \quad P_{a,b} \leqslant P_{a',b'}, P_{b,c} \leqslant P_{b',c'}, aCc \quad \text{and} \quad a'Cc' \quad \text{then} \quad P_{a,c} \leqslant P_{a',c'}. \quad (7)$$

We refer to *weak bicancellation* as the condition obtained by replacing all three inequalities in (7) by equalities.

A discrimination system (I,C,P) satisfies the *quadruple condition* iff

$$P_{a,b} \leqslant P_{a',b'} \qquad \text{iff} \qquad P_{a,a'} \leqslant P_{b,b'} \qquad (8)$$

whenever all four probabilities are defined. The *weak quadruple condition* is obtained by replacing the two inequalities in (8) by equalities.

It is clear that bicancellation implies weak bicancellation, and that the quadruple condition implies the weak quadruple condition. In the framework of a balanced discrimination system, these condition are pairwise equivalent. That is,

4.11. Theorem.   *In a balanced discrimination system:*

  (i) *Bicancellation is equivalent to weak bicancellation.*

  (ii) *The quadruple condition is equivalent to the weak quadruple condition.*

We postpone the proofs of these two propositions, which are elementary, but fairly long (see 4.15). The following strengthening of bicancellation is also useful.

4.12. Theorem.   *Let (I,C,P) be a balanced discrimination system satisfying bicancellation. If one of the two inequalities in the hypothesis of (7) is strict, the inequality in the conclusion is also strict.*

Proof.   We proceed by contradiction. Suppose for example, that $P_{a,b} < P_{a',b'}$, $P_{b,c} \leqslant P_{b',c'}$ and $P_{a,c} = P_{a',c'}$. By the symmetry of the relation C and the balance property, we derive $P_{c',b'} \leqslant P_{c,b}$, which together with $P_{a',c'} = P_{a,c}$, yields $P_{a'b'} \leqslant P_{a,b}$, a contradiction. The argument is similar in the other case. ∎

The necessity of weak bicancellation and of the weak quadruple condition for a balanced discrimination system to be Fechnerian is easily verified. Each one of these condition turns out to be sufficient.

REPRESENTATION AND UNIQUENESS THEOREM

4.13. Theorem.   *Let ψ be a balanced discrimination system. Then, the following three conditions are equivalent:*

(i) ψ is Fechnerian.

(ii) ψ satisfies weak bicancellation.

(iii) ψ satisfies the weak quadruple condition.

Moreover, suppose that (u,F), (u_0,F_0) are two Fechnerian representation of ψ, then $u_0(a) = \alpha u(a) + \beta$ and $F_0(s) = F(s/\alpha)$ for some constants $\alpha > 0$ and β.

The proof of this result, which is given in 4.17, is rather long and technical, and should probably not be examined at first reading. The impatient student may wish to glance at the preceding paragraph (4.16) where an outline of the proof is provided. Note that the balance condition can be dropped in this theorem. (See Exercises 11 to 13 in Chapter 6.)

Placed on the background of the conditions defining a balanced discrimination system, each of weak bicancellation and of the weak quadruple condition constitutes a complete solution to the Representation Problem. Or, to put it another way, any model for choice probabilities $P_{a,b}$ satisfying either weak bicancellation or the weak quadruple condition can be put in the form of Equation 4. In principle, these conditions can be tested experimentally. In practice, however, rather delicate statistical issues arise (cf. Iverson & Falmagne, 1985).

The importance given in this chapter to Equation 4 may surprise the reader. Actually, this representation has an impact beyond Fechner's scaling method. Many current models for choice probabilities are Fechnerian (in the sense of Definition 4.10). As we will see, these models differ in the specific assumptions made regarding the mechanisms of choice, which in turn determine the form of the function F in Equation 4.

The critical issue remains the status of the scale u, once it has been constructed. Does it make sense, as Fechner proposed, to consider that such a scale measures the magnitude of the "sensation" evoked by the stimulus? We postpone this discussion for the moment (see Chapter 13).

*PROOFS

4.14. Proof of Theorem 4.8. Let (I,C,P) be a discrimination system (Definition 4.7). For every $a \in I$, let $Ca = \{b|bCa\}$, and $aC = \{b|aCb\}$; thus $aC = \{b|a \in Cb\}$. By Axiom 4 of 4.7, the sets Ca and aC are open intervals, for every $a \in I$. Define a relation $\sim$ on I by

$$a \sim b \qquad \text{iff} \qquad a_i Ca_{i+1}, \qquad 1 \leqslant i \leqslant n - 1,$$

for some finite sequence $(a_i)_{1 \leqslant i \leqslant n}$ in I, with $a = a_1$, and $b = a_n$. It is clear that $\sim$ is an equivalence relation. Moreover, every equivalence class is an open set, since it is a union of open sets. Indeed, the class of $\sim$ containing a includes $\kappa_a = \bigcup_{b \in Ca} bC$. It also includes κ_b, for any $b \in \kappa_a$, etc. There can only be one such class, otherwise I could be partitioned into two open sets, contradicting the assumption that I is an (open) interval. ∎

4.15. Proof of Theorem 4.11.   Let (I,C,P) be a discrimination system.

(i) We have to show that weak bicancellation implies bicancellation. (The converse is obvious.) We proceed by contradiction. Suppose that weak bicancellation holds, but

$$P_{a,b} \leqslant P_{a',b'}, P_{b,c} \leqslant P_{b',c'}, \quad \text{and} \quad P_{a',c'} < P_{a,c}$$

for some $a, b, c, a', b', c' \in I$.

We consider six cases corresponding to the six possible orderings of $\{a',b',c'\}$: (1) $c' \leqslant b' \leqslant a'$; (2) $c' \leqslant a' \leqslant b'$; (3) $b' \leqslant c' \leqslant a'$; (4) $b' \leqslant a' \leqslant c'$; (5) $a' \leqslant c' \leqslant b'$; (6) $a' \leqslant b' \leqslant c'$. Each of the six cases leads to an absurdity. We give a detailed proof of Case 1, and sketch the proofs of Cases 2 to 6.

Case 1.   Since $c' \leqslant a'$, we obtain $P_{c,c} = \frac{1}{2} \leqslant P_{a',c'} < P_{a,c}$ yielding $c < a$, and, by continuity, there exists $a'' < a$ such that $P_{a'',c} = P_{a',c'}$. Using the inequalities

$$P_{b,c} \leqslant P_{b',c'} \leqslant P_{a',c'} < P_{a,c},$$

we get $b < a$ by Axiom 3 of 4.7; moreover, there exists similarly $b'' \geqslant b$ such that $P_{b'',c} = P_{b',c'}$. From the balance condition, we obtain $P_{a'',c} = P_{a',c'}, P_{c,b''} = P_{c',b'}$ and if $a''Cb''$, then $P_{a'',b''} = P_{a',b'}$ by weak bicancellation, yielding

$$P_{a,b} \leqslant P_{a',b'} = P_{a'',b''} < P_{a,b''} \leqslant P_{a,b}$$

a contradiction. The fact that $a''Cb''$ results, by convexity, from $b \leqslant b'' < a$ and $c \leqslant a'' < a$, with either $b \leqslant c$ or $c \leqslant b$.

Case 2. $c' \leqslant a' \leqslant b'$ and the hypothesis yield $c \leqslant a \leqslant b$, and a'',b'' exist satisfying $P_{c,a''} = P_{c',a'}, P_{a'',b''} = P_{a',b'}$ with cCb'' and $b'' < b$. Using weak bicancellation, we derive $P_{c,b''} = P_{c',b'}$ with, successively $P_{c,b} < P_{c,b''} = P_{c',b'} \leqslant P_{c,b}$.

Case 3. $b' \leqslant c' \leqslant a'$ and the hypothesis imply $b \leqslant c \leqslant a$ and a'',b'' exist satisfying $P_{a'',c} = P_{a',c'}, P_{c,b''} = P_{c',b'}$ with $a''Cb''$, aCb'' and $a'' < a$, $b \leqslant b''$. Weak bicancellation yields $P_{a'',b''} = P_{a',b'}$ with, successively, $P_{a'',b''} < P_{a,b''} \leqslant P_{a,b} \leqslant P_{a',b'} = P_{a'',b''}$.

Case 4.   From $b \leqslant a' \leqslant c'$ and the hypothesis, we derive $b < a \leqslant c$, and there exist a'',b'' such that $P_{c,b''} = P_{c',b'}, P_{a'',c} = P_{a',c'}$ with $b \leqslant b'' \leqslant a'' < a$. Thus, $a''Cb''$, aCb'' and $P_{a'',b''} = P_{a',b'}$ by weak bicancellation. Successively,

$$P_{a'',b''} < P_{a,b''} \leqslant P_{a,b} = P_{a',b'}.$$

Case 5.   From $a' \leqslant c' \leqslant b'$ and the hypothesis we derive $a \leqslant c < b$, and there exist a'',b'' such that $P_{a'',c'} = P_{a,c}, P_{c',b''} = P_{c,b}$, with $a' < a'' \leqslant c' < b'' < b'$. Thus $a''Cb''$, $a'Cb''$ and $P_{a'',b''} = P_{a,b}$ by weak bicancellation. Successively,

$$P_{a,b} \leqslant P_{a',b'} \leqslant P_{a',b''} < P_{a'',b''}.$$

Case 6.   From $a' \leqslant b' \leqslant c'$ and the hypothesis we derive $a \leqslant b \leqslant c$, and there exists a'',c'' such that $P_{a'',b} = P_{a',b'}, P_{b,c''} = P_{b',c'}$ with $a \leqslant a'' \leqslant b \leqslant c'' \leqslant c$. Thus

$a''Cc''$, aCc'' and by weak bicancellation $P_{a'',c''} = P_{a',c'}$. Successively,

$$P_{a,c} \leqslant P_{a,c''} \leqslant P_{a'',c''} = P_{a',c'} < P_{a,c}.$$

This completes the proof of part (i).

(ii) We also proceed by contradiction. Assume that the weak quadruple condition holds, but that the quadruple condition does not, since

$$P_{a,b} < P_{a',b'} \qquad \text{and} \qquad P_{b,b'} < P_{a,a'}. \tag{9}$$

Again, we consider the order of the values of the stimuli. There are $4! = 24$ orders of a, a', b, b', but half of these are not consistent with (9). For instance, we cannot have $b \leqslant a$ and $a' \leqslant b'$, since this would imply that $P_{a',b'} \leqslant \frac{1}{2} \leqslant P_{a,b}$. Similarly, we cannot have $b' \leqslant b$ and $a \leqslant a'$, in view of the second inequality in (9). Of the remaining 12 cases, 6 can be dropped because of the symmetry introduced by the balance condition. For example, the case $a \leqslant b \leqslant a' \leqslant b'$ of (9) is equivalent to the case $b' \leqslant a' \leqslant b \leqslant a$ of

$$P_{b',a'} < P_{b,a} \qquad \text{and} \qquad P_{a',a} < P_{b',b},$$

which follows from (9) by applying the balance condition. Finally, only 3 of the 6 remaining cases have to be discussed, because of the symmetry of Formula 9: for example, the case $a \leqslant b \leqslant a' \leqslant b'$ of the first inequality in (9) corresponds to the case $b \leqslant b' \leqslant a \leqslant a'$ of the second inequality. We consider 3 cases.

Case 1. $a \leqslant b \leqslant a' \leqslant b'$. By the balance condition, this implies

$$P_{a,b} < P_{a',b'} \leqslant \tfrac{1}{2} \leqslant P_{b',b}.$$

Using continuity and convexity (Axioms 3 and 4 of Definition 4.7), we can assert the existence of $a'' \in I$ satisfying $P_{a'',b} = P_{a',b'}$, with $a \leqslant a'' \leqslant b \leqslant a'$. Notice that aCa' implies aCa''; that is, $a''Ca$. Applying the weak quadruple condition, we obtain

$$P_{a'',a'} = P_{b,b'} < P_{a,a'},$$

yielding $a'' < a$, a contradiction. Cases 2 and 3 are similar, and we only sketch the argument.

Case 2. $a \leqslant b \leqslant b' \leqslant a'$. There is $b'' \geqslant b$ such that $P_{b'',b'} = P_{a,a'}$ with $b''Ca$, and thus

$$P_{a,b''} = P_{a',b'} > P_{a,b}$$

yielding $b'' < b$, a contradiction.

Case 3. $a \leqslant a' \leqslant b \leqslant b'$. There is $a'' > a$ such that $P_{a'',b} = P_{a',b'}$ with $a''Ca'$, and thus

$$P_{a'',a'} = P_{b,b'} < P_{a,a'}$$

yielding $a'' \leqslant a$, a contradiction. ■

4.16. Outline of the proof of Theorem 4.13. Let $\Psi = (I,C,P)$ be a balanced discrimination system. Our proof of Theorem 4.13 follows the pattern

$$(ii) \Rightarrow (i) \Rightarrow (iii) \Rightarrow (ii).$$

To show that (ii) implies (i), we define

$$J = \{t \mid t = P_{a,b} > \tfrac{1}{2}, a,b \in I\}, \tag{10}$$

$$B = \{(s,t) \in J \times J \mid s = P_{a,c}, t = P_{b,c} \quad \text{for some } a, c, b \in I\}. \tag{11}$$

Let M be a function mapping B into J, defined by

$$M(P_{a,c}, P_{c,b}) = P_{a,b} \tag{12}$$

In view of weak bicancellation, it is clear that M is a well-defined function. We then prove that (J,B,M) is an additive system in the sense of 3.26. Using Theorem 3.27, we can assert the existence of a function h, satisfying

$$h[M(s,t)] = h(s) + h(t),$$

or, with $s = P_{a,c}, t = P_{c,b}$

$$h(P_{a,b}) = h(P_{a,c}) + h(P_{c,b}). \tag{13}$$

The function h is only defined on part of the range of P. We extend h to a function H defined on $\mathscr{R}(P)$ by

$$H(s) = \begin{cases} h(s) & \text{if } s \in J; \\ -h(1-s) & \text{if } (1-s) \in J; \\ 0 & \text{if } s = \tfrac{1}{2}. \end{cases} \tag{14}$$

It is easily verified that H is strictly increasing and continuous, and satisfies (13). Notice that (13) has the form of Equation 51 in Chapter 3. In this connection, we show (using 3.22 and 3.23), that with $(a,b) \mapsto H(P_{a,b}) = \theta(a,b)$, the triple (I,C,θ) is a Sincov system in the sense of 3.20. From Theorem 3.21, we derive that

$$\theta(a,b) = H(P_{a,b}) = u(a) - u(b),$$

for some function u. Or, equivalently, with $F = H^{-1}$,

$$P_{a,b} = F[u(a) - u(b)],$$

and it is not difficult to check that the functions u and F satisfy the required conditions. We conclude that (I,C,P) is Fechnerian. The uniqueness properties of the functions u and F in Theorem 4.13 are easy consequences of the uniqueness of the functions in Theorem 3.27 and 3.21.

The proof that (i) implies (iii) relies on simple algebra and is very short. We leave it to the reader (Exercise 14). So far, the argument, however long and tedious, is quite elementary. The last part of the proof, that is, (iii) implies (ii), uses the so-called maximal principle (e.g., Ore, 1962), a property equivalent to the Axiom of Choice.

We begin by showing that if C is a finite union of overlapping open "squares" $(a,b)^2 \subset \mathbb{R}^2$, then the quadruple condition implies bicancellation. Such unions are called $\mathscr{S}$-coverings. Finally, in the general case, we argue that C can always be represented as a chain of such $\mathscr{S}$-coverings, and an application of the maximal principle yields the result.[6]

4.17. Proof of Theorem 4.13. Suppose that $\Psi = (I,C,P)$ is a balanced discrimination system.

(ii) *implies* (i). In view of Theorem 4.11, we assume that bicancellation holds.

Since $P_{a,a}$ is defined and equal to $\frac{1}{2}$ for all $a \in I$, it follows from the continuity of P that the J defined in (10) is an open interval. Let B and M be defined by (11) and (12), respectively.

Lemma 1. $\mathscr{R}(M) = J$.

We leave the proof of the reader.

Lemma 2. (J,B,M) *is an additive system, in the sense of* 3.26.

Proof. We successively prove Axioms 2 to 5 of 3.26, and we conclude by the associativity, Axiom 1.

2. Suppose that $s < s'$, with sBt, $s'Bt$. Say that $s = P_{a,b}$, $t = P_{b,c} = P_{b'c'}$, $s' = P_{a',b'}$ and $P_{a,b} < P_{a',b'}$. Then $M(s,t) = P_{a,c}$, $M(s',t) = P_{a',c'}$ and $P_{a,c} < P_{a',c'}$, follows from Theorem 4.12. The argument in the other case is similar.
3. Suppose that $\frac{1}{2} < s \leqslant s'$, $\frac{1}{2} \leqslant t \leqslant t'$ and $s'Bt'$. Say that $s' = P_{a,b}$, $t' = P_{b,c}$. Using Axioms 4 and 5 of a discrimination system, we derive $s = P_{a',b}$, $t = P_{b,c'}$ for some $a',c' \in I$, with necessarily $a'Cc'$ and thus, sBt.
4. Assume that $M(s,t) \leqslant s$, with $\frac{1}{2} < M(s,t) = P_{a,b} \leqslant P_{a,c} = s$, and $\frac{1}{2} = P_{b,b} < P_{c,b} = t$. By the monotonicity properties of P, we obtain $c \leqslant b$ and $b < c$, a contradiction.
5. Immediate from the continuity and monotonicity properties of P.
1. Finally, we establish the associativity of M. Suppose that rBs, $M(r,s)Bt$. Say that $r = P_{a,b}$, $s = P_{b,c}$, $M(r,s) = P_{a,c} = P_{a',c'}$, $P_{c',d} = t$, $a'Cd$. (The situation is shown in Figure 4.3.) Since $P_{a,b} < P_{a,c} = P_{a',c'}$ (Axiom 4 of an additive system established above), we have $P_{a',b'} = P_{a,b}$ for some $b' \in I$, with $b'Cc'$. The two equalities $P_{a,c} = P_{a',c'}$ and $P_{a',b'} = P_{a,b}$ yield $P_{b',c'} = P_{b,c}$, by the balance condition and weak bicancellation. We also have $b'Cd$. Thus sBt and since $a'Cd$, $rBM(s,t)$. In fact,

$$
\begin{aligned}
M[r,M(s,t)] &= M[P_{a',b'}, M(P_{b',c'}, P_{c',d})] \\
&= P_{a',d} \\
&= M(P_{a',c'}, P_{c',d}) \\
&= M[M(r,s), t].
\end{aligned}
$$

The proof in the other case is similar. ∎

6. For this part of the proof, I benefited from discussions with W. Pankey.

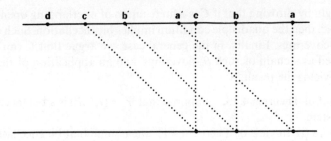

FIGURE 4.3. Lemma 2 in 4.17. The associativity of M.

Using Theorem 3.27, we can assert the existence of a function h on J, positive valued, strictly increasing, continuous, with inf $h(J) = 0$, satisfying

$$h[M(s,t)] = h(s) + h(t).$$

We extend this function h to a function H defined by (14) on the range of P, as specified in the outline of the proof. It is easily verified that H is strictly increasing and continuous. (In particular, the fact that inf $h(J) = 0$ provides the continuity of H at the point $\frac{1}{2}$.)

Define a function θ on C by

$$\theta(a,b) = H(P_{a,b}).$$

Lemma 3.   (I,C,θ) is a Sincov System (Definition 3.20).

We leave it to the reader to verify that (I,C,θ) satisfies Conditions 1 to 3 of 3.20 and Condition (ii) of Theorem 3.23. Using Theorem 3.21, we know that there is a function u mapping I into the reals, such that whenever aCb, then

$$\theta(a,b) = H(P_{a,b}) = u(a) - u(b). \tag{15}$$

Since both H and $a \mapsto P_{a,b}$ are strictly increasing and continuous functions, the function u shares these properties. Defining $F = H^{-1}$, we see that (u,F) is a Fechnerian representation of Ψ. This completes the proof that (ii) implies (i).

The uniqueness of the Fechnerian representation in Theorem 4.13 follows readily from the uniqueness the representations in Theorems 3.21 and 3.27. We only sketch the argument. Going back to Theorem 3.21, we know that if u_0 is another function satisfying (15)—for a fixed function H—then $u_0 = u + \gamma$ for some constant γ. Suppose that (u_0,F_0) is some other Fechnerian representation of Ψ. Then F_0^{-1} is a function, and with $\frac{1}{2} < s = P_{a,b}$, $\frac{1}{2} < t = P_{b,c}$ and $M(s,t) = P_{a,c}$, we have successively

$$\begin{aligned}
F_0^{-1}[M(s,t)] &= F_0^{-1}(P_{a,c}) \\
&= u_0(a) - u_0(c) \\
&= [u_0(a) - u_0(b)] + [u_0(b) - u_0(c)] \\
&= F_0^{-1}(P_{a,b}) + F_0^{-1}(P_{b,c}) \\
&= F_0^{-1}(s) + F_0^{-1}(t).
\end{aligned}$$

From Lemma 2 and Theorem 3.27, we conclude that $F_0^{-1} = \alpha F^{-1}$ for some constant $\alpha > 0$. Thus, $F_0(s) = F(s/\alpha)$, from which we easily derive $u_0/\alpha = u + \gamma$, or $u_0 = \alpha u + \beta$, $\beta = \alpha \gamma$. The above argument only concerns the upper portion of F, F_0 but is easily extended to the lower portion.

(i) *implies* (iii). This argument, which only requires elementary algebra, is left to the reader.

(iii) *implies* (ii). Applying Theorem 4.11, we assume thus that the quadruple condition holds for $\Psi = (I, C, P)$. In this part of the proof, we consider particular subsystems $\Psi^* = (I^{(A)}, A, P^{(A)})$ of Ψ, in which $I^{(A)} \subset I$ is some open interval, $A \subset C$ and $P^{(A)}$ is the restriction of P to A. For simplicity, we drop the exponent (A) in the notation and simply write $\Psi^* = (I, A, P)$. In the sequel, the notation (s, t) with $s, t \in \mathbb{R}$ may either stand for the point $(s, t) \in \mathbb{R}^2$, or represent the open interval with end points s, t (in which case, obviously, $s < t$). The context will eliminate ambiguities.

The argument establishing that weak bicancellation holds for Ψ is spelled out as a series of lemmas. We omit or only give a sketch of the proofs, which are quite simple.

Lemma 4. For any point $(s, t) \in C$, with $s < t$, the subsystem $(I, (s, t)^2, P)$ satisfies bicancellation.

Lemma 5. Let $\Psi^* = (I, \bigcup_{i=1}^{n} I_i^2, P)$ be a subsystem of Ψ such that each $I_i \subset I$ is an open interval, and for $1 \leqslant i \leqslant n - 1$, $I_i \cap I_{i+1} \neq \varnothing$. Then Ψ^* satisfies weak bicancellation.

Proof. By Lemma 4, the subsystem $\Psi_i = (I_i, I_i^2, P)$ satisfies bicancellation. Thus, by the first part of the proof of Theorem 4.13 (the implication (ii) $\Rightarrow$ (i)), each Ψ_i is Fechnerian, with a representation (u_i, F_i). Using the uniqueness of the Fechnerian representations, and the fact that the subsystems Ψ_i overlap, a Fechnerian representation for Ψ^* extending (u_1, F_1) can be constructed inductively. Since the existence of a Fechnerian representation implies weak bicancellation, the lemma follows. ∎

The union $\bigcup_{i=1}^{n} I_i^2$ in Lemma 5 will be called a *(finite)* $\mathscr{S}$-*covering*.

In the rest of the proof, we proceed to show that C can be represented as a union of a chain of $\mathscr{S}$-covering. Weak bicancellation results then from an application of the maximal principle. From a geometrical viewpoint the existence of the chain of $\mathscr{S}$-coverings is intuitively obvious. The next three lemmas should remove all doubts.

Lemma 6. For any $a, b \in I$, with $a < b$, there is an $\mathscr{S}$-covering $\bigcup_{j=1}^{n} I_j^2$ such that $\bigcup_{j=1}^{n} I_j$ is the open interval (a, b).

Proof. Use Theorem 4.8 and the openness of C: for each a_i in Theorem 4.8, there is an open square $I_i \times I_i \subset C$ containing a_i. ∎

Lemma 7. Let $S(a, b)$ be the $\mathscr{S}$-covering of Lemma 6. Take any $(s, t) \in C$ such that either $a < s < b$ or $a < t < b$. Then there is an $\mathscr{S}$-covering $S'(s, t)$ such that

$$S(a, b) \cup \{(s, t), (t, s)\} \subset S'(s, t).$$

Lemma 8.   For any $a,b \in I$, with $a < b$, the set $(a,b)^2 \cap C$ can be represented as a chain of $\mathscr{S}$-coverings.

This results readily from Lemmas 6 and 7. By Lemma 6, each $\mathscr{S}$-covering S defines a subsystem (I,S,P) satisfying weak bicancellation. Using Lemma 8 and the maximal principle, we can assert that any subsystem $(I, (a,b)^2 \cap C, P)$ also satisfies weak bicancellation. Noticing that

$$C = \bigcup_{a < b} [(a,b)^2 \cap C],$$

still another application of the maximal principle yields that weak bicancellation holds for all of Ψ.

This completes the proof of Theorem 4.13. ■

REFERENCE NOTES

The discussion of Fechner's scaling methods given here, even though perfectly compatible with Fechner's own presentation, was strongly influenced by the developments of measurement theory, as given for example in Krantz et al. (1971) or Roberts (1979). In this context, Fechner's problem is a case of "difference measurement." The notions of a representation problem, representation theorem, and uniqueness theorem are standard in measurement theory.

This modern viewpoint regarding Fechner's enterprise is due to Luce and his collaborators (Luce, 1959; Luce & Edwards, 1958; Luce & Galanter, 1963). The solution to the representation problem given here is mostly due to Doignon and Falmagne (1974; see also Falmagne, 1971a, 1974). Related references are Levine (1971, 1972) and Krantz (1971, 1972). Equation 4 also appears in the general context of choice theory where it is dubbed the strong utility model (Luce & Suppes, 1965). The quadruple condition has been investigated by Marschak (1960) and Debreu (1960).

As indicated, statistical issues regarding the empirical testing of axioms such as bicancellation or the quadruple condition, which raise difficult problems, are discussed in Iverson and Falmagne (1983).

EXERCISES

1. Refine the criterion embodied in Equation 1, to fully justify the numerical assignment given in Table (3).
2. Let (I,C,P) be a balanced discrimination system (Definition 4.7). Suppose that $P_{a,b} = P_{\xi a,\xi b}$, whenever aCb, $\xi aC\xi b$. (This is a version of Weber's law.) Give two proofs that bicancellation must hold.
*3. Consider the equation

$$P_{a,b} = \Phi\left[\frac{a - b}{(a + b)^{1/2}}\right] = F[u(a) - u(b)] \qquad (*)$$

of 4.9. Assume that both F and u are differentiable functions, with positive derivatives. Show that (*) cannot hold.

4. Consider the probabilities $P_{s,t}$ defined by the following matrix. Thus, with $A = \{a,b,c,d,e\}$, we have $\mathcal{D}(P) = A \times A$, with $P_{a,b} = .6$, etc. Do there exist functions u,F, with F strictly increasing, satisfying $P_{s,t} = F[u(s) - u(t)]$ for all $s,t \in A$? (If the answer is yes, give a constructive proof, that is, define such functions. In the other case, find a contradiction.)

	a	b	c	d	e
a	.50	.40	.25	.20	.15
b	.60	.50	.30	.25	.20
c	.75	.70	.50	.40	.25
d	.80	.75	.60	.50	.30
e	.85	.80	.75	.70	.50

5. Analyze the following matrix in the style of Exercise 4. Discuss this example from the viewpoint of the uniqueness of the functions u,F of Equation 4 (cf. Theorem 4.13): can you find two pairs of functions (u,F), (u_0,F_0) satisfying (4), for such data that are not related by the transformations: $u_0 = \alpha u + \beta$, $F_0(s) = F(s/\alpha)$?

	a	b	c	d	e
a	.50	.45	.15	.10	.05
b	.55	.50	.45	.15	.10
c	.85	.55	.50	.45	.15
d	.90	.85	.55	.50	.45
e	.95	.90	.85	.55	.50

6. (*Continuation.*) In the preceding exercises, the matrix defining the data has an interesting "diagonal" property. Is that diagonal property necessary for the existence of the functions u,F satisfying Equation 4? Prove your answer by modifying one pair of cells in the matrix of Exercise 4.

7. Prove that a discrimination system is a probabilistic low order, in the sense of Exercise 21 in Chapter 1.

*8. Let (A,C,P) be a probabilistic low order, satisfying the following multiplication condition:

$$\frac{P_{a,b}}{P_{b,a}} \cdot \frac{P_{b,c}}{P_{c,b}} \cdot \frac{P_{c,a}}{P_{a,c}} = 1,$$

whenever the probabilities are defined. Show that both bicancellation and the quadruple condition hold, but that the reverse implications do not hold. That is, bicancellation and (or) the quadruple condition may be satisfied while the multiplication condition fails.

9. Let P be a function defined on the open, unit square $(0,1)^2$ by the equation $P_{a,b} = a^2(a^2 + b)^{-1}$. Show that the triple $((0,1), (0,1)^2, P)$ satisfies all but one of the defining conditions of a balanced discrimination system in 4.7. Which is the missing condition?

*10. The preceding exercise concerns an argument establishing the independence of one of the defining conditions of a balanced discrimination system, from the remaining ones. Show by a counterexample that the assumption that C is an open subset of $\mathbb{R}^2$ is also independent of the other conditions. Analyze the role of this condition and of Axiom 4. Are they necessary for the existence of a Fechnerian representation? For the uniqueness stated in Theorem 4.13? Does Theorem 4.13 still hold if these assumptions are dropped?

11. Prove Lemma 1 in 4.17.

12. Prove Lemma 3 in 4.17.

13. Prove Lemma 4 in 4.17.

14. Prove that (i) implies (iii) in Theorem 4.13.

5

Models of Discrimination

In Chapter 4, we considered a forced-choice paradigm, in which a subject is presented with pairs (a,b) of stimuli (a,b are real numbers, representing the stimulus values on some physical scale). The subject's task is to select one of the two stimuli as exceeding the other, in terms of some subjective attribute such as loudness or perceived weight, depending on the nature of the stimuli. The basic theoretical notion was a probability $P_{a,b}$ that the subject chooses a over b.

A detailed theoretical analysis was made of the representation

$$P_{a,b} = F[u(a) - u(b)] \tag{1}$$

for these choice probabilities. In this equation, u and F are assumed to be real-valued, continuous, strictly increasing functions, but are otherwise unspecified. Such representation says little regarding the details of the mechanism of choice. Certainly, the choice of a stimulus is the final stage of a complex process, involving physiological and psychological components. All these aspects are somehow captured by the functions u and F. This rather abstract viewpoint is open to criticisms, particularly regarding the interpretation of the functions u and F. Suppose, for example, that the subject is under time pressure. Say that the choice response must be made within t sec after the presentation of the stimuli, with t varying across conditions (e.g., $t = 1, 3, 10$). Assuming that Equation 1 holds in each condition, will the value of t affect u,F, or both of these functions? Without a more explicit model, it is difficult to guess. One could obviously *assume* for instance, that only F will vary across conditions. However, some may feel uneasy about the (absence of) rationale for such a position. To take another example, suppose that the stimuli a,b etc. are pure tones, presented on a background n of noise (say, n is the sound pressure of a Gaussian noise). The values of n, if their range is chosen appropriately, will certainly affect the choice probabilities. Again, however, the impact of n on u or F is difficult to predict. In turn, one may argue, this uncertainty regarding the role of u and F in these experiments casts some doubt on the interpretation of u as a "sensation scale" (cf. Chapter 4).

In psychophysical theory, such objections are met by postulating specific mechanisms underlying the psychophysical choices. When translated into mathematical terms, these mechanisms are often consistent with Equation 1. In many cases, the resulting models turn out to be special cases of (1). Such models may then provide useful guidelines for the interpretation of the Fechnerian representation, and more generally, regarding the notion of a "sensation scale."

This chapter discusses a number of examples.

RANDOM VARIABLE MODELS

We assume that to each stimulus a corresponds a random variable $\mathbf{U}_a$ symbolizing the effect of the stimulus on the subject's sensory apparatus. We also assume that when a subject is presented with a pair (a,b) of stimuli, his or her response is based on a comparison of the sample values of $\mathbf{U}_a$ and $\mathbf{U}_b$. More precisely:

5.1. Definition.   Let $\Psi = (I,C,P)$ be a discrimination system. Let $\mathscr{U} = \{\mathbf{U}_a | a \in I\}$ be a collection of jointly distributed random variables.[1] Then $\mathscr{U}$ is a *random representation* of Ψ iff whenever aCb, and $a \neq b$ then[2]

$$P_{a,b} = \mathbb{P}\{\mathbf{U}_a \geqslant \mathbf{U}_b\}. \tag{2}$$

If the random variables in $\mathscr{U}$ are independent, we say that $\mathscr{U}$ is an *independent random representation of* Ψ.

In the literature of choice theory, this model is often referred to as the *random utility model* (Block & Marschak, 1960; Luce & Suppes, 1965; Marschak, 1960; more complete references are given in the last section of this chapter). Since no assumptions are made regarding the joint distribution of the random variables $\mathbf{U}_a$, one may ask whether this model sets any constraint on the data. An example of such constraint is given in Theorem 5.3. The impact on this model of the balance condition

$$P_{a,b} + P_{b,a} = 1$$

(Definition 4.9) is specified below.

5.2. Theorem.   *Let* $\{\mathbf{U}_a | a \in I\}$ *be a random representation of a discrimination system* $\Psi = (I,C,P)$. *Then* Ψ *is balanced iff*

$$\mathbb{P}\{\mathbf{U}_a = \mathbf{U}_b\} = 0$$

whenever aCb.

Proof.   Generally,

$$\mathbb{P}\{\mathbf{U}_a > \mathbf{U}_b\} + \mathbb{P}\{\mathbf{U}_a = \mathbf{U}_b\} + \mathbb{P}\{\mathbf{U}_b > \mathbf{U}_a\} = 1, \tag{3}$$

since the three events are exhaustive and mutually exclusive. But Ψ is balanced iff

$$\mathbb{P}\{\mathbf{U}_a \geqslant \mathbf{U}_b\} + \mathbb{P}\{\mathbf{U}_b \geqslant \mathbf{U}_a\} = 1,$$

that is, iff

$$\mathbb{P}\{\mathbf{U}_a > \mathbf{U}_b\} + 2\mathbb{P}\{\mathbf{U}_a = \mathbf{U}_b\} + \mathbb{P}\{\mathbf{U}_b > \mathbf{U}_a\} = 1. \tag{4}$$

---

1. We recall that the random variables in the collection $\mathscr{U}$ are said to be *jointly distributed* iff for any finite sequence $a_1, a_2, \ldots, a_n \in I$, and any real numbers $\xi_1, \xi_2, \ldots, \xi_n$, the quantity $\mathbb{P}\{\mathbf{U}_{a_1} \leqslant \xi_1, \mathbf{U}_{a_2} \leqslant \xi_2, \ldots, \mathbf{U}_{a_n} \leqslant \xi_n\}$ is defined.
2. For rather trivial reasons (the fact that $\mathbb{P}\{\mathbf{U}_a \geqslant \mathbf{U}_a\} = 1$) this model does not predict the probabilities $P_{a,a}$. A slightly more complicated machinery is required to accommodate these cases, in which several "copies" of the random variables $\mathbf{U}_a$ are available (cf. Remark 5.4(4)).

In view of (3) and (4), Ψ is balanced iff

$$2\mathbb{P}\{U_a = U_b\} = \mathbb{P}\{U_a = U_b\}.$$

The result follows. ∎

Thus, in the case of a balanced discrimination system, (2) is equivalent to

$$P_{a,b} = \mathbb{P}\{U_a > U_b\}.$$

5.3. Theorem. *In a balanced discrimination system $\Psi = (I,C,P)$, the four conditions below are equivalent. Whenever the probabilities are defined,*

(i) $P_{a,c} \leqslant P_{a,b} + P_{b,c}$;
(ii) $1 \leqslant P_{a,b} + P_{b,c} + P_{c,a}$;
(iii) $P_{a,b} + P_{b,c} + P_{c,a} \leqslant 2$;
(iv) $P_{a_1,a_2}, P_{a_2,a_3} + \cdots + P_{a_{n-1},a_n} + P_{a_n,a_1} \leqslant n - 1$.

Moreover, each of these conditions follows from the assumption that Ψ has a random representation.

Proof. We leave to the reader to verify the equivalence between (i), (ii), and (iii). Notice that (iii) is a special case of (iv). Conversely, suppose that (iii) holds, and that (iv) holds for a particular value of $n \geqslant 3$. If $a_n C a_{n+1}$ and $a_{n+1} C a_n$, we have, by (iii),

$$P_{a_1,a_n} + P_{a_n,a_{n+1}} + P_{a_{n+1},a_1} \leqslant 2.$$

Adding this inequality to (iv), we obtain

$$\sum_{i=1}^{n} P_{a_i,a_{i+1}} + P_{a_n,a_1} + P_{a_1,a_n} + P_{a_{n+1},a_1} \leqslant n + 1.$$

Using the balance condition, and subtracting 1 on both sides, yields

$$\sum_{i=1}^{n} P_{a_i,a_{i+1}} + P_{a_{n+1},a_1} \leqslant n,$$

and (iv) follows by induction.

Let $\{U_a | a \in I\}$ be a random representation of Ψ. We show that (ii) holds. For any $r,s,t \in I$, we write

$$\alpha(r,s,t) = \mathbb{P}\{U_r > U_s > U_t\}.$$

Suppose that aCb, bCc, and cCa. Notice that the event

$$\{U_a = U_b > U_c\}$$

has probability zero, since it is included in the event $\{U_a = U_b\}$, which has probability zero by Theorem 5.2. Generalizing this observation, we obtain

$$1 = \alpha(a,b,c) + \alpha(a,c,b) + \alpha(b,a,c)$$
$$+ \alpha(b,c,a) + \alpha(c,a,b) + \alpha(c,b,a). \tag{5}$$

Obviously,

$$0 \leqslant \alpha(a,b,c) + \alpha(c,a,b) + \alpha(b,c,a), \tag{6}$$

since the three terms in the right member are nonnegative. Adding (5) and (6) and grouping terms, we have

$$
\begin{aligned}
1 \leqslant\ & [\alpha(a,b,c) + \alpha(a,c,b) + \alpha(c,a,b)] \\
& + [\alpha(a,b,c) + \alpha(b,a,c) + \alpha(b,c,a)] \\
& + [\alpha(c,a,b) + \alpha(c,b,a) + \alpha(b,c,a)] \\
= \ & P_{a,b} + P_{b,c} + P_{c,a}. \quad\blacksquare
\end{aligned}
$$

5.4. Remarks. (1) Condition (ii) of Theorem 5.4 is referred to as the *triangle condition* by Luce & Suppes (1965). The appeal of this condition, which Guilbaud (1953) first formulated, is that it is essentially a "blurred" version of the transitivity of a binary relation. If the choice probabilities $P_{a,b}$ take only the values 0 or 1, then the 1 values define a binary relation which is transitive iff the triangle condition holds.

(2) Note that the triangle condition is not sufficient to guarantee the existence of a random representation. A counterexample can be found in McFadden & Richter (1971; see also Cohen and Falmagne, 1978).

(3) Many special cases of the general random utility model defined in 5.1 are consistent with a random representation. Examples will be given in a moment. On the other hand, it is not true that a Fechnerian representation of a discrimination system is necessarily consistent with *some* random variable representation (Exercise 5).

(4) A more general random utility model may be postulated, which does not necessarily obey the constraints expressed in Theorem 5.3. Corresponding to each pair (a,b) of stimuli is a pair of random variables $(\mathbf{U}_{a,\{a,b\}}, \mathbf{U}'_{b,\{a,b\}})$ such that

$$P_{a,b} = \mathbb{P}\{\mathbf{U}_{a,\{a,b\}} \geqslant \mathbf{U}'_{b,\{a,b\}}\}.$$

The prime notation indicates the random variable attached to the second term in a pair (a,b). We assume that $\mathbf{U}_{a,\{a,b\}}$ is identically distributed as, but not necessarily identical to, $\mathbf{U}_{a,\{a,c\}}$ or $\mathbf{U}'_{a,\{a,b\}}$. This model is reasonable. It assumes that the outcome of a discrimination involving a pair (a,b) is decided by the result of a joint sampling of the random variables $\mathbf{U}_{a,\{a,b\}}$ and $\mathbf{U}'_{b,\{a,b\}}$. These random variables need not be independent. If they are independent, then the constraints of Theorem 5.3 follow, but not in general (see Exercise 13).

THURSTONE'S LAW OF COMPARATIVE JUDGMENTS

This title refers to a well-known model for a discrimination system, which is obtained when one assumes that the random variables $\mathbf{U}_a$ and $\mathbf{U}_b$ in (2) are normally distributed. The most frequently used case (the only one considered here), arises when the random variables are pairwise independent.

5.5. The constant variance assumption.   More specifically, suppose that U_a and U_b are independent and normally distributed, with respective means and variances $\mu(a), \mu(b), \sigma(a)^2, \sigma(b)^2$. Thus, $U_a - U_b$ is normally distributed, with mean $\mu(a) - \mu(b)$ and variance $\sigma(a)^2 + \sigma(b)^2$. We obtain, from (2), if $a \neq b$,

$$P_{a,b} = \mathbb{P}\{U_a - U_b \geqslant 0\} \tag{7}$$

$$= \Phi\left\{\frac{\mu(a) - \mu(b)}{[\sigma(a)^2 + \sigma(b)^2]^{1/2}}\right\} \tag{8}$$

where Φ is the distribution function of a unit normal random variable (i.e., a normal random variable with a mean equal to 0 and a variance equal to 1). Suppose, moreover, that the random variables have equal variances, say $\sigma^2(c) = \alpha^2/2$ for all stimuli c. Then, writing $u(c) = \mu(c)/\alpha$ in (8) yields, after simplification,

$$P_{a,b} = \Phi[u(a) - u(b)], \tag{9}$$

a special case of Equation 1, with $F = \Phi$. The models embodied in Equations 8 and 9 are usually referred to as *Case III and V*, respectively, of the *law of comparative judgment* (Thurstone, 1927a, 1927b; a very complete discussion of Thurstone's theory can be found in Bock & Jones, 1968). Thurstone's Case V has been given a special interpretation in a psychoacoustic context, and has been applied to an impressive body of data by Durlach, Braida, and their co-workers (Braida & Durlach, 1972; Durlach & Braida, 1969; Jesteadt & Bilger, 1974; Jesteadt & Sims, 1975; Lim, Rabinowitz, Braida, & Durlach, 1977; Pynn, Braida, & Durlach, 1972).

5.6. Dropping the normality assumption.   Notice that the normality assumption is not critical in the above discussion. Suppose that in (7), the random variables U_a, U_b are independent, and identically distributed except for a "shift" parameter. That is, suppose that for any stimulus c, U_c has the same distribution as $u(c) + \xi$, where u is a real-valued function, and ξ is a fixed random variable. From (7), we have, with ξ, ξ' independent and identically distributed,

$$P_{a,b} = \mathbb{P}\{u(a) + \xi - [u(b) + \xi'] \geqslant 0\}$$
$$= \mathbb{P}\{\xi' - \xi \leqslant u(a) - u(b)\}$$
$$= G[u(a) - u(b)]$$

where G is the distribution function of $\xi' - \xi$. This is a special case of (1), generalizing Case V of the law of comparative judgment.

5.7. Dropping the constant variance assumption.   The constant variance assumption used in the two preceding examples is not essential. Suppose that in (8) μ varies linearly with σ:

$$\mu(c) = \alpha\sigma(c) + \beta, \tag{10}$$

for some constants $\alpha > 0$ and β. Successively, from (8) and (10),

$$
\begin{aligned}
P_{a,b} &= \Phi\left\{\frac{\alpha[\sigma(a) - \sigma(b)]}{[\sigma(a)^2 + \sigma(b)^2]^{1/2}}\right\} \\
&= \Phi\left\{\frac{\alpha[(\sigma(a)/\sigma(b)) - 1]}{[(\sigma(a)/\sigma(b))^2 + 1]^{1/2}}\right\}
\end{aligned}
\tag{11}
$$

Thus, $P_{a,b}$ only depends on the ratio $\sigma(a)/\sigma(b)$. Defining

$$u(a) = \ln \sigma(a),$$

we rewrite the ratios $\sigma(a)/\sigma(b)$ in (11) as differences $u(a) - u(b)$, obtaining

$$P_{a,b} = F[u(a) - u(b)], \tag{12}$$

where

$$F(s) = \Phi[\alpha(e^s - 1)/(e^{2s} + 1)^{1/2}]. \tag{13}$$

It is easy to check that F is strictly increasing. This model is sometimes referred to as Case VI of Thurstone's law of comparative judgment (Bock & Jones, 1968; S. S. Stevens, 1959b). Again, the normality assumption is not critical in the above derivation (Exercise 7).

5.8. A timing model.   The linearity assumption (10) linking the mean and standard deviation of a random variable U_c may seem arbitrary. Actually, the above model arises quite naturally in psychoacoustics. Let a and b denote the sound pressure levels of two pure tones of the same frequency, say 1000 cps, presented successively and monaurally. Fairly detailed hypotheses will be made regarding the neural coding of physical sound intensity. We assume that a tone of level c applied in the auditory channel gives rise to a homogeneous Poisson process $L_t(c)$ of neural points events, with mean $\lambda(c)$. The interarrival times of these events (the interspike intervals) are thus independent and distributed exponentially, with expectation $\lambda(c)^{-1}$. Along lines explored by Luce and Green (1972, 1974), suppose that a sample average $S_{n,c}$ of these interarrival times is used as the basis for loudness discrimination (where n denotes the size of the sample). Stimulus a will be judged at least as loud as stimulus b if $S_{n,a} \leqslant S_{n,b}$; that is,

$$P_{a,b} = \mathbb{P}\{S_{n,a} \leqslant S_{n,b}\}.$$

Since n can be assumed to be large ($n > 100$), $s_{n,c}$ is distributed very nearly normally, with expectation $\lambda(c)^{-1}$ and variance $\lambda(c)^{-2}/n$. The standard deviation is thus a linear function of the expection, as in (10). We obtain

$$
\begin{aligned}
P_{a,b} &= \Phi\left\{\frac{n^{1/2}[\lambda(b)^{-1} - \lambda(a)^{-1}]}{[\lambda(b)^{-2} + \lambda(a)^{-2}]^{1/2}}\right\} \\
&= \Phi\left\{\frac{n^{1/2}\left[\dfrac{\lambda(a)}{\lambda(b)} - 1\right]}{\left[\left(\dfrac{\lambda(a)}{\lambda(b)}\right)^2 + 1\right]^{1/2}}\right\},
\end{aligned}
$$

a special case of (11). In particular, (12) and (13) follow with $u(a) = \ln \lambda(a)$, and $\alpha = n^{1/2}$.

In the next section, we discuss an entirely different mechanism consistent with an independent random representation, and implying the existence of a Fechnerian representation. Since the developments often rely on more advanced techniques, we star the whole section.

*EXTREME VALUE DISTRIBUTIONS AND THE LOGISTIC MODEL

We assume that the neutral coding of a stimulus of level c results from the combined effects of a large number $n(c)$ of independent, parallel channels. This number $n(c)$ of excited channels varies with the intensity of the stimulus. Let us denote by $\mathbf{X}_{c,i}$ the effect of stimulus c on channel i, with $i = 1,2,\ldots,n(c)$. We suppose that the $\mathbf{X}_{c,i}$ are independent, identically distributed random variables, with a common distribution function F that does not depend on c. The critical neural information regarding stimulus c is assumed to be the maximum of the effects of c in the $n(c)$ channels. That is, this information is represented by a random variable

$$\mathbf{U}_c = \max\{\mathbf{X}_{c,1},\mathbf{X}_{c,2},\ldots,\mathbf{X}_{c,n(c)}\}.$$

The choice probabilities are then specified by the equation

$$P_{a,b} = \mathbb{P}\{\mathbf{U}_a \geqslant \mathbf{U}_b\},$$

where $\mathbf{U}_a$, $\mathbf{U}_b$ are independent random variables.

Notice that the asymptotic distribution function G of $\max\{\mathbf{X}_{c,1},\mathbf{X}_{c,2},\ldots,\mathbf{X}_{c,n}\}$ as $n \to \infty$ is of little interest, if it exists at all. Indeed,

$$\begin{aligned}
\mathbb{P}\{\max\{\mathbf{X}_{c,1},\mathbf{X}_{c,2},\ldots,\mathbf{X}_{c,n}\} \leqslant x\} &= \mathbb{P}\{\mathbf{X}_{c,1} \leqslant x, \mathbf{X}_{c,2} \leqslant x,\ldots, \mathbf{X}_{c,n} \leqslant x\} \\
&= \mathbb{P}\{\mathbf{X}_{c,1} \leqslant x\}\mathbb{P}\{\mathbf{X}_{c,2} \leqslant x\} \cdots \mathbb{P}\{\mathbf{X}_{c,n} \leqslant x\} \\
&= [F(x)]^n,
\end{aligned}$$

yielding

$$G(x) = \lim_{n\to\infty} [F(x)]^n = \begin{cases} 1 & \text{if } F(x) = 1, \\ 0 & \text{if } F(x) < 0. \end{cases}$$

For example, if the random variables $\mathbf{X}_{c,i}$ are normally distributed, then $G(x) = 0$ for all x; thus G is not a distribution function. At best (if $F(x) = 1$ for some x), G is a step function. Of importance to the sequel is the asymptotic distribution of the "normalized" maxima

$$\mathbf{Y}_{c,n} = \max\{\mathbf{X}_{c,1},\mathbf{X}_{c,2},\ldots,\mathbf{X}_{c,n}\} - \beta_{c,n}$$

when $(\beta_{c,n})$ is a sequence of appropriate constants.

It will be shown that if the asymptotic distribution function of $\mathbf{Y}_{c,n}$ exists and is strictly increasing, then approximately for large $n(a)$, $n(b)$

$$P_{a,b} = \frac{n(a)}{n(a) + n(b)} \tag{14}$$

$$= \{1 + e^{-[\ln n(a) - \ln n(b)]}\}^{-1}. \tag{15}$$

These results are based on somewhat far-fetched speculations regarding the neural codes of psychophysical stimuli and must be regarded, for the time being, as suggestive curiosities. This material is included here since these speculations have an undeniable appeal in some circles and may also contain a speck of truth. The rest of this section is devoted to precise statements, proofs, and references.

5.9. Definition.   A sequence (X_n) of random variables is called *stable* iff there exists a sequence (β_n) of constants such that

$$H(x) = \lim_{n \to \infty} \mathbb{P}\{\max\{X_1, X_2, \ldots, X_n\} - \beta_n \leqslant x\} \tag{16}$$

defines a strictly increasing distribution function. It can be shown in such a case that, if the random variables are independent and identically distributed, then

$$[H(x)]^n = H(x - \beta_n) \tag{17}$$

for all $x \in \mathbb{R}$ and $n \in \mathbb{N}$ (Fréchet, 1927). No proof of this fact will be given here (see, however, footnote 3).

5.10. Theorem.   *Let (X_n) be a stable sequence of independent and identically distributed random variables; let (β_n) and H be as in Definition 5.9. Then, there are constants $\theta > 0$ and ξ such that*

$$\beta_n = \theta \ln n \tag{18}$$

and

$$H(x) = \exp\left[-e^{\frac{-(x-\xi)}{\theta}} \right]. \tag{19}$$

This theorem summarizes results due to Fréchet (1927), Fisher and Tippett (1928), von Mises (1939), and Gnedenko (1943).[3] The distribution function defined by (19) is sometimes called the *double exponential* distribution (Johnson & Kotz, 1970).

---

3. See Gumbel (1958) or Galambos (1978) for a general presentation of this topic. Actually, the notion of "stability" analyzed by Fréchet and others is a more general one than that given in Definition 5.9, in which (16) and (17) are replaced by

$$H(x) = \lim_{n \to \infty} \mathbb{P}\{\alpha_n \max\{X_1, X_2, \ldots, X_n\} - \beta_n \leqslant x\} \tag{*}$$

and

$$[H(x)]^n = H(\alpha_n x - \beta_n) \tag{**}$$

where (α_n) and (β_n) are sequences of appropriately chosen constants. The last equation, which is occasionally called the *stability postulate*, was derived by Fréchet (1927). An informal argument which is sometimes used to obtain (**) from (*) (e.g., Fisher & Tippett, 1928) is based on the observation that the maximum Y'_{nm} of nm random variables $Y_1, Y_2, \ldots, Y_{nm}$ is also the maximum of the n random variables $Y''_{i,m} = \max\{Y_{(i-1)m+1}, Y_{(i-1)m+2}, \ldots, Y_{im}\}, (i = 1, 2, \ldots, n)$. As $m \to \infty$, each of the $Y''_{i,m}$ must have the same asymptotic distribution as Y'_{nm}, provided that this asymptotic distribution exists.

Proof.   Equation 17 can be regarded as a functional equation in two unknown functions H and β. From (17) we derive successively

$$H(x - \beta_{nm}) = [H(x)]^{nm}$$
$$= [H(x - \beta_n)]^m$$
$$= [H(x - \beta_n - \beta_m)],$$

yielding

$$\beta_{nm} = \beta_n + \beta_m.$$

Since $0 < H(x) < 1$ for some x, β_n is strictly increasing in n. Using Theorem 3.5, we obtain (18), with $\theta > 0$.

Taking logarithms in (17) and replacing β_n by its expression in (18), gives

$$n \ln H(x) = \ln H(x - \theta \ln n)$$

or more simply

$$ng(y) = g(y/n) \tag{20}$$

with

$$y = e^{x/\theta}, \tag{21}$$

$$g(y) = \ln [H(\theta \ln y)], \tag{22}$$

with $g < 0$, strictly increasing and defined on the positive reals. Setting successively $y = 1$ and $y = n/m$, $n, m \in \mathbb{N}$, in (20) we obtain

$$ng(1) = g(1/n)$$

$$ng(n/m) = g(1/m) = g(1)m,$$

yielding

$$g(n/m) = g(1)(m/n),$$

for every rational number n/m. Since g is strictly increasing, we derive, with $\gamma = g(1) < 0$,

$$g(x) = \gamma/x \tag{23}$$

for all $x \in \mathbb{R}_+$. From (21), (22), and (23), we get

$$H(x) = H(\theta \ln y)$$
$$= \exp(\gamma/y)$$
$$= \exp(\gamma e^{-x/\theta}),$$

yielding (19) with $\xi = \theta \ln(-\gamma)$. ∎

Except for details of formulation, our next result is due to Thompson and Singh (1967).

5.11. Theorem. *Let (I,C,P) be a psychophysical system. For $a,b \in I$ let $(\mathbf{X}_{a,n})$, $(\mathbf{X}_{b,n})$ be two stable sequences of independent, identically distributed random variables, such that for any positive integers n, m, $\mathbf{X}_{a,n}$ is independent of, and identically distributed as, $\mathbf{X}_{b,m}$. Suppose that whenever aCb, then*

$$P_{a,b} = \mathbb{P}\left\{\max\left\{\mathbf{X}_{a,1}, \mathbf{X}_{a,2}, \ldots, \mathbf{X}_{a,n(a)}\right\} \geqslant \max\left\{\mathbf{X}_{b,1}, \mathbf{X}_{b,2}, \ldots, \mathbf{X}_{b,n(b)}\right\}\right\}$$

where $n(a)$, $n(b)$ are fixed integers. Then, approximately, for large $n(a)$, $n(b)$,

$$P_{a,b} = \frac{n(a)}{n(a) + n(b)}.$$

In the proof of this theorem, we use the fact that if two random variables $\mathbf{Z}_a$, $\mathbf{Z}_b$ are independent and have the same double exponential distribution specified by (19), then their difference is a logistic distribution (Gumbel, 1958). In particular, with $\xi = 0$ and $\theta = 1$ in (19),

$$\mathbb{P}(\mathbf{Z}_b - \mathbf{Z}_a \leqslant x) = (1 + e^{-x})^{-1}. \tag{24}$$

Proof. We write

$$X'_{a,n} = \max\left\{\mathbf{X}_{a,1}, \mathbf{X}_{a,2}, \ldots, \mathbf{X}_{a,n}\right\},$$

$$X'_{b,n} = \max\left\{\mathbf{X}_{b,1}, \mathbf{X}_{b,2}, \ldots, \mathbf{X}_{b,n}\right\}.$$

Notice that each of the two sequences $(\mathbf{X}_{a,n})$, $(\mathbf{X}_{b,n})$ satisfies the conditions of Theorem 5.10. Let $(\beta_{a,n})$, $(\beta_{b,n})$ be the two sequences of constants defining $(\mathbf{X}_{a,n})$ and $(\mathbf{X}_{b,n})$, respectively, as stable sequences (cf. Definition 5.9).

By Theorem 5.10,

$$\beta_{a,n} = \theta_a \ln n, \qquad \beta_{b,n} = \theta_b \ln n,$$

and since for any $n, m \in \mathbb{N}, \mathbf{X}_{a,n}$ is identically distributed as $\mathbf{X}_{b,m}$, we have successively, for all $x \in \mathbb{R}$,

$$\exp\left[-e^{\frac{-(x-\xi_a)}{\theta_a}}\right] = \lim_{n \to \infty} \mathbb{P}\left\{X'_{a,n} - \beta_{a,n} \leqslant x\right\}$$

$$= \lim_{n \to \infty} \mathbb{P}\left\{X'_{b,n} - \beta_{b,n} \leqslant x\right\}$$

$$= \exp\left[-e^{\frac{-(x-\xi_b)}{\theta_b}}\right],$$

yielding $\theta_a = \theta_b$, $\xi_a = \xi_b$ and thus $\beta_{a,n} = \beta_{b,n}$ for all $n \in \mathbb{N}$. In the sequel, we write

$$\theta = \theta_a = \theta_b, \qquad \xi = \xi_a = \xi_b \qquad \text{and} \qquad \beta_n = \beta_{a,n} = \beta_{b,n}.$$

This implies

$$\exp(-e^{-x}) = \lim_{n \to \infty} \mathbb{P}\left\{\theta^{-1}(X'_{a,n} - \beta_n - \xi) \leqslant x\right\}$$

$$= \lim_{n \to \infty} \mathbb{P}\left\{\theta^{-1}(X'_{b,n} - \beta_n - \xi) \leqslant x\right\}.$$

Using standard results on the convergence of sequence of random variables (Feller, 1968, Chapter 8), this indicates that, as $n \to \infty$, $m \to \infty$,

$$\mathbb{P}\{(\theta\sqrt{2})^{-1}(\mathbf{X}'_{b,n} - \mathbf{X}'_{a,m}) - (\beta_n - \beta_m) \leqslant x\} \to \mathbb{P}\{\mathbf{Z}_b - \mathbf{Z}_a \leqslant x\sqrt{2}\}$$

where $\mathbf{Z}_a$, $\mathbf{Z}_b$ are independent random variables, with

$$\mathbb{P}\{\mathbf{Z}_a \leqslant x\} = \mathbb{P}\{\mathbf{Z}_b \leqslant x\} = \exp(-e^{-x}),$$

for all $x \in \mathbb{R}$. From (24), we conclude that, approximately, for large $n(a)$, $n(b)$

$$\mathbb{P}\{(\theta\sqrt{2})^{-1}[\mathbf{X}'_{b,n(b)} - \mathbf{X}'_{a,n(a)}] - [\beta_{n(b)} - \beta_{n(a)}] \leqslant x\} = (1 + e^{-x\sqrt{2}})^{-1}.$$

Remarking that, by hypothesis, $P_{a,b} = \mathbb{P}\{\mathbf{X}'_{a,n(a)} \geqslant \mathbf{X}'_{b,n(b)}\}$, the theorem follows. ∎

BRADLEY-TERRY-LUCE REPRESENTATIONS

Theorem 5.11 points to the following representation for a balanced discrimination system (I,C,P):

$$P_{a,b} = \frac{v(a)}{v(a) + v(b)}, \qquad v > 0 \tag{25}$$

$$= \{1 + e^{-[\ln v(a) - \ln v(b)]}\}^{-1}.$$

We have thus here a Fechnerian representation $(\ln v, F)$, with F the distribution function of a standard logistic random variable; that is, $F(t) = (1 + e^{-t})^{-1}$, (cf. Johnson & Kotz, 1970, Chapter 22). This representation is very popular, which is certainly due to the simple form of (25). It must be realized that it can be obtained from assumptions apparently very different from those entertained in the last section. Let us demonstrate this.

5.12. Definition. Let $\Psi = (I,C,P)$ be a discrimination system. We say that Ψ satisfies the *product rule* iff whenever aCb, bCb, and aCc, then

$$\frac{P_{a,b}}{P_{b,a}} \cdot \frac{P_{b,c}}{P_{c,b}} \cdot \frac{P_{c,a}}{P_{a,c}} = 1.$$

(We recall that $P > 0$ by Definition 4.7.)

Let v be a function mapping I into the positive reals. Then v is called a *B.T.L. representation* of Ψ if whenever aCb, then

$$P_{a,b} = \frac{v(a)}{v(a) + v(b)}. \tag{26}$$

Let $\mathcal{U} = \{\mathbf{U}_a | a \in I\}$ be a collection of random variables, defined by

$$\mathbb{P}\{\mathbf{U}_a \leqslant t\} = \begin{cases} e^{v(a)t} & \text{if } t \leqslant 0; \\ 1 & \text{if } t > 0. \end{cases} \tag{27}$$

The function $v > 0$ on I implicitly defined by (27) is called the *parameter of $\mathcal{U}$*. We say that $\mathcal{U}$ is an *(independent) negative exponential random representation* of Ψ iff $\mathcal{U}$ is a (independent) random representation of Ψ.

The model defined by (26) has been investigated by Bradley and Terry (1952), Luce (1959a) and Suppes and Zinnes (1963), among others. Theorem 5.13 summarizes results of Luce (1959), Suppes and Zinnes (1963), and Holman and Marley (cited by Luce & Suppes, 1965).

5.13. Theorem. *In a balanced discrimination system Ψ, the following three conditions are equivalent.*

  (i) *Ψ satisfies the product rule.*
 (ii) *Ψ has a B.T.L. representation.*
(iii) *Ψ has a negative exponential random representation $\mathcal{U}$.*

Moreover, the B.T.L. representation in (ii) *can be taken to be the parameter of $\mathcal{U}$ in* (iii) *and this function is necessarily strictly increasing and continuous. Finally, if v and v_0 are two B.T.L. representations of Ψ, then $v_0 = \gamma v$ for some constant $\gamma > 0$.*

Proof. We begin by establishing the equivalence of (ii) and (iii). Let $\mathcal{U} = \{U_a | a \in I\}$ be a negative exponential random representation of a balanced discrimination system $\Psi = (I, C, P)$. Suppose that aCb. Successively,

$$P_{a,b} = \mathbb{P}\{U_a \geqslant U_b\}$$

$$= \int_{-\infty}^{+\infty} \mathbb{P}\{U_a \geqslant U_b | U_b = t\}\, d\mathbb{P}\{U_b \leqslant t\}$$

$$= \int_{-\infty}^{+\infty} \mathbb{P}\{U_a \geqslant t\}\, d\mathbb{P}\{U_b \leqslant t\}$$

$$= \int_{-\infty}^{0} [1 - e^{v(a)t}] v(b) e^{v(b)t}\, dt$$

$$= \left[1 - \frac{v(b)}{v(a) + v(b)}\right] \int_{-\infty}^{0} [v(a) + v(b)]\, e^{[v(a) + v(b)]t}\, dt$$

$$= \frac{v(a)}{v(a) + v(b)},$$

yielding (ii). Reversing the argument used above, we immediately obtain that (ii) implies (iii). The correspondence between the B.T.L. representation and the parameter of $\mathcal{U}$ is clear, and the monotonicity and continuity properties of v follow from that of P. The equivalence between (i) and (ii) is left to the reader (Exercise 8).

Finally, the uniqueness of the B.T.L. representation is a consequence of the uniqueness of a Fechnerian representation in Theorem 4.13. Indeed, if v and v_0 are two B.T.L. representations, then $(\ln v, F)$ and $(\ln v_0, F)$ are two Fechnerian representations (with F the distribution function of a standard logistic random variable). By 4.13,

$$\ln v_0(a) = \ln v(a) + \beta,$$

and thus $v_0(a) = \gamma v(a)$, with $\gamma = e^{\beta} > 0$. ∎

5.14. Remarks.   (1) The diversity of the models discussed so far in this chapter, many of which lead to Equation 1, justifies the place given here to this equation. This diversity also carries an important lesson. In each of these examples, a key role is played for each stimulus c, by a basic random variable $\mathbf{U}_c$ formalizing the neural coding of the stimulus. The discrimination probabilities are symbolized by the equation

$$P_{a,b} = \mathbb{P}\{\mathbf{U}_a \geq \mathbf{U}_b\}.$$

Assuming that such a theoretical device is warranted, and that the particular form of (the distribution function of) these random variables is taken seriously, it may seem sensible to assign a fundamental role to a central location index of these random variables. This would suggest adopting $E(\mathbf{U}_c)$—the expectation of the random variable $\mathbf{U}_c$—as a measure of the magnitude of the sensation evoked by the stimulus c. Notice, however, that $E(\mathbf{U}_c)$ does not necessarily coincide with $u(c)$ in Equation 1. Such coincidence is obtained in 5.5 and 5.6, but not in other models, such as 5.7 where for example, we have $u(c) = \ln E(\mathbf{U}_c)$.

Thus, even though Equation 1 may play a fundamental role, the theoretical status of the scale u entering in this equation is not necessarily clear.

It is natural to ask if there are reasonable models incompatible with Equation 1. The example in 5.15 provides an answer.

(2) There is another lesson to be derived from these examples. Comparing the extreme value model (5.11) with the law of comparative judgment—Case V (5.5)—we must conclude that the mechanisms postulated are very different.

Nevertheless, these models are very difficult to distinguish from an empirical viewpoint. The extreme value model predicts that the choice probabilities will satisfy the equation

$$P_{a,b} = F[u(a) - u(b)]$$

where F is the distribution function of a standard logistic random variable, while in Thurstone's Case V, the same equation is obtained except that F is replaced by Φ, the distribution function of a standard normal random variable. It turns out that F and Φ are close approximations to each other (see Johnson & Kotz, 1970, for details on this matter). So close, in fact, that choosing one model over the other by some empirical test is practically hopeless.

The reason for this paradox—drastically different assumptions but indistinguishable predictions—is that these models consist of very elaborate constructions concerning unobservable choice mechanisms for a relatively scarce data base. There are simply not enough data to support the edifice. This is especially true for the extreme value model.

It is certainly tempting to model the unobservable details of the choice mechanisms and it may even be useful to do so, since this may provide insightful interpretations of the data and suggest useful experiments. The lesson is, however, that such detailed assumptions should probably not be taken too seriously, except in cases in which the data base is much richer, relative to the theoretical construction, than was assumed here.

A MODEL INCONSISTENT WITH
A FECHNERIAN REPRESENTATION

Most of the models encountered in this chapter turn out to be consistent with Equation 1. This might suggest that any reasonable assumption is likely to lead to that equation. The model discussed in this section dispels that notion.

5.15. A neural Poisson counting model. As in 5.8, suppose that a tone of level c generates an homogeneous Poisson process of spike events $L_t(c)$, of mean $\lambda(c)$. Suppose now, however, that intensity discrimination, rather than being based on the average spike intervals as in 5.8, relies on a count of the number of spikes during a fixed interval τ. Let $\mathbf{N}_a$, $\mathbf{N}_b$ be two random variables representing the number of spikes counted for each of the two stimuli a,b. Thus $\mathbf{N}_a$, $\mathbf{N}_b$ are two independent Poisson random variables, with expectations $\mu(a) = \lambda(a)\tau$, $\mu(b) = \lambda(b)\tau$, respectively. (We recall that the variance of a Poisson random variable is equal to its expectation.) Assume further that

$$P_{a,b} = \mathbb{P}\{\mathbf{N}_a \geqslant \mathbf{N}_b\}.$$

For large $\lambda(a)\tau$, $\lambda(b)\tau$, the random variables $\mathbf{N}_a$, $\mathbf{N}_b$ are nearly normal (Cramér, 1963, p. 250), yielding approximately

$$P_{a,b} = \Phi\left[\frac{\mu(a) - \mu(b)}{\sqrt{\mu(a) + \mu(b)}}\right].$$

This model which, as far as we know, was proposed by Strackee and van der Gon (1962; see also Luce & Green, 1972, 1974; McGill & Goldberg, 1968) is incompatible with Equation 1: there are no (continuous, monotonic) functions μ, u, and F satisfying the equation

$$\Phi\left[\frac{\mu(a) - \mu(b)}{\sqrt{\mu(a) + \mu(b)}}\right] = F[u(a) - u(b)]. \tag{28}$$

Rather than proving this fact directly, we derive it as a consequence of the following more general result (Iverson, 1979).

5.16. Theorem. *Let I be a real, open interval. Suppose that*

$$\frac{\mu(a) - \mu(b)}{[\sigma(a)^2 + \sigma(b)^2]^{1/2}} = G[u(a) - u(b)] \tag{29}$$

for all a,b ∈ I, where u, μ, σ, and G are real-valued continuous functions, with σ > 0 and u, μ, and G strictly increasing. Then, either σ is constant or μ = ασ + β for some constants α > 0 and β.

This theorem effectively rules out (28) as a special case of (29) by setting $\mu(a) = \sigma(a)^2$ and $\Phi^{-1} \circ F = G$. It also shows, in particular, that 5.5 and 5.7 are the only special cases of Thurstone's Case III,

$$P_{a,b} = \Phi\left[\frac{\mu(a) - \mu(b)}{\sqrt{\sigma^2(a) + \sigma^2(b)}}\right]$$

compatible with Equation 1.

For a proof of this result, see Iverson (1979).

STATISTICAL ISSUES

5.17. Remarks. The models discussed in this section can usually be tested empirically by standard statistical techniques. A likelihood ratio method is sketched below for the logistic model, the principle of which is easily extended to other cases.

According to the logistic model defined by (26), the choice probabilities must satisfy the equation

$$P_{a,b} = (1 + e^{-\theta_{ab}})^{-1}, \tag{30}$$

with

$$\theta_{ab} = u(a) - u(b). \tag{31}$$

Notice that (31) implies—in fact, is equivalent to—the condition

$$\theta_{ab} + \theta_{bc} + \theta_{ca} = 0, \tag{32}$$

for all stimuli a, b, and c. In particular,

$$\theta_{aa} = 0,$$

$$\theta_{ba} = -\theta_{ab}.$$

There is a good reason for this reparametrization of the model. The new parameters θ_{ab} have to be estimated from the data, subject to the linear constraint (32). This is a standard situation in statistics, which leads naturally to a likelihood ratio procedure. Let n_{ab} be the number of choices of stimulus a observed in the course of $n_{ab} + n_{ba}$ trials. Let Θ be the vector of all the parameters θ_{ab}. Under the usual conditions concerning the independence of trials, the likelihood of the data is the product

$$\ell(\Theta) = \prod_{(a,b)} (1 + e^{-\theta_{ab}})^{-n_{ab}}(1 + e^{-\theta_{ba}})^{-n_{ba}}. \tag{33}$$

The unconstrained maximum likelihood estimates of the parameters θ_{ab} are given by

$$\hat{\theta}_{ab} = \ln(n_{ab}/n_{ba}). \tag{34}$$

(This corresponds to estimating the probabilities $P_{a,b}$ by their relative frequencies.) Let ℓ_1 be the value of the likelihood function ℓ in (33), when the parameters θ_{ab} are replaced by their unconstrained maximum likelihood estimates. Let ℓ_2 be the value of the likelihood function ℓ, when the parameters θ_{ab} are replaced by their maximum likelihood estimates, obtained under the linear constraint (32). A classical result is that the ratio

$$-2\ln(\ell_1/\ell_2),$$

is asymptotically (i.e., for a large number of trials) distributed as a chi-square random variable with a degree of freedom equal to the number of independent parameters remaining in ℓ_2 (cf. e.g., Wilks, 1962, or any standard statistical text).

This procedure can be applied in principle to any model for a discrimination system, consistent with the Fechnerian equation

$$P_{a,b} = F[u(a) - u(b)] \tag{35}$$

in which the function F is specified exactly. This function being strictly increasing, its inverse F^{-1} exists, and (35) gives immediately

$$F^{-1}(P_{a,b}) + F^{-1}(P_{b,c}) + F^{-1}(P_{c,a}) = 0, \tag{36}$$

generalizing (32).

SELECTED REFERENCES

Some papers of general interest are Luce and Suppes (1965) and Luce (1977a, 1977b). Even though centered on applications in economics, the review paper by McFadden (1976) is a useful reference, in which a special attention is payed to statistical matters. Bock and Jones (1968) discuss Thurstone's discrimination models very thoroughly. Gumbel (1958) and Galambos (1978) are introductory texts on extreme value distributions. Other useful titles are listed below, organized by topics.

General Random Utility Models   Marschak (1960); Block and Marschak (1960); McFadden and Richter (1970, 1971), Manski (1977); Falmagne (1978).

Thurstone's Law of Comparative Judgments   Thurstone (1927a, 1927b); Braida and Durlach (1972); Durlach and Braida (1969); Jesteadt and Bilger (1974); Jesteadt and Sims (1975); Lim, Rabinowitz, Braida, and Durlach (1977); Pynn, Braida, and Durlach (1972).

Extreme Value Model   Fisher and Tippett (1928); Fréchet (1927); Gnedenko (1943); Thompson and Singh (1967); von Mises (1939); Wandell and Luce (1978).

Logistic Model B.T.L. systems   Bradley (1954a, 1954b; 1955); Bradley and Terry (1952); Luce (1959a, 1959b); Suppes and Zinnes (1963); Yellott (1977). (As indicated by its title, Yellott's paper could also be placed in either of the two above categories.)

Timing and Counting Models   Luce and Green (1972, 1974); Strackee and van der Gon (1962); McGill and Goldberg (1968).

The complete literature on probabilistic choice theory is huge, and the above list should not be taken as exhaustive. Only references of general interest, or having a potential relevance to psychophysics were included.

Finally, a generally useful source for facts regarding the distribution function of commonly encountered random variables is Johnson and Kotz (1969, 1970, 1972).

EXERCISES

1. Considering Theorem 5.2, is it the case that the random variables of a random representation of a balanced discrimination system are not independent? Is there a paradox here?
2. Show that Condition (i), (ii), and (iii) in Theorem 5.3 are equivalent.
3. In the conditions of Theorem 5.3, prove that any of Conditions (i) to (iv) is equivalent to:

   (v) $1 \leqslant \min \{P_{a,b}, P_{a,c}\} + \min \{P_{b,c}, P_{b,a}\} + \min \{P_{c,a}, P_{c,b}\},$

   whenever the probabilities are defined.
4. How would you test the conditions of Theorem 5.3 statistically? For example, design a statistical test of the hypothesis: $P_{a,c} \leqslant P_{a,b} + P_{b,c}$.
*5. Find sufficient conditions on a Fechnerian representation (u, F) that guarantee the existence of a random representation of a (balanced) discrimination system. Investigate the necessity of such conditions (Luce & Suppes, 1965).
6. Give an example of a random representation of a balanced discrimination system, with nonindependent random variables, which is consistent with a Fechnerian representation.
7. Check that the normality assumption is not critical in the argument given in 5.7. Specify the more general condition required.
8. Prove the equivalence of the product rule, and of the existence of a B.T.L. representation in Theorem 5.13.
9. Let A, X be two real, open intervals; let $(a, x) \mapsto P_{a,x}$ be a function, mapping $A \times X$ into the open interval $(0,1)$, continuous, strictly increasing in the first

variable, and strictly decreasing in the second variable. Prove the equivalence of the two following conditions:

(i) There exist two strictly increasing, continuous functions h, g mapping, respectively, A, X into the positive reals, satisfying

$$P_{a,x} = \frac{h(a)}{h(a) + g(x)}.$$

(ii) $\dfrac{P_{a,x}}{1 - P_{a,x}} \cdot \dfrac{1 - P_{b,x}}{P_{b,x}} = \dfrac{P_{a,y}}{1 - P_{a,y}} \cdot \dfrac{1 - P_{b,y}}{P_{b,y}}$

for all $a, b \in A$ and $x, y \in X$. (Andersen, 1973; Rasch, 1960.)

10. (*Continuation.*) Extending the above result, state and prove a Theorem in the style of 5.13.

11. Suppose that $\mathscr{U} = \{U_a | a \in I\}$ is an independent random representation of a discrimination system Ψ. Let f be a strictly increasing, continuous function mapping $\mathbb{R}$ into itself. Prove that $\mathscr{U}^* = \{f \circ U_a | a \in I\}$ is another independent random representation of Ψ (two lines).

12. (*Continuation.*) Show that the above situation does not exhaust the possibilities. In other words, the existence of one independent random representation of Ψ does not imply that all the random representations are independent.

13. Under which conditions does the model described in Remark 5.4(4) satisfy the conditions (i) to (iv) of Theorem 5.3?

6

Psychometric Functions[†]

For a fixed stimulus b, let $p_b(a)$ be the probability that stimulus a is judged as exceeding b from the viewpoint of some sensory attribute, such as loudness or brightness. (As in Chapters 4 and 5, both a and b are numbers denoting the intensities of the stimuli on some physical scale.) A typical experimental finding is that $p_b(a)$ increases continuously with the value of a. A somewhat idealized graph of a function p_b, which is consistent in its main features with many data, is shown in Figure 6.1.

Except for a change of notation, the function of two variables $(a,b) \mapsto p_b(a)$ is just the choice probability $(a,b) \mapsto P_{a,b}$ discussed in the two preceding chapters. As we will see, however, the change of notation is indicative of a change of viewpoint, which in turn leads to new theoretical insights.

Such a function p_b is traditionally referred to as a *psychometric function*. This term is also used in a different situation, when $p_b(a)$ denotes the probability of detecting a stimulus a embedded in some "noisy" background b. In this case, a and b may denote different kinds of physical variables. Occasionally, we encounter the term in an even broader context, when the empirical measure under investigation is not a probability of discrimination or detection, but some other variable, such as a reaction time, or a count of neural spike firing. Our discussion will cover all these cases.

In this chapter, we examine in detail the notion that two or more psychometric functions are "parallel," that is, they can be made to coincide by a "rigid" shift along the horizontal axis. The rationale for this question is that parallelism is a criterion for an important class of models represented by the equation

$$p_b(a) = F[a - g(b)] \tag{1}$$

in which the functions F and g are specified by the particular model being studied. In other words, any model satisfying this equation must predict parallel psychometric functions. The exact correspondence between (1) and parallelism will be described. A more general situation will also be considered, corresponding to the equation

$$p_b(a) = F[u(a) - g(b)]. \tag{2}$$

[†] This chapter and the next are based on "Psychometric Functions Theory" by Jean-Claude Falmagne, *Journal of Mathematical Psychology*, Vol. 25, No. 1, February 1982, Academic Press. Copyright © 1982.

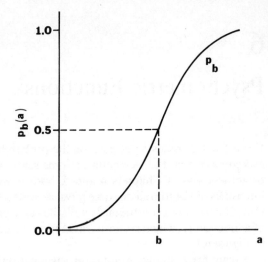

FIGURE 6.1. Idealized graph of a
psychometric function.

INTENSITY (in physical units)

As specified by this equation, the psychometric functions are not (necessarily) parallel, but they may be rendered so by some appropriate rescaling of the physical variable *a*. Obviously, (2) generalizes the Fechnerian representation

$$p_b(a) = F[u(a) - u(b)] \qquad (3)$$

discussed at length in Chapters 4 and 5.

Besides parallelism, other properties of psychometric functions will be investigated, such as *symmetry* (in a sense germane to that used in statistics for distribution functions) or *balance*, a condition encountered earlier and corresponding here to the equation

$$p_a(b) + p_b(a) = 1.$$

In this connection, the following question may interest the practitioner. Consider a discrimination experiment, in a two-alternative-forced-choice design (cf. 6.1(b)). In this situation, the order or the position of the alternatives is typically of little interest, and the experimenter often averages the frequencies (which automatically realizes balance). What is the theoretical impact, if any, of this standard practice, in particular with regard to Equation 2? The answer contained in this chapter will be a warning to the "careful experimenter" addicted to this procedure.

We begin by considering a few empirical examples, leading to a basic definition.

6.1. Examples.   (a) In an experiment reported by Engen (Kling & Riggs, 1971, p. 24) a subject was required to compare by inspection the length of two lines projected successively on a screen, from a viewing distance of about 2.3 m. In the course of the experiment, five lines 61, 62, 63, 64, and 65 mm long were to be compared to a fixed line 63 mm long. Thus, in the above notations, $b = 63$ mm and a takes on five values. The pairs (a,b) were presented randomly, with 100 trials per pair. On half of the trials, b was presented first. The subject was asked whether the perceived length of the first line exceeded that of the second. No feedback was given. Denote by $f_b(a)$ the relative frequency of the judgment that the perceived length of a exceeds that of b. The values of $f_b(a)$ are displayed in Figure 6.2. Such data are consistent with Figure 6.1 and suggest that p_b is a smooth function, strictly increasing on an interval bracketing b, and such that $p_b(b) = .5$. The method employed in this experiment is usually referred to as the method of *constant stimuli*. The fixed stimulus b is called the *standard stimulus*.

(b) In a commonly used psychoacoustic detection situation (cf. Pavel, 1980), the stimulus is a narrow-band signal embedded in a wide-band noise. On each trial the subject is given two successive interval presentations of the noise signal, one of which also contained the stimulus. The task of the subject is to identify the interval containing the stimulus. The assignment of the stimulus to the first or second interval is random. This paradigm is often referred as the *two-alternative-forced choice* (2AFC). Let b denote the noise, and let a be the intensity of the stimulus. Let $f_b(a)$ be the proportion of correct identifications. Typical data support the assumption of a probability $p_b(a)$ of correct identification, which increases smoothly as a function of a, and has an S-shape reminiscent of Figure 6.1. Two differences with the preceding example are noteworthy however.

1. There is no reason here to expect $p_b(a)$ to approach 0 for small values of the variable a. Indeed, when stimulus a is not detectable over the noisy background b, we should expect $p_b(a)$ to be at chance (or guessing) level (e.g., $p_b(a) = .5$).

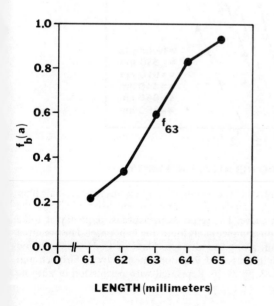

FIGURE 6.2. Proportion of "longer" judgment as a function of line length obtained with the method of constant stimuli (Example 6.1(a); cf. Engen, 1971). From "Psychophysics: Discrimination and Detection" by T. Engen, 1971, in *Experimental Psychology* by J. W. Kling and L. A. Riggs. New York: Holt, Rinehart and Winston. Adapted and reprinted with permission of author and editor.

2. This example evokes the possibility that in some experiment, the background b may be evaluated on a different physical scale (for instance, the background could involve a different sensory modality). A more extreme situation is that the background may be of a different nature than the stimulus. In some cases, it may be appropriate to represent the background by a spectral density function, or even by a stochastic process.

(c) In an unpublished experiment of Graham and Hartline (1933; reported in Sirovich & Abramov, 1977), the frequency of spike firing of a single fiber in the lateral eye of the horseshoe crab, *Limulus*, was recorded as a function of the intensity of a visual stimulus for various monochromatic lights. The data (frequency of spike firing in the initial portion of the response immediately following the stimulus) are plotted in Figure 6.3, which is reproduced from Sirovich & Abramov (1977). The wavelength of the monochromatic light (in nanometers) is the parameter. It is clear that the five curves underlying the data in Figure 6.3 contain essentially the same information as traditional psychometric functions. Notice a difference, however, which concerns the ranges of the frequency of firing functions. As suggested by the data, these are real intervals bounded by, say, 0 and 80. This is easily taken care of. Any number of transformations would yield ranges bounded by 0 and 1. For example, with $\Psi_b(a)$

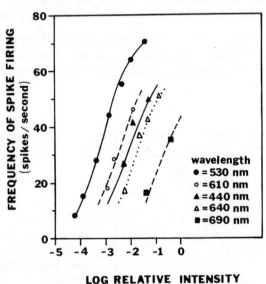

FIGURE 6.3. Response versus log intensity (quantum basis) functions from a single fiber in the lateral eye of the horseshoe crab, *Limulus*. Stimuli were monochromatic lights; the wavelength is indicated next to each curve. The response measure is frequency of spike firing in the initial portion of the response immediately following light onset. The five fitted curves are identical, except for a shift along the abscissa. Data of C. H. Graham and H. K. Hartline, 1933. From "Photopigments and Pseudopigments" by L. Sirovich and I. Abramov, 1977, *Vision Research*, *17*, pp. 5–16. Reprinted with permission of authors and publisher.

denoting the frequency of spike firing, for a stimulus b of intensity a, either of the two transformations below would be adequate.

$$\Psi_b(a) \mapsto p_b(a) = \Psi_b(a)/80$$

or

$$\Psi_b(a) \mapsto p_b(a) = \frac{\Psi_b(a)}{\Psi_b(a) + k'} \tag{4}$$

where k is a positive constant. Such transformations would not affect an important property suggested by the data of Figure 6.3: the frequency of firing functions appear to be parallel when plotted as functions of the logarithm of intensity. In fact, this parallelism would not be altered by any transformation

$$\Psi_b(a) \mapsto g[\psi_b(a)],$$

where g is any continuous, strictly increasing function mapping the ranges of the functions Ψ_b into $(0,1)$. For good reasons, much is made of this parallelism by Sirovich and Abramov, who point out that it supports (actually is essentially equivalent to) the representation

$$\Psi_b(a) = R[a\mu(b)] \tag{5}$$

where μ, R are real-valued functions, with R strictly increasing. The product $a\mu(b)$ is regarded as measuring the number of light quanta absorbed by the photoreceptor (cf. Naka & Rushton, 1966a, 1966b, 1966c). This representation of the function Ψ is usually referred to as "univariance" in visual psychophysics. Notice that, with $p_b(a)$ as in (4) and $F(s) = R(e^s)/[R(e^s) + k]$, (5) can be rewritten as

$$p_b(a) = F\{\ln a - \ln [1/\mu(b)]\},$$

a special case of (2).

In this example, a complete description of the stimulus involves a pair (b,a) where b denotes the wavelength and a the intensity. Thus, the role of the background in Example (b) is played here by one coordinate of the stimulus. In the sequel, however, "background" will often be used as a generic term denoting the index of a psychometric function. For the sake of consistency, we shall also occasionally speak about the "masking effect" of the background even though such language only refers to a particular application.

(d) In the experiment described above, Graham and Hartline also recorded the latency from light onset to first spike (cf. Figure 6.4). Most of the comments made concerning Example (c) remain applicable here. To force the (average) latency $\ell_b(a)$ (where a,b are as in Example (c)) into our theoretical framework, we can—to take an example among many—adopt the transformation

$$\ell_b(a) \mapsto p_b(a) = \frac{k}{k + \ell_b(a)}$$

where $k > 0$ is an appropriately chosen constant.

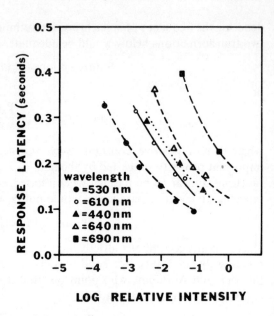

FIGURE 6.4. Response versus log intensity (quantum basis) functions from a single fiber in the lateral eye of the horseshoe crab, *Limulus*. Stimuli were monochromatic lights. This set of records is identical to that of Figure 6.3, except that the response measure is the latency of the response from light onset to first spike. The five fitted curves are identical except for a shift along the abscissa. Data of C. H. Graham and H. K. Hartline, 1933. From "Photopigments and Pseudopigments" by L. Sirovich and I. Abramov, 1977, *Vision Research*, *17*, pp. 5–16. Reprinted with permission of authors and publisher.

PSYCHOMETRIC FAMILIES

Except if one is concerned with predicting their exact mathematical form, psychometric functions are of little interest if considered in isolation. Typically, the psychophysicist wishes to investigate how the shape of the psychometric function is affected by variation of the background (or standard). Accordingly, the definition below specifies the concept of a *family* of psychometric functions. The examples of 6.1 naturally suggest a definition of such family, in which the background is assumed to vary in some subset of a mathematical space—say, a vector space over the real numbers—equipped with a suitable distance function. This is reasonable since we should expect the change of shape of the psychometric functions, say from p_a to p_b, to be related to the distance between a and b. (If a and b are close, the shapes of p_a and p_b should not be very different and their domain may overlap.) We suspect (and hope) however, that the main thrust of this chapter will interest readers who may not be thoroughly familiar with the topology of metric spaces. We thus postpone the metric space assumptions until the admittedly more difficult Chapter 7, and simply suppose here that the backgrounds vary in some abstract, uncountable set I. Definition 6.2 must be regarded as a temporary compromise adopted for readability's sake. The temporary character of the definitions will be marked by the "†" (dagger) symbol.

Notice the switch in notation, from $p_b(a)$ to $p_b(x)$, to emphasize that b,x may belong to different physical domains.

6.2. Definition. Let I be a set of backgrounds. For each background b in I, let C_b be a subset of the reals, and let p_b be a real-valued function defined on C_b.

Suppose that for some $b \in I$, the following axioms are satisfied:

1. C_b is an open interval.
2. $0 < p_b < 1$.
3. The function $x \mapsto p_b(x)$ is strictly increasing and continuous.

Then p_b is called a †-*psychometric function*. The index b of a †-psychometric function p_b will be referred to as the *standard* or the *background*. A set $\{p_b | b \in I\}$ of †-psychometric functions is called *well-linked* iff

4. for all $a,b \in I$, there exists a finite sequence $a_1 = a, a_2, \ldots, a_n = b$, such that

$$C_{a_i} \cap C_{a_{i+1}} \neq 0, \qquad \text{for } 1 \leqslant i \leqslant n.$$

A well-linked set $\{p_b | b \in I\}$ of †-psychometric functions in which I is an uncountable set is a †-*psychometric family*. The "†" (dagger) symbol will be dropped in the sequel for simplicity.[1]

6.3. Remarks. (1) Notice that, as defined in 6.2, a psychometric function resembles a distribution function (in the sense of statistics) but does not necessarily satisfies all the properties of this concept. Specifically, we do not require in general that

$$\sup_{x \in C_b} p_b(x) = 1,$$

nor

$$\inf_{x \in C_b} p_b(x) = 0.$$

Such properties are not essential in most of our developments. More important, they would be a source of difficulty with various kind of data. One example was provided in the detection experiment described in 6.1(b), where we argued that $.5 \leqslant p_b \leqslant 1$ was a reasonable hypothesis, .5 being the probability of guessing the correct interval.

A different kind of difficulty may arise at the upper end of the stimulus scale. For example, if the background value is very near the threshold of pain, the experimenter may be reluctant to present a stimulus highly detectable above this background. The upper part of the corresponding psychometric function may thus be truncated. Similar remarks apply in the case of a "discrimination family," which is defined in 6.8 as a special case of a psychometric family.

(2) The conditions defining a psychometric family should appear quite acceptable in many empirical situations. Axioms 1 and 2 are straightforward. Axiom 3 states that a psychometric function is strictly increasing and continuous. (This presupposes that the possibly constant upper and lower portions have been deleted.) This seems reasonable. (See, however, Falmagne, 1982.) The role of Axiom 4 should be appreciated. This axiom states that any two psychometric functions can be linked by a finite sequence of psychometric functions, such

---

1. The definition given in 7.2 will be more satisfying and more demanding, and require that $p_b(x)$ is continuous in the variable b, and that I is a connected, thus uncountable, set.

that any two successive psychometric functions in the sequence have overlapping domains. This requirement is very natural, both from an empirical and, especially, theoretical standpoint. A particular psychometric function provides precise, but highly local, information regarding the detectability (or discriminability) of the stimulus in a neighborhood of the stimulus scale. Axiom 4 ensures that these local informations can be pieced together to provide an overall picture of the subject sensitivity, for example in the form of a psychophysical scale.

Examples of psychometric families are not difficult to manufacture, for example by generalizing the models of discrimination discussed in Chapter 5. Other examples will be found later in this chapter and in Chapter 7.

PARALLEL PSYCHOMETRIC FAMILIES

Two empirical examples of "parallel" psychometric families were provided in 6.1(c) and 6.1(d). Intuitively, a psychometric family is parallel if any two psychometric functions can be made to coincide by a horizontal "rigid" shift of one toward the other. This suggests that, given one psychometric function, say p_a, any other psychometric function p_b is completely characterized by the value of one parameter depending on b, which we denote by $g(b)$, expressing the length and direction of the "rigid" shift ($g(b)$ may be negative). This intuition is basically sound, but slightly misleading in its details. For instance, one or both of the psychometric functions p_a, p_b may be "truncated," and if both are, their "truncation" may be of a different kind, so that the coincidence after shift may not be complete (cf. Fig. 6.5). Definition 6.4 takes care of this situation, and is, in fact, consistent with a case in which, for two particular psychometric functions p_a, p_b,

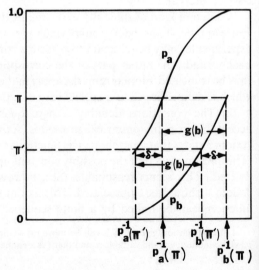

FIGURE 6.5. Two psychometric functions in a parallel psychometric family. The figure illustrates the notion of truncation, and the concepts of Definition 6.4 and Theorem 6.5. Notice that, in the situation of the figure, $g(b)$ is positive and δ negative.

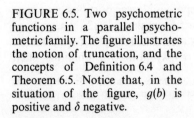

no shift would achieve coincidence because the ranges of p_a, p_b do not overlap.[2]

The concept of parallelism is important since it offers an easily testable criterion of the fact that the effects of the stimulus and the background combine "subtractively" (or "additively" as the case may be).

6.4. Definition. A psychometric family $\mathscr{F}$ is called *parallel* iff for any two psychometric functions $p_a, p_b \in \mathscr{F}$,

$$p_a[p_a^{-1}(\pi) + \delta] = p_b[p_b^{-1}(\pi) + \delta] \tag{6}$$

for all $\pi \in (0,1)$ and $\delta \in \mathbb{R}$ such that both members of the equation are defined. (We recall that we write f^{-1} for the inverse function of a one-to-one function f.)

The following simple result will help the reader to grasp the correspondence between this definition and Figure 6.5.

6.5. Theorem. *A psychometric family $\mathscr{F}$ is parallel iff for all $p_a, p_b \in \mathscr{F}$,*

$$p_a^{-1}(\pi) - p_a^{-1}(\pi') = p_b^{-1}(\pi) - p_b^{-1}(\pi') \tag{7}$$

whenever all four terms are defined.

This means, in particular, that if p_a, p_b are parallel distribution functions, their interquartile range must span the same distance:

$$p_a^{-1}(.75) - p_a^{-1}(.25) = p_b^{-1}(.75) - p_b^{-1}(.25).$$

Proof. Suppose that $\mathscr{F}$ is parallel, with

$$p_a^{-1}(\pi) - p_a^{-1}(\pi') = \delta, \qquad p_b^{-1}(\pi) - p_b^{-1}(\pi') = \delta'.$$

This implies

$$\pi = p_a[p_a^{-1}(\pi) + \delta] = p_b[p_b^{-1}(\pi') + \delta']$$

which, since $\mathscr{F}$ is parallel, leads easily to $\delta = \delta'$.

Conversely, suppose that (7) holds whenever its terms are defined, but

$$\pi' = p_a[p_a^{-1}(\pi) + \delta] < p_b[p_b^{-1}(\pi) + \delta] = \pi''.$$

Suppose also that $\delta \geqslant 0$. This implies that $\pi \leq \pi' < \pi''$. Since the range of p_b is an interval, $p_b^{-1}(\pi')$ is defined, yielding successively

$$\begin{aligned} \delta &= p_a^{-1}(\pi') - p_a^{-1}(\pi) \\ &= p_b^{-1}(\pi') - p_b^{-1}(\pi) \\ &< p_b^{-1}(\pi'') - p_b^{-1}(\pi) \\ &= \delta, \end{aligned}$$

a contradiction.

The argument is similar in the case $\delta < 0$. ∎

---

2. At this point, the reader may wonder whether a psychometric family could not be "vacuously" parallel, that is, Equation 6 would never fail since its members would never be simultaneously defined. This conjecture is false: no such psychometric family can exist (see Exercise 4 in this connection.)

As mentioned earlier, the definition of a parallel psychometric family does not preclude the possibility that the ranges of some psychometric functions would not overlap. In a special case where such situation does not arise, a useful representation of a psychometric family is available: the psychometric functions satisfy the equation

$$p_a(x) = F[x - g(a)],$$

for some functions F, g where F is strictly increasing and continuous. This case is analyzed in Definition 6.6 and Theorem 6.7.

6.6. Definition.   A psychometric family $\mathscr{F} = \{p_a | a \in I\}$ is called *anchored* iff there exists a number $\xi \in (0,1)$ such that:

1. For all $a \in I$ there is an x satisfying $p_a(x) = \xi$.
2. For all $x \in \bigcup_{a \in I} C_a$, there is an $a \in I$ such that $p_a(x) = \xi$.

(We recall that C_a denotes the domain of the psychometric function p_a.) In words, Conditions 1 and 2 mean that for every background a there is a stimulus x, and for every stimulus x there is a background a, such that $p_a(x) = \xi$. A number $\xi \in (0,1)$ satisfying these conditions will be called an *anchor* of $\mathscr{F}$.

These conditions are not very demanding. Suppose, for example, that the psychometric functions are defined from the choice probabilities $P_{a,b}$ of a balanced discrimination system (cf. 4.9), by the equation $p_a(b) = P_{b,a}$. It follows then that .5 is an anchor. Indeed, $p_a^{-1}(.5) = a$ is the identity function on I.

6.7. Theorem.   *An anchored psychometric family $\mathscr{F} = \{p_a | a \in I\}$ is parallel iff it has a representation*

$$p_a(x) = F[x - g(a)], \tag{8}$$

where F is a continuous, strictly increasing function.

Proof.   Suppose that representation (8) holds for some functions g and F satisfying the required conditions. For any $a \in I$ and $\pi \in (0, 1)$, with $p_a(x) = \pi$, we have

$$p_a^{-1}(\pi) = x = F^{-1}(\pi) + g(a).$$

If $p_a(x') = \pi'$, we have thus
$$p_a^{-1}(\pi) - p_a^{-1}(\pi') = F^{-1}(\pi) - F^{-1}(\pi'),$$

independent of a. Applying Theorem 6.5, the parallelism of $\mathscr{F}$ follows.

Conversely, suppose that $\mathscr{F}$ is a parallel, anchored psychometric family. Let ξ be an anchor of $\mathscr{F}$; let J be the set of all real numbers δ such that $[p_a^{-1}(\xi) + \delta] \in C_a$ for some $a \in I$. Define a function F on J by

$$F(\delta) = p_a[p_a^{-1}(\xi) + \delta].$$

Since $\mathscr{F}$ is parallel, F is a well-defined function; notice that it is also strictly increasing and continuous. Define a function g on I by

$$g(a) = p_a^{-1}(\xi).$$

We obtain

$$p_a(x) = p_a[p_a^{-1}(\xi) + (x - p_a^{-1}(\xi))]$$
$$= F[x - p_a^{-1}(\xi)]$$
$$= F[x - g(a)]. \quad \blacksquare$$

It must be realized that the property of parallelism of a psychometric family depends critically of the scale used to measure the stimulus, and would not be preserved under nonlinear transformation of that scale. Consider, for example, an anchored, parallel psychometric family $\mathcal{F} = \{p_a | a \in I\}$ admitting a representation

$$p_a(x) = F[x - g(a)]$$

as in Theorem 6.7. Let v be a real-valued, strictly increasing, continuous function defined on the interval of variation of x. Notice that, with $t = v(x)$, the equation $p_a^*(t) = p_a(x)$ defines a new anchored, psychometric family $\mathcal{F}^* = \{p_a^* | a \in I\}$. But $\mathcal{F}^*$ need not be parallel. In fact, it is easy to show that $\mathcal{F}^*$ is parallel if and only if v is a function of the form $v(x) = \mu x + \theta$, where $\mu > 0$ and θ are constants. In general—that is, when v is not necessarily linear—the transformation of the stimulus scale generates a new psychometric family $\mathcal{F}^*$ satisfying a "subtractive" representation

$$p_a^*(t) = F[u(t) - g(a)]. \tag{9}$$

(Thus, $u = v^{-1}$.) This suggests that we reverse the process.

We shall ask: Under which conditions on a psychometric family does there exist a transformation of the stimulus scale that renders the psychometric functions parallel? Or in other terms: When does a psychometric family $\mathcal{F}^* = \{p_a^*\}$ have a "subtractive" representation of the form (9)? These and related matters are discussed in the next two sections.

SUBTRACTIVE FAMILIES

6.8. Definition. A psychometric family $\mathcal{F} = \{p_a | a \in I\}$ is *subtractive* or a *subtractive family* iff there are three real-valued functions g, u, and F, the latter two being continuous and strictly increasing, such that

$$p_a(x) = F[u(x) - g(a)]$$

for all $a \in I$ and $x \in C_a$. In such case, we will occasionally say that (g, u, F) is a *subtractive representation* of $\mathcal{F}$.

A special case of this representation has, of course, been encountered before, in the framework of a Fechnerian discrimination system (Definition 4.10). It makes sense to adopt a terminology consistent with the earlier one. Suppose thus that the psychometric family $\mathcal{F}$ has, in fact, been obtained from a discrimination system (I,C,P), through the equation

$$p_a(b) = P_{b,a}.$$

In this situation, $\mathscr{F}$ will be referred to as a *discrimination family*, which will be called *balanced* iff (I,C,P) is balanced, that is, iff

$$p_a(b) + p_b(a) = 1.$$

Thus, when $\mathscr{F}$ is a discrimination family, the functions g and u in (9) have the same domain. In the special case where $g = u$, $\mathscr{F}$ will be called *Fechnerian*, or a *Fechner family*, and (u,F) will be labeled a *Fechnerian representation* of $\mathscr{F}$.

6.9. Remarks.   (1) A discrimination family $\mathscr{F} = \{p_a | a \in I\}$ can be subtractive without being Fechnerian. (Say that Equation 9 is satisfied but u is not linearly related to g. An example is provided in 6.11(a).) If, however, $\mathscr{F}$ is a balanced discrimination family, then it is subtractive only if it is Fechnerian. Indeed, for all $a \in I$,

$$p_a(a) = F[u(a) - g(a)] = .5,$$

yielding, with $\alpha = F^{-1}(.5)$,

$$u(a) = g(a) + \alpha.$$

Defining $G(s) = F(s - \alpha)$, we obtain

$$\begin{aligned} p_b(a) &= F[u(a) - g(b)] \\ &= G\{u(a) - [g(b) + \alpha]\} \\ &= G[u(a) - u(b)]. \end{aligned}$$

This indicates that our usage of the term Fechnerian is consistent with that in 4.10. (Notice in passing that the above argument only uses the fact that $p_a(a) = .5$.)

(2) If a discrimination family $\mathscr{F} = \{p_b\}$ is unbalanced, it can always be rendered balanced by a normalization such as

$$p_b^*(a) = p_b(a)/[p_b(a) + p_a(b)].$$

More generally, any real valued continuous function Ψ of two real variables, strictly increasing in the first variable and strictly decreasing in the second, satisfying

$$0 < \Psi < 1, \tag{10}$$

$$\Psi(s,t) + \Psi(t,s) = 1 \tag{11}$$

achieves a similar normalization. The reader can check that the family $\mathscr{F}^* = \{p_b^*\}$ defined from family $\mathscr{F}$ by the equation

$$p_b^*(a) = \Psi[p_b(a), p_a(b)] \tag{12}$$

is indeed a balanced discrimination family. However, as demonstrated by the model in 6.11(a), it is not generally the case that if $\mathcal{F}$ is subtractive, then the normalized family $\mathcal{F}^*$ is subtractive. What is true, and easy to show, is that if $\mathcal{F}$ is Fechnerian, then $\mathcal{F}^*$ is also Fechnerian (see Exercise 1).

(3) In some experimental situations, the order of presentation of the stimuli has an effect on the (probability of the) response. Such effect is often of little interest, and the "careful experimenter" sometimes adopts a normalization procedure, which suffers from the drawback just mentioned. That is, it does not necessarily preserve the subtractive character of a discrimination family. Let us demonstrate this. Denote by $n[a,(a,b)]$ the number of times stimulus a is chosen in the set $\{a,b\}$ when this set is presented in the order (a,b). Let $N(a,b)$ be the number of times $\{a,b\}$ is presented in the order (a,b). To simplify the argument, we identify probabilities and relative frequencies, in the sense that

$$p_b(a) = n[a,(a,b)]/N(a,b).$$

We also assume that $N(a,b) = N(b,a)$. The standard normalization is

$$\begin{aligned} p_b^*(a) &= \{n[a,(a,b)] + n[a,(b,a)]\}/[N(a,b) + N(b,a)] \\ &= \tfrac{1}{2}[p_b(a) + 1 - p_a(b)], \end{aligned} \tag{13}$$

which indeed defines a balanced discrimination family $\mathcal{F}^* = \{p_b^*\}$, if $\mathcal{F} = \{p_b\}$ is a discrimination family. If we assume that both $\mathcal{F}$ and $\mathcal{F}^*$ are subtractive, then (by Remark 1) $\mathcal{F}^*$ is Fechnerian, and we must have for some continuous, strictly increasing functions u, g, F, h, and H,

$$p_b(a) = F[u(a) - g(b)],$$

$$p_b^*(a) = H[h(a) - h(b)],$$

which, together with (13), yields an equation of the form

$$F[u(a) - g(b)] - F[u(b) - g(a)] = K[h(a) - h(b)] \tag{14}$$

(where the constants $\tfrac{1}{2}$ and 1 of (13) have been absorbed in the function K).

This functional equation (cf. Chapter 3) severely restricts the relation between the functions u, g, or the form of the function F. In general, the normalization is ill-advised since a subtractive model will not survive it. However, in cases in which F is approximately linear, this normalization may not create difficulties.

6.10. Definition. In the sequel, any function $(p,p') \mapsto \Psi(p,p')$ defined on the unit square $(0,1) \times (0,1)$, real-valued, continuous, strictly increasing in the first variable, strictly decreasing in the second variable, and satisfying

$$0 < \Psi < 1,$$

and

$$\Psi(s,t) + \Psi(t,s) = 1$$

will be called a *balancing function*.

6.11. Examples of subtractive discrimination families.   (a) Consider the family of functions $\mathscr{F} = \{p_b | b > 0\}$, defined by

$$p_b(a) = e^{-(b^\eta/a^\mu)}$$

for each $a > 0$, where $\eta, \mu > 0$ are constants. This expression is closely related to a model frequently encountered in the vision literature (Green and Luce, 1975; Nachmias, 1981; Quick, 1974).

It is easily checked that $\mathscr{F}$ satisfies all the conditions of an unbalanced discrimination family, which is subtractive since

$$p_b(a) = \exp\left[-e^{-(\mu \log a - \eta \log b)}\right]. \tag{15}$$

Let us balance $\mathscr{F}$. Since for every positive real number s, we have (denoting as usual by Φ the distribution function of a standard, normal random variable),

$$0 < \Phi(\log s) < 1$$

and

$$\Phi(\log s) + \Phi(\log \tfrac{1}{s}) = 1,$$

it follows that the function $(p, p') \mapsto \Phi[\log(p/p')]$ is a balancing function. This yields the balanced family $\mathscr{F}^* = \{p_b^* | b > 0\}$, defined by

$$p_b^*(a) = \Phi\left\{\log\left[\frac{p_b(a)}{p_a(b)}\right]\right\},$$

that is,

$$p_b^*(a) = \Phi[(ab)^{-\mu}(a^{\eta+\mu} - b^{\eta+\mu})].$$

Since $\mathscr{F}^*$ is balanced, the assumption that it is subtractive would lead (using Remark 6.9(1)) to the equation

$$(ab)^{-\mu}(a^{\eta+\mu} - b^{\eta+\mu}) = \Phi^{-1}\{G[u(a) - u(b)]\}, \tag{16}$$

for some strictly increasing, continuous functions u and $\Phi^{-1} \circ G$. This functional equation has no solution. We leave the proof of this fact to the reader (Exercise 3).

(b) For another example of an unbalanced discrimination family, take $\mathscr{F}^* = \{p_s^* | -\infty < s < +\infty\}$ with

$$p_s^*(t) = \exp(-e^{\eta s - \mu t}) \quad (-\infty < t < +\infty), \tag{17}$$

where $\eta, \mu > 0$ are parameters. A comparison between (15) and (17) suggests that $\mathscr{F}$ and $\mathscr{F}^*$ have striking similarities. The exact correspondence between $\mathscr{F}$ and $\mathscr{F}^*$ is examined in Chapter 7 (see 7.15(a) and (b)).

(c) *The ideal observer model (for the stimulus a sample of Gaussian noise).* Suppose that the background is a sample of so-called *Gaussian noise* with power density b, presented for T units of time, and that the stimulus itself is also a sample of Gaussian noise, of the same duration, of power density $x = b + \gamma$, $\gamma \geqslant 0$. Each of the stimuli and the background, is then a stochastic process which, to a good approximation,[3] has a Fourier series representation

$$\sum_{k=1}^{WT} [\alpha_k \cos(2\pi kt(T) + \beta_k \sin(2\pi kt/T)],$$

where W is the bandwidth, and α_k, β_k are independent, normal random variables with mean 0, and variance σ_k^2 depending on the signal presented. It can be shown (see, for example, Green & Swets, 1974) that in such case, the energy in the stimulus and the background are respectively distributed as

$$Wx\chi_{(2WT)}^2, \quad Wb\chi_{(2WT)}^{2'}$$

where $\chi_{(2WT)}^2$ and $\chi_{(2WT)}^{2'}$ are two independent chi-square random variables with $2WT$ degrees of freedom. Let us suppose that the decision of some (ideal) subject is based on a comparison of the energies in the stimulus and the background. More precisely, we assume that

$$p_b(x) = \mathbb{P}\{Wx\chi_{(2WT)}^2 \geq Wb\chi_{(2WT)}^{2'}\}.$$

If $2WT$ is large, each of the two chi-square random variables is approximately normally distributed. Since $E(\chi_{(n)}^2) = n$ and $\mathrm{var}(\chi_{(n)}^2) = 2n$, we obtain, after simplification, approximately

$$p_b(x) = \Phi\left[\frac{WT(x-b)}{\sqrt{x^2 WT + b^2 WT}}\right]$$

$$= \Phi\left[\sqrt{WT}\,\frac{(x/b)-1}{\sqrt{(x/b)^2+1}}\right]$$

$$= G(\log x - \log b),$$

with

$$G(s) = \Phi\left[\frac{\sqrt{WT}(e^s - 1)}{\sqrt{e^{2s}+1}}\right]$$

Thus $\{p_b\}$ is a subtractive family.

(d) We recall briefly here Examples 6.1(c) and (d), concerning the frequency and latency of spike of a single fiber in the lateral eye of the horseshoe crab, *Limulus* (Graham & Hartline, 1933; see Sirovich & Abramov, 1977). "Parallel" psychometric functions were observed, which gave support to the assumption of a representation

$$p_b(a) = R[a\mu(b)]$$

for these psychometric functions ($R, \mu > 0$ are real-valued functions). Clearly, such a representation is equivalent to a subtractive one, since it can be rewritten

$$p_b(a) = F[\log a - g(b)],$$

---

3. See, however, Levitt (1972) for some cautionary remarks on this approximation; also see Green & Swets (1974).

with

$$F = R \circ \exp \quad \text{and} \quad g(b) = -\log \mu(b).$$

In this case, parallel psychometric functions are obtained after a suitable transformation—here logarithmic—of the physical variable measuring the intensity of the stimulation. A generalization of this idea is considered in the next section.

NECESSARY CONDITIONS FOR THE EXISTENCE OF A SUBTRACTIVE REPRESENTATION

6.12. Problem. Under which conditions does a psychometric family

$$\mathscr{F} = \{p_a | a \in I\}$$

have a subtractive representation?

This problem generalizes Fechner's problem discussed in 4.4 and 4.5. Necessary conditions are not difficult to find. For example, suppose that $\mathscr{F}$ is subtractive, with a representation (g,u,F), and that

$$p_a(x) \leqslant p_{a'}(x') \tag{18}$$

$$p_{a'}(y') \leqslant p_a(y) \tag{19}$$

$$p_b(y) \leqslant p_{b'}(y') \tag{20}$$

are simultaneously satisfied. Since the function F in the subtractive representation of $\mathscr{F}$ is strictly increasing, this yields

$$u(x) - g(a) \leqslant u(x') - g(a')$$

$$u(y') - g(a') \leqslant u(y) - g(a)$$

$$u(y) - g(b) \leqslant u(y') - g(b').$$

Adding these inequalities, we obtain

$$u(x) - g(b) \leqslant u(x') - g(b'),$$

or equivalently, assuming that $x \in C_b$, $x' \in C_{b'}$,

$$p_b(x) \leqslant p_{b'}(x'). \tag{21}$$

6.13. Definition. A psychometric family $\mathscr{F} = \{p_b | b \in I\}$ satisfies *triple cancellation* iff (18), (19), and (20) together imply (21), for all $a, a', b, b' \in I$ and $x,y \in C_a \cap C_b$ and $x',y' \in C_{a'} \cap C_{b'}$.

This condition is well known in the measurement literature (cf. Krantz et al., 1971). The above argument shows thus that a psychometric family has a subtractive representation only if it satisfies triple cancellation. Another necessary condition in the same vein is stated in Definition 6.14.

6.14. Definition. A psychometric family $\mathscr{F} = \{p_b | b \in I\}$ satisfies *double cancellation* iff

$$p_a(x) \leqslant p_b(y)$$

and

$$p_b(z) \leqslant p_c(x)$$

together imply

$$p_a(z) \leqslant p_c(y),$$

whenever all six probabilities are defined. The verification of the necessity is left to the reader.

In the framework of appropriate side conditions, each of triple cancellation and double cancellation is actually sufficient to guarantee the existence of a subtractive representation. The exact statement of these results and their proofs are contained in Chapter 7.

The scales u and g are usually specified up to a linear transformation. For example, the following uniqueness result follows (cf. Theorem 7.26) from a slight strengthening of the conditions defining an anchored psychometric family. If (u,g,F) and (u^*,g^*,F^*) are two subtractive representations of the same psychometric family, then

$$g(t) = \beta_0 g^*(t) + \beta_1,$$

$$u(t) = \beta_0 u^*(t) + \beta_1 + \beta_2,$$

$$F(t) = F^*\left(\frac{t - \beta_2}{\beta_0}\right),$$

for some constants $\beta_0 > 0$, β_1, and β_2.

SYMMETRIC FAMILIES

Occasionally, strong assumptions are made regarding the shape of the psychometric functions p_a in a psychometric family $\mathscr{F}$. For example, it is sometimes assumed that p_a is the distribution function of a normal random variable.[4] Notice that, in such a case, p_a must be symmetric, in the sense that

$$p_a[\mu(a) + \delta] + p_a[\mu(a) - \delta] = 1 \tag{22}$$

---

4. This is traditionally referred to as the "phi-gamma hypothesis," a term due to the particular notation used by the early psychophysicists who wrote

$$\Phi(\gamma) = \frac{1}{\sqrt{2\pi}} \int_{-\infty}^{\gamma} e^{x^2/2} \, dx$$

to define the normal integral.

for every real number δ, with $\mu(a)$ denoting the expectation of the normal random variable. The rationale for the term "symmetric" in connection with this equation is that if p_a is differentiable, then (22) yields

$$p_a'[\mu(a) + \delta] = p_a'[\mu(a) - \delta],$$

that is, the derivative p_a' is "symmetric around" $\mu(a)$. Since the assumption of normality has been extensively investigated elsewhere (Bock & Jones, 1968), we only consider here this more general property, which is easy to test and has important consequences.

6.15. Definition.   A function p_a in a psychometric family $\mathscr{F}$ will be called *symmetric* iff there exist a number $\mu(a) \in C_a$ such that (22) holds whenever $[\mu(a) + \delta]$, $[\mu(a) - \delta] \in C_a$. The psychometric family $\mathscr{F}$ is *symmetric* iff all its psychometric functions are symmetric.

Setting $\delta = 0$ in (22), we obtain $\mu(a) = p_a^{-1}(.5)$. That is, if p_a is a distribution function, then $\mu(a)$ is its median. This implies that if $\mathscr{F}$ is a balanced discrimination family, then (22) is equivalent to

$$p_a(a + \delta) + p_a(a - \delta) = 1, \tag{23}$$

since $p_a[\mu(a)] = p_a(a) = .5$, yielding $\mu(a) = a$. Actually, the equivalence between (22) and (23) only depends on the fact that $p_a(a) = .5$. This property will be used in the sequel. A psychometric function p_a in a discrimination family will be called *centered* iff $p_a(a) = .5$. A discrimination family is *centered* iff all its psychometric functions are centered. Clearly, a discrimination family is centered if it is balanced, but the reverse implication does not necessarily hold (see 6.16).

It is sometimes suggested that parallelism and symmetry are logically related. Specifically (Guilford, 1954), Weber's law—a special case of nonparallelism— would imply that the psychometric functions are positively skewed.[5] Even though this statement is incorrect (cf. Exercise 10), the underlying intuition is fruitful, in the sense that in the framework of assumptions which may be judged empirically reasonable, symmetry may imply parallelism (cf. Exercise 9). Generally, however, parallelism and symmetry are independent properties:

6.16. Examples.   Let $\mathscr{F} = \{p_a | a \in \mathbb{R}\}$ be a discrimination family, with

$$p_a(b) = \frac{1}{\sqrt{2\pi}} \int_{-\infty}^{\frac{b-a+k}{\sigma(a)}} e^{z^2/2}\, dz$$

for all $b \in \mathbb{R}$, where k is a constant, and $\sigma > 0$ a real-valued function on $\mathbb{R}$. If $\sigma(a) = 1$ for all $a \in \mathbb{R}$, and $k \neq 0$, then $\mathscr{F}$ is parallel but neither symmetric nor balanced. If $k = 0$ and σ is not a constant function, then $\mathscr{F}$ is symmetric and centered, but neither balanced, nor parallel.

---

5. Actually, Guilford writes "negatively skewed." The context makes it clear however that, in the language of contemporary statistics (Cramér, 1963), and considering a psychometric function p_a as a distribution function, "positively skewed" is what he meant.

Some connections between parallelism, symmetry, and balance are stated in Theorem 6.18.

6.17. Definition. A psychometric function p_ξ in a family $\mathscr{F} = \{p_a | a \in I\}$ is called a *major* of $\mathscr{F}$ iff $\pi, (1 - \pi) \in \mathscr{R}(p_\xi)$ whenever $p_a(x) = \pi$ for some $a \in I$ and $x \in C_a$.

In Example 6.16, all the psychometric functions are majors, since $\mathscr{R}(p_a) = (0,1)$ for all $a \in \mathbb{R}$.

6.18. Theorem. *Let $\mathscr{F}$ be a discrimination family with a major. The properties of balance, symmetry, and parallelism are pairwise independent. However, if $\mathscr{F}$ is parallel, then $\mathscr{F}$ is balanced iff it is symmetric and centered.*

Proof. In 6.16, we gave two examples of discrimination families with a major, which were, respectively,

(a) Symmetric without being balanced or parallel.
(b) Parallel without being symmetric or balanced.

To establish pairwise independence, a third counterexample is required. Suppose that $\mathscr{F} = \{p_a | a \in \mathbb{R}\}$ with $p_a(b) = \Phi(b^3 - a^3)$ for any $a,b \in \mathbb{R}$. Then any psychometric function in $\mathscr{F}$ is a major, and $\mathscr{F}$ is balanced but neither parallel nor symmetric.

Let $\mathscr{F} = \{p_a | a \in I\}$ be a parallel discrimination family, and let p_ξ be a major of $\mathscr{F}$. It is easy to show (cf. Exercise 6) that if $\mathscr{F}$ is centered $p_a(b) = F(b - a)$ for $a \in I$, $b \in C_a$, where F is a strictly increasing, continuous function. Take any $\delta \in \mathscr{D}(F)$. This implies that $p_a(b) = F(b - a) = F(\delta)$ for some $a \in I$ and $b \in C_a$, yielding for some $x \in C_\xi$,

$$p_\xi(x) = F(x - \xi) = F(\delta) = p_\xi(\xi + \delta).$$

Thus, if $\delta, -\delta \in \mathscr{D}(F)$ and $\mathscr{F}$ is symmetric and centered,

$$F(\delta) + F(-\delta) = p_\xi(\xi + \delta) + p_\xi(\xi - \delta) = 1.$$

Consequently, if $a \in C_b$ and $b \in C_a$,

$$p_b(a) + p_a(b) = F(a - b) + F(b - a) = 1,$$

and we conclude that $\mathscr{F}$ is balanced.

Conversely, suppose that $\mathscr{F}$ is balanced and let $(a + \delta), (a - \delta) \in C_a$. Successively,

$$1 = p_a(a + \delta) + p_{a+\delta}(a)$$
$$= p_a(a + \delta) + F(-\delta)$$
$$= p_a(a + \delta) + p_a(a - \delta),$$

which establishes the facts that $\mathscr{F}$ is symmetric and centered. ∎

Further connections between these properties are explored in the exercises.

REFERENCE NOTES

The material in this chapter and in Chapter 7 is largely based on a paper by Falmagne (1982).

As far as I know, the term "psychometric function" was first used by Urban (1907), even though the notion was in use by Fechner and Wundt. Despite its importance in psychophysical research, this notion has prompted exceptionally few theoretical investigations. Three papers by Levine (1971, 1972, 1975) must be mentioned. His general approach to the analysis of a family of psychometric functions is similar in spirit to that of this chapter. Rather than focusing on specific models or processes, general conditions are sought that guarantee the existence and uniqueness properties of some abstract (e.g., subtractive) representation. Levine's side conditions are different from those used here, however, which were tailored for applications in psychophysics. In his 1972 paper, Levine analyzes a problem that was not considered here, involving a generalization of the notion of a subtractive representation. In the notation of this chapter, this representation is symbolized by the equation

$$p_b(x) = F[k(b)u(x) - g(b)].$$

EXERCISES

1. Show that if $\mathscr{F} = \{p_a | a \in I\}$ is a Fechnerian discrimination family, then the balanced family $\mathscr{F}^* = \{p_a^* | a \in I\}$, $p_a^*(b) = \Psi[p_a(b), p_b(a)]$, where Ψ is the balancing function, is also Fechnerian (cf. 6.9(2)).

2. Let $p_a(x) = F[x - g(a)]$ be the representation of Theorem 6.7 for the anchored, parallel psychometric family $\mathscr{F} = \{p_a\}$. Let v be a real-valued, strictly increasing, continuous function defined on the interval of variation of x. With $t = v(x)$, define a psychometric family by the equation $p_a^*(t) = p_a(x)$. Then $\mathscr{F}^* = \{p_a^*\}$ is also anchored. Show that $\mathscr{F}^*$ is parallel iff v is of the form $v(x) = \mu x + \theta$, for some constants $\mu > 0$ and θ.

*3. Prove that the discrimination family $\mathscr{F}^* = \{p_a^* | a > 0\}$, defined by

$$p_a^*(b) = \Phi\left[\frac{a^{n+\mu} - b^{n+\mu}}{(ab)^\mu}\right]$$

is not Fechnerian (cf. 6.11(a)).

*4. Prove that in any psychometric family $\mathscr{F} = \{p_b | b \in 1\}$, there are some $a, b \in I$ and $x \in C_a$, $y \in C_b$, such that $p_a(x) = p_b(y)$. Use this fact to argue that a psychometric family cannot be vacuously parallel (cf. footnote 1).

5. Check that the double cancellation condition is necessary for the existence of a subtractive representation.

6. Show that any parallel discrimination family $\{p_b\}$ is Fechnerian, with a representation $p_b(a) = F(a - b)$, for some strictly increasing, continuous function F.

7. Is it true that if a psychometric family has one anchor, then it necessarily has (i) more than one anchor? (ii) Uncountably many anchors? Provide proofs or counterexamples.

8. Let $\mathscr{F} = \{p_a | \alpha < a < \infty\}$ be a discrimination family, such that for all $a > \alpha$, $(a + \delta) \in C_a$ implies $(b + \delta) \in C_b$ whenever $b \geqslant a$. Prove that if $\mathscr{F}$ is symmetric and balanced, then $p_a(a + \delta) = p_{a+m\delta}[a + (m + 1)\delta]$, whenever $(a + \delta) \in C_a$, for all $m \in \mathbb{N}$.

9. (*Continuation.*) Prove that, in the conditions of the preceding exercise, $\mathscr{F}$ is parallel if the function $p_a(a + \delta)$ is monotonic in a for every δ.

10. Guilford (1954, p. 146) writes: "Thurstone has pointed out that the phi-gamma hypothesis [i.e., the hypothesis that the psychometric functions are normal integrals] is in violation of Fechner's law or any similar psychophysical law. The distribution of observed proportions of judgments should theoretically not be normally distributed if plotted against equal stimulus interval on the abscissa." Confront Guilford's statement with the following example. Let $\mathscr{F} = \{p_a | -\infty < a < \infty\}$ be a psychometric family, defined by

$$p_a(b) = \frac{1}{\sqrt{2\pi}} \int_{-\infty}^{\frac{b-a}{\sigma(a)}} e^{-z^2/2} \, dz,$$

where σ is a nondecreasing function. Thus, $\mathscr{F}$ satisfies the phi-gamma hypothesis, even though, when σ is strictly increasing, $\mathscr{F}$ is not parallel. Show, however, that if $\mathscr{F}$ is a balanced family, then it is a parallel family (i.e., $\sigma = 1$). Notice in particular that if $\sigma(a) = \alpha a, \alpha > 0$, then $p_{\xi a}(\xi b) = p_a(b)$, that is, Weber's law holds (cf. Chapter 8).

Thurstone's result, alluded to by Guilford, is as follows (Thurstone, 1959, p. 82): "*Theorem*: If the absolute limen increases as the stimulus increases, then the psychometric curve for two categories of judgment is positively skewed." Taken literally, this "theorem" is clearly false, in view of the above counterexample. Examination of Thurstone's proof indicates, however, that he has a balanced discrimination family in mind.

11. Let $\mathscr{F} = \{p_a\}$ be a discrimination family, and let Ψ be a balancing function. As in Exercise 1, define the balanced family $\mathscr{F}^* = \{p_a^*\}$, $p_a^*(b) = \Psi[p_a(b), p_b(a)]$. Show that $p_a(b) \leqslant p_c(d)$ iff $p_a^*(b) \leqslant p_c^*(d)$. Use this fact to argue that there is a strictly increasing, continuous function K, such that $p_a(b) = K[p_a^*(b)]$.

12. (*Continuation.*) Show that the weak quadruple condition (respectively, the weak bicancellation condition) holds for $\mathscr{F}$ iff it holds for $\mathscr{F}^*$.

13. Use the results of the two preceding exercises to show that the balance condition can be dropped in Theorem 4.13.

7

*Further Topics on Psychometric Functions[1]

We suppose here that the background b indexing a psychometric function p_b can be identified with a point in some metric space. This assumption is in line with the examples of psychometric families described in 6.1(c) and 6.1(d), and is also compelling on psychological grounds: if the distance function of the metric space is suitably chosen, that is, if it is consistent with the sensory aspects of the situation (more about this in a moment), then we should expect the shape and other characteristics of the psychometric functions to vary smoothly with the distance. For example, if two backgrounds a and b are close enough, the domains of the psychometric functions p_a and p_b should overlap (Theorem 7.4). A number of consequences of such a definition will be explored.

We will also investigate in detail the representation

$$p_b(x) = H[x, \mu(b)], \tag{1}$$

in which μ is a function mapping the set of backgrounds into the reals, and H is a function that is strictly increasing in its first variable and strictly decreasing in its second variable. Equation 1 captures the notion that the backgrounds can be ordered in terms of their "masking" effects. These effects are then measured by the function μ in (1). This representation is a natural generalization of the subtractive representation

$$p_b(x) = F[u(x) - g(x)] \tag{2}$$

considered in Chapter 6. Sufficient conditions for both (1) and (2) will be obtained, and various examples will be given.

Finally, pursuing briefly an idea encountered in 5.1, a "random utility" model for a psychometric family will be considered, corresponding to the representation

$$p_b(x) = \mathbb{P}\{\mathbf{U}_x \geqslant \mathbf{V}_b\}, \tag{3}$$

in which $\mathbf{U}_x$ and $\mathbf{V}_b$ are random variables. This equation formalizes explicitly the notion that both the stimulus and the background have a random effect on the subject's sensory system. The subject reports a detection whenever the momentary effect of the stimulus exceeds the momentary masking effect of the background. A necessary condition for (3) will be stated.

---

1. This chapter can be omitted without loss of continuity. We recall that the asterisk (*) symbol in front of a chapter, section, or paragraph indicates that its content is more difficult than the remainder of the text.

We begin by recalling a number of standard definitions regarding the topology of metric spaces. Our discussion is self-contained, but intended for readers having some familiarity with notions such as "interior point," "open set," "connected set," etc. For a detailed presentation of these notions, consult such basic texts as Rudin (1964) or Choquet (1966).

7.1. Definition.   A *metric space* is a set S equipped with a *distance*, that is, a function d mapping $S \times S$ into $\mathbb{R}$ and satisfying, for all $a,b,c \in S$:

1. $d(a,b) \geqslant 0$.
2. $d(a,b) = 0$ iff $a = b$.
3. $d(a,b) = d(b,a)$.
4. $d(a,c) \leqslant d(a,b) + d(b,c)$.

An expression such as "Let S be a metric space" thus means implicitly that there is a particular real-valued function d defined on $S \times S$ and satisfying (1) to (4). Occasionally, when specificity is required, the pair (S,d) rather than the set S, will be referred to as the metric space. Let (S,d) be a metric space. The *open ball* with *center* $a \in S$ and *radius* $r > 0$ is the set

$$B(a,r) = \{b \in S \mid d(a,b) < r\}.$$

A point $a \in A \subset S$ is an *interior point of A* iff there exists an open ball $B(a,r) \subset A$. A subset of S is called *open* iff all its points are interior points. It follows easily from this definition that arbitrary unions of open sets are open, and that finite intersections of open sets are also open. Since (as can be checked without difficulty)

$$B[b, r - d(a,b)] \subset B(a,r)$$

for any $a \in S, r > 0$ and $b \in B(a,r)$, any open ball is an open set. We conclude that a set is open iff it is a union of open balls. For example, the open sets of the set $\mathbb{R}$ of real numbers (equipped with the Euclidean distance $d(a,b) = |a - b|$), are those sets which are unions of open intervals.

A set $A \subset S$ is called *connected* iff there do not exist two disjoint open sets $A',A'' \subset S$ such that

$$A \cap A' \neq \varnothing, \qquad A \cap A'' \neq \varnothing$$

and

$$A \subset A' \cup A''.$$

It is evident that if S is finite, every subset of S is open, but the only connected subsets of S are S itself, and $\varnothing$. In the case of the Euclidean space $\mathbb{R}^n$, it can be shown that an open subset A is connected iff any two points of A belong to a polygonal line, whose segments are parallel to the coordinate axes, and which is contained in A. It follows that the only connected subsets of $\mathbb{R}$ are the real intervals (open, half open, or closed).

Let f be a function mapping a metric space S into a metric space S^*. Then f is *continuous* iff for any open set $A^* \subset S^*$ the inverse image

$$f^{-1}(A^*) = \{a \in S \mid f(a) \in A^*\}$$

of the set A^* is an open set of S. (This is equivalent to the $\varepsilon - \delta$ definition of calculus.) This implies that the image of a connected set by a continuous function is connected. As an application of this result, we have *Bolzano's theorem*: If f is a continuous function mapping a connected subset A of a metric space into the reals, and $f(a) < s < f(b)$, then there exists $c \in A$ such that $f(c) = s$.

REDEFINING PSYCHOMETRIC FAMILIES

7.2. Definition.   Let I be a subset of a metric space. For each $b \in I$, let p_b be a function mapping a nonempty subset C_b of the reals into the reals. Then

$$\mathscr{F} = \{p_b \mid b \in I\}$$

is a *partial psychometric family* iff for all $b \in I$:

1. I is connected.
2. C_b is an open interval.
3. $0 < p_b < 1$.
4. The function $(b,x) \mapsto p_b(x)$ is continuous in both variables, and strictly increasing in x.

Each $p_b \in \mathscr{F}$ will be called a *psychometric function*. The partial psychometric family $\mathscr{F}$ is said to be *well-linked* iff

5. for all $a,b \in I$, there exists a finite sequence $a_1 = a, a_2, \ldots, a_n = b$, such that

$$C_{a_i} \cap C_{a_{i+1}} \neq \varnothing, \qquad \text{for} \qquad 1 \leqslant i \leqslant n - 1.$$

A well-linked partial psychometric family is called a *psychometric family*. Examples of psychometric families will be given in 7.7. The sets

$$I_x = \{b \in I \mid x \in C_b\}$$

will be of importance in our developments. Thus, I_x is the set of all backgrounds that could be used for a given stimulus x. We will refer to I_x as the *background set* of x. Clearly,

$$I = \bigcup_{x \in \mathbb{R}} I_x.$$

(However, since not all real numbers necessarily denote stimuli, some of the sets I_x may be empty.)

7.3. Remarks.   (1) Notice that a psychometric family contains uncountably many psychometric functions. This results from the fact that the index set of the family is a connected set in a metric space: such sets are uncountable. Thus, the definition of a psychometric family given here is consistent with that of a †-psychometric family in 6.2, but more demanding, since no topological assumptions were formulated in 6.2. This strengthening of the assumptions seems reasonable to us. With regard to Axiom 1 in particular, there is no reason to suspect that the set of backgrounds that *could* be used in an experiment is divided into two or more "unconnected" regions. On the other hand, we do not generally require that the backgrounds sets are connected. An example showing that such requirement may not hold is given in 7.7(a). (Occasionally, in the case of particular results, this condition will be assumed.)

(2) The role of the distance, say *d*, on the set *I* of backgrounds must be appreciated. We have indicated that this distance should be consistent with the sensory aspects of the situation. We may suppose however that the choice of *d* will be made a priori, based on physical considerations. The reader may ask how critical such a choice may be. How do we know which distance function on the set of backgrounds makes sense from a sensory viewpoint? Actually, as a close examination of the axioms indicates, the only role of *d* is to define the open sets (which define the continuous functions). This means that the choice of a particular distance is much less critical than it may seem at first. For the distance *d* to be consistent with some underlying sensory topology, it is sufficient that the backgrounds that are physically close are also close in the underlying sensory space.[2]

The importance of the topological assumptions and the role of the distance *d* is illustrated in Theorems 7.4 and 7.5, in which an interesting strengthening of the assumptions is introduced. Theorem 7.5 generalizes Theorem 4.8. Its proof is left to the reader (Exercise 1).

7.4. Theorem.   Let $\{p_b | b \in I\}$ *be a partial psychometric family in which the background sets are open sets; let d be the distance. Then for every* $b \in I$, *there exist* $\varepsilon > 0$ *such that*

$$d(a,b) < \varepsilon \text{ implies } C_a \cap C_b \neq \varnothing.$$

In words: any two psychometric functions have overlapping domains provided their respective backgrounds are close enough.

2. The following examples illustrate these remarks. Consider the set S of all real-valued, bounded continuous functions on an interval (s,t). Each of the equations

$$d(g,f) = \left[\int_s^t [g(x) - f(x)]^2 \, dx \right]^{1/2},$$

$$d'(g,f) = \sup_{s < x < t} |g(x) - f(x)|,$$

$$d''(g,f) = \int_s^t |g(x) - f(x)| \, dx$$

defines a distance on S. It turns out that the open sets defined by these distances are identical (cf. Choquet, 1966).

Proof. Notice that the set

$$K_b = \{a \in I \,|\, C_a \cap C_b \neq \varnothing\} = \bigcup_{x \in C_b} I_x$$

is an open set, since it is a union of background sets, which are open by assumption. Moreover, $b \in K_b$, since $C_b \neq \varnothing$. Thus, b is an interior point of K_b. The theorem follows. ∎

7.5. Theorem. *A partial psychometric family in which all the background sets are open is well-linked; thus, it is a psychometric family.*

In view of these theorems, the assumption that the background sets are open is appealing. However, many useful results can be obtained without this assumption, and it will be used only sparingly in the sequel. The following result is of interest.

7.6. Theorem. *In a psychometric family, the union of the domains of the psychometric functions is a real, open interval. Moreover, if the background sets are connected, then the union of the ranges of the psychometric function is also a real, open interval.*

Proof. Let $\mathscr{F} = \{p_b \,|\, b \in I\}$ be a psychometric family. Let us show that

$$J = \bigcup_{b \in I} C_b$$

is a real, open interval. As a union of open intervals, J is an open set. Suppose that $s, t \in J$ and $s \leqslant x \leqslant t$. We have $s \in C_a$, $t \in C_b$ for some $a, b \in I$. Let $(a_i)_{1 \leqslant i \leqslant n}$ be the finite sequence of Axiom 5 of a psychometric family. Since $C_{a_i} \cap C_{a_{i+1}} \neq \varnothing$ for $1 \leqslant i \leqslant n - 1$ with $a_1 = a$, $a_n = b$, it follows that

$$\bigcup_{i=1}^{n} C_{a_i}$$

is an open interval containing both s and t. It must also contain x.

Since each psychometric function p_b is strictly increasing, continuous and defined on an open interval, its range $\mathscr{R}(p_b)$ is an open interval. Thus,

$$V = \bigcup_{b \in I} \mathscr{R}(p_b)$$

is an open set. Suppose that V is not an interval. Then, there is $\pi \in (0,1)$ and a partition $\{I', I''\}$ of I such that

$$I' = \{b \in I \,|\, p_b(x) < \pi \text{ for all } x \in C_b\},$$

$$I'' = \{b \in I \,|\, p_b(x) > \pi \text{ for all } x \in C_b\}.$$

Since $\mathscr{F}$ is well-linked, however, we have $a' \in I'$, $a'' \in I''$ satisfying $C_{a'} \cap C_{a''} \neq \varnothing$. Take $x \in C_{a'} \cap C_{a''}$. Since I_x is connected, the image $p_{I_x}(x)$ of I_x by the function $b \mapsto p_b(x)$ is an interval, with $p_{a'}(x) < \pi < p_{a''}(x)$, a contradiction. ∎

Realistic, nontrivial examples of psychometric families are not difficult to manufacture, but tend to require a somewhat heavy machinery, as we shall see. We shall ease our way into such examples by considering first a simple case, in which I is a real, open interval.

7.7. Examples. (a) *A Thurstone-type model.* Let $I = (0,\alpha)$, where $\alpha > 0$ is a constant. For every $a \in I$, define

$$C_a = \{x > 0 | g(a) < u(x) < g(a) + \beta\},$$

where $\beta > 0$ is a constant and u, g are real-valued, positive, continuous functions, with u strictly increasing. We assume that u, g are such that $C_a \neq \varnothing$. For any $a \in I$ and $x \in C_a$, define

$$p_a(x) = \frac{1}{\sqrt{8\pi}} \int_{g(a)}^{u(x)} e^{-z^2/2}\, dz + .5.$$

It is clear that I and C_a (for all $a \in I$) are real intervals, that $0 < p < 1$ and that $p_a(x)$ is continuous in both variables and strictly increasing in x. Since g is continuous, $g^{-1}(u(x) - \beta, u(x))$ is an open set. Thus

$$I_x = (0,\alpha) \cap g^{-1}(u(x) - \beta, u(x))$$

is also an open set. Since the background sets are open, $\mathscr{F} = \{p_a | a \in I\}$ is well-linked by Theorem 7.5. We conclude that $\mathscr{F}$ satisfies all the conditions of a psychometric family.

A couple of features of this example are worth noticing. First, the function g, which captures the effects of the background, is not assumed to be a strictly increasing function of the physical scale (represented here by the interval I). In fact, g can be regarded as realizing a "reordering" of I in terms of the intensity of the impact of the background on the detection of the stimulus. Consequently, the background sets are not necessarily connected. Second, the Euclidean distance (on the interval I) is only used implicitly here, through the continuity properties of the functions p, v, g, and Φ (the normal integral). No essential change would result in this example if we replace the Euclidean distance by another, which would leave p, u, g and Φ continuous. This reiterates on earlier remark (7.3(2)). Finally, this model belongs to a general class of models represented by the equation

$$p_a(x) = F[u(x) - g(a)]. \tag{4}$$

(b) *The automatic gain control model.* Let S be the set of all real-valued, continuous functions a defined on an interval $(0,\mu)$. Suppose that S is equipped with the distance

$$d(a,b) = \int_0^\mu |a(t) - b(t)|\, dt.$$

Let $I \subset S$ be defined by

$$I = \{a \in S | 0 < a < \alpha\},$$

where α is a positive constant. Thus, I is the subset of S containing all those positive functions a bounded above by the number α. Clearly, I is a connected subset of S. For instance, I might be the set of all spectral density functions that characterize background noises, in a psychoacoustic experiment. For any $a \in I$, define

$$C_a = \left\{ x \in \mathbb{R} | \theta_1 < \frac{v(x)}{h(x) + f(a)} < \theta_2 \right\},$$

where θ_1, θ_2 are positive constants and v, h and f are real-valued, positive, continuous functions, such that v and v/h are strictly increasing. These conditions imply that C_a is a real, open interval, which we assume to be nonempty for every $a \in I$. Finally, suppose that

$$p_a(x) = G\left[\frac{v(x)}{h(x) + f(a)} \right] \tag{5}$$

for some strictly increasing, continuous function G, the range of which is included in $(0,1)$. The reader can verify that $\{p_a | a \in I\}$ is a psychometric family. We point out in passing a connection between the classes of models defined by (4) and (5): if the functions v and h in (5) are linearly related, that is, if for some constants $\gamma > 0$ and ξ,

$$h(x) = \gamma v(x) + \xi, \tag{6}$$

Equation 5 is equivalent to (4) and can thus be rewritten in the form of a difference. Indeed,

$$p_a(x) = G\left[\frac{v(x)}{\gamma v(x) + \xi + f(a)} \right]$$

$$= G\left\{ \frac{1}{\gamma + \exp - [\log v(x) - \log(\xi + f(a))]} \right\}$$

$$= F|u(x) - g(a)],$$

with

$$F(s) = G[(\gamma + e^{-s})^{-1}],$$

$$u(x) = \log v(x)$$

$$g(a) = \log[\xi + f(a)].$$

Actually, it can be shown that (4) and (5) define equivalent models only if (6) holds. This model, which has been investigated by Iverson and Pavel (1980, 1981; see also Pavel, 1980; Pavel & Iverson, 1981), is sometimes referred to as the *automatic gain control model* by analogy to devices that achieve gain control by setting their gain inversely proportional to total input power.

(c) *A stochastic model.* The above model can be given an interpretation in terms of an explicit stochastic process modeling the information flow in this situation. Suppose that, in a psychoacoustic paradigm, x denotes the intensity of a 1000-Hz tone, and a the spectral density of a narrow band noise. As in the paradigm of Example 6.1(b), the subject is given on each trial two successive presentations of the noise signal, one of them also containing the 1000-Hz stimulus. Assume that the presentation of the stimulus generates, at some neural location, a Poisson process $U_t(x)$ of spike pulses, of intensity $v(x)$ (where $t > 0$ denotes time). Similarly, the noise generates at the same neural location a Poisson process $G_t(a)$ of intensity $f(a)$. We suppose that these two Poisson processes are independent, and that when the stimulus is presented embedded in the noise, the resulting neural chain of events involves a sum

$$U_t(x) + G_t(a),$$

which is thus itself a Poisson process, of intensity $v(x) + f(a)$. The idea here is that the effect of the masking noise is to flood the neural location responsible for the detection of the 1000-Hz stimulus with irrelevant spikes. The subject's decision regarding which interval contains the stimulus involves a comparison of the two Poisson processes $U_t(x) + G_t(a)$ and $G'_t(a)$ (a Poisson process independent of $G_t(a)$ but having the same intensity.) Note that the interspike intervals in each of these Poisson processes are exponentially distributed, with respective means $[v(x) + f(a)]^{-1}$ and $f(a)^{-1}$. Suppose that the subject's decision is based on comparing two sample averages $S_n(x,a)$, $S'_n(a)$ of n of these interspike intervals, where n is large ($n > 50$). Specifically, consider the following decision rule, where $\beta \geqslant 1$ is a criterion parameter, and y a guessing parameter, $0 \leqslant \gamma \leqslant 1$.

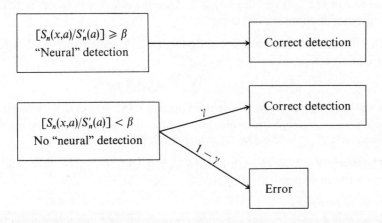

Notice that both $S_n(x,a)$ and $S'_n(a)$ are approximately normal. Denoting the probability of a correct detection by $p_a(x)$, we have successively (leaving the filling of some gaps to the reader), with $\mathbb{P}$ the probability measure,[3]

$$p_a(x) = \mathbb{P}\{[S_n(x,a)/S'_n(a)] \geqslant \beta\} + \mathbb{P}\{S_n(x,a)/S'_n(a)] < \beta\}\gamma$$
$$= \mathbb{P}\{\beta S'_n(a) - S_n(x,a) \leqslant 0\}(1 - \gamma) + \gamma$$
$$\approx \Phi\left\{\frac{\sqrt{n}[\beta - 1 + v(x)/(v(x) + f(a))]}{\sqrt{\beta^2 + [1 - v(x)/(v(x) + f(a))]^2}}\right\}(1 - \gamma) + \gamma$$
$$= G\left[\frac{v(x)}{v(x) + f(a)}\right] \tag{7}$$

with

$$G(s) = \Phi\left[\frac{\sqrt{n}(\beta - 1 + s)}{\sqrt{\beta^2 + (1 - s)^2}}\right](1 - \gamma) + \gamma.$$

This model is thus a special case of that of Example (b), which can, if one wishes, be put in the form of the difference representation, Equation 4.

ORDERING THE BACKGROUNDS

Each of the models discussed in the preceding paragraph is a special case of the equation

$$p_a(x) = H[x, \mu(a)], \tag{8}$$

where μ maps the set of backgrounds into the reals, and H is a continuous function, strictly increasing in the first argument, and strictly decreasing in the second. Thus, μ is a scale measuring the effectiveness of the background in masking the stimulus. It is clear that not all psychometric families can be represented in the form of Equation 8. One necessary condition is that the psychometric functions do not cross.

7.8. Definition.   A psychometric family $\{p_a | a \in I\}$ is called *uncrossed* iff for all $a, b \in I$ and $x, y \in C_a \cap C_b$,

$$p_a(x) \leqslant p_b(x) \qquad \text{iff} \qquad p_a(y) \leqslant p_b(y).$$

We will investigate this condition in some detail. In particular, we show that in the presence of some reasonable side conditions, a psychometric family is uncrossed only if (8) holds. The following result will be useful.

7.9. Theorem.   *In a psychometric family $\mathscr{F} = \{p_b | b \in I\}$, the following four conditions are equivalent:*

(i) *$\mathscr{F}$ is uncrossed.*
(ii) *$p_a(x) \geqslant p_b(x)$ iff $p_a^{-1}(\pi) \leqslant p_b^{-1}(\pi)$ whenever all four quantities are defined.*

---

3. As is customary, we denote by Φ the distribution function of a standard normal, random variable.

(iii) $p_a^{-1}(\pi) \leqslant p_b^{-1}(\pi)$ *iff* $p_a^{-1}(\pi') \leqslant p_b^{-1}(\pi')$ *whenever all four quantities are defined.*

(iv) *For any two finite sequences* $(a_i)_{1 \leqslant i \leqslant n}$ *and* $(x_i)_{1 \leqslant i \leqslant n}$ *of backgrounds and of stimuli, respectively, whenever*

$$p_{a_i}(x_i) \leqslant p_{a_{i+1}}(x_i), \qquad for \qquad 1 \leqslant i \leqslant n-1$$

and $x_n \in C_{a_1} \cap C_{a_n}$, *then* $p_{a_1}(x_n) \leqslant p_{a_n}(x_n)$. *Moreover, the presence of a strict inequality in any of the n antecedent inequalities implies a strict inequality in the conclusion.*

The equivalence of (i), (ii) and (iii) being geometrically obvious, we skip this part of the proof. (The reader is invited to draw a picture.)

Proof that (i) *is equivalent to* (iv). Since (i) is a special case of (iv), it remains to show that (i) implies (iv). We use induction. The case $n = 1$ in (iv) is vacuous, while in the case $n = 2$, (iv) clearly holds since it reduces to (i). Assume that (iv) holds for all $n \leqslant m$ and consider the case $n = m + 1$. Suppose that

$$p_{a_i}(x_i) \leqslant p_{a_{i+1}}(x_i), \qquad i \leqslant 1 \leqslant m,$$

with

$$p_{a_{m+1}}(x_{m+1}) < p_{a_1}(x_{m+1}).$$

We shall use in this proof the abbreviation

$$\beta(r,s,t) \qquad \text{iff} \qquad (r \leqslant s \leqslant t \text{ or } t \leqslant s \leqslant r)$$

for any real numbers r,s,t. Notice that if, for some $1 < j \leqslant m$, $\beta(x_j, x_{j-1}, x_{j+1})$ or $\beta(x_{j-1}, x_{j+1}, x_j)$ then the result follows from the induction hypothesis. Indeed, since $C_{a_{j+1}}$ is a real interval containing both x_j and x_{j+1}, $\beta(x_j, x_{j-1}, x_{j+1})$ implies $x_{j-1} \in C_{a_{j+1}}$. Using the fact that $\mathcal{F}$ is uncrossed, we obtain

$$p_{a_{j-1}}(x_{j-1}) \leqslant p_{a_j}(x_{j-1}) \leqslant p_{a_{j+1}}(x_{j-1})$$

and the terms a_j, x_j can be deleted from their respective sequences, yielding a contradiction by the induction hypothesis. Similarly, $\beta(x_{j-1}, x_{j+1}, x_j)$ implies $x_{j+1} \in C_{a_j}$, leading to delete a_{j+1}, x_j, with a similar argument. We conclude that we must have $\beta(x_1, x_m, x_{m+1})$, which forces $x_m \in C_{a_1}$, and

$$p_{a_m}(x_m) \leqslant p_{a_{m-1}}(x_m) < p_{a_1}(x_m),$$

so that a_{m+1}, x_{m+1} can be removed. The result follows by the induction hypothesis. ∎

We turn to the main result of this section. A preliminary definition is needed.

7.10. Definition. A psychometric family $\{p_b | b \in I\}$ is called *conditionally overlapping* iff for all $a,b,c \in I$, whenever

$$p_a(x) \leqslant p_b(x) \qquad \text{and} \qquad p_a(y) \leqslant p_c(y)$$

or

$$p_b(x) \leqslant p_a(x) \quad \text{and} \quad p_c(y) \leqslant p_a(y),$$

for some $x \in C_a \cap C_b$ and $y \in C_a \cap C_c$, then $C_b \cap C_c \neq \varnothing$.

If one assumes that the backgrounds can indeed be ordered in terms of their masking effects on the stimulus, this condition appears quite natural. It means that if b and c are on the same side of a (with respect to masking effects) then b and c should be at least as close to each other as they are from a. Since C_a overlaps with both C_b and C_c, then C_b and C_c should overlap. The importance of this definition with regard to Equation 8, our main concern here, is made clear in our next theorem.

7.11. Theorem. *A conditionally overlapping psychometric family*

$$\mathscr{F} = \{p_a | a \in I\}$$

is uncrossed iff there exist a function μ mapping I into the reals, and a function H, strictly increasing in its first argument and strictly decreasing in its second argument, such that

$$p_a(x) = H[x, \mu(a)] \tag{9}$$

for all $a \in I$ and $x \in C_a$. Moreover, if the background sets are connected, then μ, H can be chosen to be continuous.

It is clear that if Equation 9 holds for the required functions μ, H, then $\mathscr{F}$ must be uncrossed. The converse is less obvious. Our proof consists in constructing an order on I which can be embedded in the reals in a suitable manner. A glance at (10) and at the statement of the four lemmas will make the basic ideas of the proof fairly transparent.

Note that the fact that I is connected is not used in this proof.

7.12. Proof. Suppose that $\mathscr{F}$ is uncrossed. Define

$$a \precsim b \quad \text{if} \quad p_a(x) \geqslant p_b(x) \tag{10}$$

for some $x \in C_a \cap C_b$ and let $\precsim^t$ be the transitive closure of $\precsim$ (cf. 1.20).

Lemma 1. $\precsim^t$ *is a weak order on I, that is, $\precsim^t$ is transitive and order-connected on I.*

The proof of these facts is simple, and we leave it to the reader.
We now show that a function μ exists, mapping I into the reals, and satisfying

$$\mu(a) \leqslant \mu(b) \quad \text{if} \quad a \precsim^t b,$$

To establish this, we prove the equivalent property: I has an order dense subset I^*, such that the partition Λ^* of I^* induced by $\precsim^t$ is at most countable (cf. Theorem 1.17).

Let us proceed to construct I^*. For any rational number ξ, let I_ξ be the background set of ξ, and let $\precsim_\xi$ be the restriction of $\precsim^t$ to I_ξ. For a particular rational number ξ, both I_ξ and $\precsim_\xi$ may be empty. We have clearly, however,

$$I = \bigcup_{\xi \in \mathbb{Q}} I_\xi,$$

$$\precsim = \bigcup_{\xi \in \mathbb{Q}} \precsim_\xi,$$

where $\mathbb{Q}$ denotes the set of rational numbers.
Since

$$a \precsim_\xi b \quad \text{iff} \quad p_a(\xi) \geqslant p_b(\xi)$$

for all $a,b \in I_\xi$, we can assert, using Theorem 1.39, that $\precsim_\xi$ is a weak order on I_ξ and that there exists an order dense subset I_ξ^* of I_ξ, such that the partition Λ_ξ^* of I_ξ^* induced by $\precsim_\xi$ is at most countable. (This fact concerning Λ_ξ^* must be remembered for later use.) Define

$$I^* = \bigcup_{\xi \in \mathbb{Q}} I_\xi^*.$$

Lemma 2. I^* is order dense in I (cf. Definition 1.37).

Proof. Suppose that $a \prec^t b$. Since $\precsim^t$ is the transitive closure of $\precsim$, there exist a sequence $a_1 = a, a_2, \ldots, a_n = b$ such that $a_i \prec a_{i+1}$ for $1 \leqslant i \leqslant n - 1$. For the remainder of this proof, we fix the index i to some arbitrary value. By definition of $\precsim$, it follows that

$$p_{a_i}(x) > p_{a_{i+1}}(x) \quad \text{for some } x \in C_{a_1} \cap C_{a_{i+1}}.$$

Since $C_{a_i} \cap C_{a_{i+1}}$ is a nonempty, open interval, there is a rational number $\xi \in C_{a_i} \cap C_{a_{i+1}}$. This yields, $\mathscr{F}$ being uncrossed,

$$p_{a_i}(\xi) > p_{a_{i+1}}(\xi)$$

and therefore, by definition of $\precsim_\xi$,

$$a_i \prec_\xi a_{i+1}.$$

Using the fact that I_ξ^* is order dense in I^*, we have

$$a_i \precsim_\xi a' \precsim_\xi a_{i+1}.$$

for some $a' \in I_\xi^*$, which implies

$$a \precsim^t a' \precsim^t b,$$

for some $a' \in I^*$, as required. ∎

Lemma 3. The partition Λ^* of I^* induced by $\precsim^t$ is at most countable.

Proof. Notice first that, as a countable union of sets which are at most countable, the set

$$\Lambda' = \bigcup_{\xi \in \mathbb{Q}} \Lambda_\xi^*$$

is at most countable. For any $a \in I^*$, we denote by $[a]$ the equivalence class of Λ^* containing a; similarly, we denote $[a]_\xi$ the equivalence class of Λ_ξ^* containing a. We prove that each $[a] \in \Lambda^*$ is a union of classes $[b]_\xi (b \in I_\xi^*, \xi \in \mathbb{Q})$. To establish this fact, it suffices to show that

$$[a] \cap [b]_\xi \neq \varnothing \text{ implies } [b]_\xi \subset [a],$$

(since any $c \in I^*$ must satisfy $c \in I_\xi^*$ for some $\xi \in \mathbb{Q}$). Suppose that $c \in [a] \cap [b]_\xi$. This gives

$$p_b(\xi) = p_c(\xi) \quad \text{and} \quad p_a(\xi') = p_c(\xi'),$$

for some $\xi' \in \mathbb{Q}$. Since $\mathscr{F}$ is conditionally overlapping and uncrossed, we obtain, using also Theorem 7.9 ((i) implies (iv)), $p_a(x) = p_b(x)$ for some $x \in C_a \cap C_b$. The set $C_a \cap C_b$ being a nonempty open interval, contains a rational number ξ'', which yields $p_a(\xi'') = p_b(\xi'')$. Thus $b \in [a]$ and for any $d \in [b]_\xi$, we have $p_b(\xi) = p_d(\xi)$, which together with $p_a(\xi'') = p_b(\xi'')$ gives $p_a(\xi''') = p_d(\xi''')$ for some $\xi''' \in \mathbb{Q}$, by the same argument as above, that is, $d \in [a]$. We conclude that $[b]_\xi \subset [a]$. Thus, as asserted, any class $[a] \in \Lambda^*$ is a union of classes $[b]_\xi$. This shows that there exists a 1–1 correspondence between Λ^* and a partition of Λ', which implies, using the Axiom of Choice, that the cardinal number of Λ^* cannot exceed that of Λ'. In other words, Λ^* is at most countable. ∎

From Lemmas 2 and 3, we conclude that there is a real-valued function μ defined on I, such that

$$\mu(a) \leqslant \mu(b) \quad \text{if} \quad a \precsim^t b.$$

For any $s = \mu(a)$, $a \in I$ and any $x \in C_a$, we define

$$H[x, \mu(a)] = p_a(x).$$

It is clear that H is well defined and satisfies the monotonicity conditions of the theorem.

Finally, we turn to the matter of the continuity of μ, H and assume that the background sets of $\mathscr{F}$ are connected, that is, each of the sets $\{a \in I \mid x \in C_a\}$, for every real number x, is connected.

Lemma 4. $\precsim^t$ *is Dedekind complete (cf. Definition 2.16).*

Proof. Let (I', I'') be a cut of $(I, \precsim^t)$. Say, $a' \prec^t a''$ for all $a' \in I', a'' \in I''$. Since $\mathscr{F}$ is well-linked, there exist $b' \in I', b'' \in I''$ such that $x \in C_{b'} \cap C_{b''}$ for some x. This implies $b' \prec b''$, which yields $p_{b'}(x) > p_{b''}(x)$ by definition of $\precsim$. Defining

$$q = \sup\{p_c(x) \mid c \in I''\},$$

we observe that $p_{b'}(x) \geqslant q \geqslant p_{b''}(x)$, and by Bolzano's theorem we must have $c \in I$ such that $q = p_c(x)$ (we use here the fact that $I_x = \{a \in I \mid x \in C_a\}$ is connected). It is easy to check that c is a separating point of the cut $\{I', I''\}$. ∎

We can assume that the range of μ is a real interval. Since for any real number x, the function $a \mapsto p_a(x)$ (assuming it exists) is a continuous mapping of a connected set, the range of this function is also an interval. This means that $s \mapsto H(x,s)$ is a strictly decreasing function mapping an interval onto another. In other words, H is continuous in its second argument. By the continuity of $p_a(x)$ in the variable x, $H(x,t)$ is continuous in x. To show that μ is continuous, we prove that any restriction μ_x of μ to the set $\{a \in I \,|\, x \in C_a\}$ is continuous. Let H_x^{-1} be the continuous inverse of the function $s \mapsto H(x,s)$. We have

$$\mu_x(a) = H_x^{-1}[p_a(x)].$$

Thus, as a composition of two continuous functions, μ_x is continuous. Since $\mu = \bigcup_{x \in \mathbb{R}} \mu_x$, μ is also continuous. ∎

7.13. Remarks. (1) An almost trivial way of obtaining the function μ in Theorem 7.11 arises when we assume that the psychometric family $\mathscr{F} = \{p_a \,|\, a \in I\}$ satisfies the following condition: there is a particular number $\pi \in (0,1)$ such that for all $a \in I$, $p_a(x) = \pi$ holds for some $x \in C_a$. In such case, $\mathscr{F}$ being uncrossed, we have by Theorem 7.9,

$$p_a(x) \geqslant p_b(x) \qquad \text{iff} \qquad p_a^{-1}(\pi) \leqslant p_b^{-1}(\pi),$$

and we can define $\mu(a) = p_a^{-1}(\pi)$. Theorem 7.11 remains true, with a much shorter proof, without having to assume that $\mathscr{F}$ is conditionally overlapping. Notice, however, that the function $a \mapsto p_a^{-1}(\pi)$ is not necessarily continuous. If continuous functions μ, H are required, μ may have to be chosen distinct from $a \mapsto p_a^{-1}(\pi)$.

(2) The uncrossing property (Definition 7.8), has been used by Levine (1971) in a situation similar to that investigated here (see also Krantz et al., 1971). Levine's conditions are quite different from ours, however. He considers the case of a finite number of functions, each of which maps the reals onto the reals. A stronger result than Theorem 7.11 follows in such a case: essentially, a subtractive representation is obtained, in a sense germane to that of our Definition 6.8.

HOMOMORPHIC FAMILIES

The psychophysicist naturally expects that psychometric functions inferred from empirical data will reveal some critical features of the underlying sensory mechanisms. The shape of the psychometric functions, however, is affected by the physical scale, the choice of which is dictated by physical considerations.[4] This means that the revealing features of the psychometric function must be somewhat abstract. They should not depend, in particular, on the particular (reasonable) physical scale adopted. The following definition captures this idea.

7.14. Definition. A psychometric family $\mathscr{F}^* = \{p_s \,|\, s \in I\}$ is *homomorphic* to a psychometric family $\mathscr{F} = \{p_a \,|\, a \in I\}$ iff there exists a pair (g,u) of continuous

---

4. And also psychophysical considerations. Transformations of scales are frequent in psychophysical research. In vision, the multiplicity of scales and units is staggering. The situation is less dramatic in psychoacoustics, where power, sound pressure, and decibels are the most frequently used scales.

functions, with u strictly increasing, mapping respectively I onto I^* and $\bigcup_{a \in I} C_a$ onto $\bigcup_{s \in I^*} C_s^*$ (with $C_s^* = \mathscr{D}(p_s^*)$), satisfying

$$u[C_a] = C_{g(a)}^* \tag{11}$$

and

$$p_a(x) = p_{g(a)}^*[u(x)], \tag{12}$$

for all $a \in I$ and $x \in C_a$. The pair (g,u) is called a *homomorphism* of $\mathscr{F}$ onto $\mathscr{F}^*$.

By definition, the function u in a homomorphism (g,u) is one-to-one and strictly increasing. If g is also one-to-one with a continuous inverse, then we say that $\mathscr{F}^*$ is *isomorphic* to $\mathscr{F}$, and (g,u) will be called an *isomorphism* of $\mathscr{F}$ onto $\mathscr{F}^*$. When $\mathscr{F}$ and $\mathscr{F}^*$ are discrimination families, then the functions g, u in a homomorphism (g,u) have the same domain $I = \bigcup_{a \in I} C_a$. In such cases, it is of interest to consider the possibility that $u = g$. Since I is an (open) interval, u^{-1} is continuous and (u,u) is an isomorphism. We shall simplify our language and call u a 1-*isomorphism* of $\mathscr{F}$ onto $\mathscr{F}^*$. We also say that $\mathscr{F}^*$ is 1-*isomorphic* to $\mathscr{F}$. When a psychometric family $\mathscr{F}^*$ is homomorphic to a psychometric family $\mathscr{F}$, we occasionally say that $\mathscr{F}^*$ is a *homomorphic image* of $\mathscr{F}$. A similar convention applies to isomorphic and 1-isomorphic families. The situation concerning a homomorphism (g,u) of a psychometric family $\mathscr{F}$ onto a psychometric family $\mathscr{F}^*$ will often be compactly described by the notation

$$\mathscr{F} \xmapsto{\ (g,u)\ } \mathscr{F}^*$$

or

$$\mathscr{F} \xmapsto{\ u\ } \mathscr{F}^*$$

in the case of a 1-isomorphism. Clearly

$$\mathscr{F}^* \xmapsto{\ (g^{-1},u^{-1})\ } \mathscr{F}$$

if (g,u) is an isomorphism of $\mathscr{F}$ onto $\mathscr{F}^*$. Notice also that if (g_1,u_1) is a homomorphism of $\mathscr{F}$ onto $\mathscr{F}^*$, and (g_2,u_2) is a homomorphism of $\mathscr{F}^*$ onto $\mathscr{F}'$, then $(g_2 \circ g_1, u_2 \circ u_1)$ is a homomorphism of $\mathscr{F}$ onto $\mathscr{F}'$, or compactly:

$$\mathscr{F} \xmapsto{\ (g_1,u_1)\ } \mathscr{F}^*$$
$$(g_2 \circ g_1, u_2 \circ u_1) \searrow \quad \swarrow (g_2,u_2)$$
$$\mathscr{F}'$$

7.15. Examples.   An example of a pair $\mathscr{F}, \mathscr{F}^*$ of 1-isomorphic discrimination families was given in 6.11(a) and (b), when we had:

(a) $\mathscr{F} = \{p_b | b > 0\}$; $p_b(a) = \exp(-e^{\eta \log b - \mu \log a})$ for any $a > 0$.

(b) $\mathscr{F}^* = \{p_s^* | -\infty < s < \infty\}$; $p_s^*(t) = \exp(-e^{\eta s - \mu t})$ for $-\infty < t < \infty$.

We have

$$\mathscr{F} \xmapsto{\ \log\ } \mathscr{F}^*.$$

Indeed:

$$\log(C_b) = \log(0,\infty) = (-\infty,\infty) = C^*_{\log b}$$

and

$$p_b(a) = \exp(-e^{\eta \log b - \mu \log a}) = p^*_{\log b}(\log a),$$

specializing (11), (12).

(c) On the other hand, the family of functions

$$\mathscr{F}' = \{p'_b | b > 0\}, \, p'_b(a) = \exp(-e^{\eta \log b - a})$$

for $-\infty < a < \infty$, is a psychometric family, but not a discrimination family. However, both $\mathscr{F}$ and $\mathscr{F}^*$ are isomorphic images of $\mathscr{F}'$. In particular, writing = for the identify function, we obtain

$$\mathscr{F}' \xrightarrow{\ (=,e^{1/\mu})\ } \mathscr{F}^*,$$

since

$$[\exp(C'_b)]^{1/\mu} = [e^{(-\infty,\infty)}]^{1/\mu} = (0,\infty) = C_b$$

and

$$p'_b(a) = \exp(-e^{\eta \log b - a}) = p_b(e^{a/\mu}).$$

(What is the isomorphism of $\mathscr{F}'$ onto $\mathscr{F}^*$?)

(d) In Theorem 7.11, we concerned ourselves with obtaining a representation

$$p_a(x) = H[x, \mu(a)],$$

for a psychometric family $\mathscr{F} = \{p_a | a \in I\}$, where H, μ are real-valued, continuous functions. This theorem can be regarded as providing a sufficient set of conditions for the existence of a homomorphism of $\mathscr{F}$ onto a psychometric family $\mathscr{F}^* = \{p^*_s | s \in I^*\}$, where I^* is a real interval. (See Theorems 7.17 and 7.18 in this connection.)

7.16. Remarks. Notice a couple of useful facts regarding two homomorphic discrimination families $\mathscr{F} = \{p_a\}$, $\mathscr{F}^* = \{p^*_s\}$. Suppose that

$$\mathscr{F} \xrightarrow{\ (g,u)\ } \mathscr{F}^*.$$

1. If $\mathscr{F}$ is balanced, then $\mathscr{F}^*$ is balanced iff $\mathscr{F}$, $\mathscr{F}^*$ are 1-isomorphic. Indeed, if $\mathscr{F}^*$ is balanced, then

$$.5 = p_a(a) = p^*_{g(a)}[u(a)] = p^*_{g(a)}[g(a)],$$

yielding $u(a) = g(a)$, since $p^*_{g(a)}$ is a strictly increasing function. The sufficiency is clear.

2. If $\mathscr{F}$, $\mathscr{F}^*$ are unbalanced, one may wish to balance these families. It is natural to ask whether two balanced families $\mathscr{F}^\dagger$, $\mathscr{F}^{*\dagger}$ obtained respectively from $\mathscr{F}$, $\mathscr{F}^*$ by the balancing functions ψ, ψ^* are still homomorphic. The answer is: yes, if (and only if) $\mathscr{F}$, $\mathscr{F}^*$ are actually 1-isomorphic and the balancing functions

are the same. Suppose that $u = g$ and $\psi = \psi^*$. Since balancing does not affect the domains of the psychometric functions, we have

$$u(C_a^\dagger) = C_{u(a)}^{*\dagger}.$$

Moreover,

$$p_a^\dagger(b) = \psi[p_a(b), p_b(a)]$$
$$= \psi\{p_{u(a)}^*[u(b)], p_{u(b)}^*[u(a)]\} = p_{u(a)}^{*\dagger}[u(b)],$$

making clear, from Remark 1, that the converse also holds.

The following result will soon come in handy.

7.17. Theorem.   *If $\mathscr{F} = \{p_a | a \in I\}$ is a psychometric family and S^* is a metric space, then any pair (g,u) of continuous functions, mapping respectively I into S^* and $\bigcup_{a \in I} C_a$ into $\mathbb{R}$, with u strictly increasing, defines a psychometric family $\mathscr{F}^*$ homomorphic to $\mathscr{F}$, with*

$$\mathscr{F}^* = \{p_s^* | s \in g(I)\}$$

and

$$p_s^*(t) = p_a[u^{-1}(t)],$$

where $s = g(a)$. In particular, if $\mathscr{F}$ is a discrimination family and $u = g$, then $\mathscr{F}^*$ is a discrimination family which is 1-isomorphic to $\mathscr{F}$.

Proof.   Clearly,

$$u(C_a) = \mathscr{D}[p_{g(a)}^*] = C_{g(a)}^*. \tag{13}$$

Thus, if $\mathscr{F}^*$ is a psychometric family, it is surely homomorphic to $\mathscr{F}$, by definition of p_s^*, since g, u are continuous and u is strictly increasing. Let us show that $\mathscr{F}^*$ is a psychometric family. We check successively Axioms 1 to 5 in Definition 7.2.

1. $g(I)$ is connected by the continuity of g.
2. The sets $C_{g(a)}^* = u(C_a)$ must be open intervals, since the sets C_a are open intervals and both u, u^{-1} are continuous.
3. Obvious.
4. Obvious.
5. Assume that $\mathscr{F}$ is well-linked, and take any $s,t \in I^*$. Then $s = g(a)$, $t = g(b)$ for some $a,b \in I$ and there is a finite sequence $a_1 = a, a_2, \ldots, a_n = b \in I$ such that $C_{a_i} \cap C_{a_{i+1}} \neq \emptyset$ for $1 \leqslant i \leqslant n - 1$. By (13),

$$x \in C_{a_i} \cap C_{a_{i+1}} \text{ implies } u(x) \in C_{g(a_i)}^* \cap C_{g(a_{i+1})}^*.$$

With $s_i = g(a_i)$ for $1 \leqslant i \leqslant n$, we have thus a sequence $s_1 = s$, $s_2, \ldots, s_n = t \in I^*$ such that $C_{s_i}^* \cap C_{s_{i+1}}^* \neq \emptyset$ for $1 \leqslant i \leqslant n - 1$. We conclude that $\mathscr{F}^*$ is well-linked.

Assume that $u = g$ and $\mathscr{F}$ is a discrimination family. The fact that $\mathscr{F}^*$ is also a discrimination family follows immediately from the two observations (cf.

Theorem 7.20):

1. $s \in C_s^*$ since $u^{-1}(s) \in C_{u^{-1}(s)} = u^{-1}(C_s^*)$.
2. $s \in C_t^*$ iff $u^{-1}(s) \in u^{-1}(C_t^*) = C_{u^{-1}(t)}$
    iff $u^{-1}(t) \in C_{u^{-1}(s)}$
    iff $t \in C_s^*$. ∎

As a by-product of this result, we have:

7.18. Theorem. *If a homomorphic image of a psychometric family $\mathscr{F}$ is a discrimination family, then there exists necessarily a homomorphism $(g, =)$ onto a discrimination family.*

In other words, the conclusion of this theorem states that a discrimination family homomorphic to $\mathscr{F}$ can be obtained without transforming the stimulus scale.

Proof. Suppose that (h, u) is a homomorphism of $\mathscr{F} = \{p_a | a \in I\}$ onto a discrimination family $\mathscr{F}' = \{p_s' | s \in h(I)\}$. Define a psychometric family $\mathscr{F}^* = \{p_z^* | z \in u^{-1} | h(I)]\}$, satisfying

$$\mathscr{F}' \overset{u^{-1}}{\longmapsto} \mathscr{F}^*$$

with

$$p_a(x) = p_{h(a)}'[u(x)] = p_{u^{-1}[h(a)]}^*(x).$$

By Theorem 7.17, u^{-1} is a 1-isomorphism of $\mathscr{F}'$ onto the discrimination family $\mathscr{F}^*$. With $g = u^{-1} \circ h$, we have

$$\mathscr{F} \overset{(g, =)}{\longmapsto} \mathscr{F}^*. ∎$$

In Theorem 7.17, we gave a set of sufficient conditions for the existence of a representation

$$p_a(x) = H[x, \mu(a)]$$

of a psychometric family $\mathscr{F} = \{p_a\}$, where H and μ are real-valued, continuous functions. In Theorem 7.21, we go one step further and obtain a homomorphism of $\mathscr{F}$ onto a discrimination family. A couple of preliminary notions are needed.

7.19. Definition. In Chapter 6, we defined the notion of an *anchor* of a psychometric family $\mathscr{F} = \{p_a | a \in I\}$ as a number $\xi \in (0,1)$ satisfying:

1. for all $a \in I$, there is an x such that $p_a(x) = \xi$;
2. for all $x \in \bigcup_{a \in I} C_a$, there is an $a \in I$ such that $p_a(x) = \xi$.

A psychometric family having an anchor was called *anchored*. By abuse of language, we say here that ξ is a *continuous anchor* iff the function $a \mapsto p_a^{-1}(\xi)$ is continuous.

For example, .5 is a continuous anchor of any balanced discrimination family since $a \mapsto p_a^{-1}(.5) = a$ is the identity function.

Notice that an anchor remains an anchor under homomorphism, in the sense that if $\mathcal{F}^*$ is a homomorphic image of $\mathcal{F}$ and ξ is an anchor of $\mathcal{F}$, then it is also an anchor of $\mathcal{F}^*$.

As an immediate consequence of 6.8, we have the following theorem.

7.20. Theorem. *A psychometric family* $\mathcal{F} = \{p_a | a \in I\}$ *is a discrimination family iff for all* $a,b \in I$,

    1. $a \in C_a \subset I$ *(thus* $I = \bigcup_{a \in I} C_a$*).*
    2. $a \in C_b$ *iff* $b \in C_a$.

The proof is left to the reader.

7.21. Theorem. *Let* $\mathcal{F} = \{p_a | a \in I\}$ *be an uncrossed psychometric family. Suppose that* $\mathcal{F}$ *has a continuous anchor* ξ *satisfying*

$$p_a^{-1}(\xi) \in C_b \qquad \text{iff} \qquad p_b^{-1}(\xi) \in C_a. \tag{14}$$

Then $\mathcal{F}$ *has a homomorphic image* $\mathcal{F}^*$, *which is a discrimination family. Specifically, we can define* $\mathcal{F}^*$ *by*

$$\mathcal{F} \xrightarrow{(\mu, =)} \mathcal{F}^*,$$

with $\mu(a) = p_a^{-1}(\xi)$ *for all* $a \in I$.

The hypothesis involving (14), obviously tailor made to yield Condition 2 in Theorem 7.20, is not unrealistic. However, since this hypothesis is not necessary for the conclusion, there is room for improvement here.

Proof. Since $\mu(a) = p_a^{-1}(\xi)$ is continuous, by Theorem 7.17 $(\mu, =)$ is a homomorphism of $\mathcal{F}$ onto a psychometric family $\mathcal{F}^* = \{p_x | x \in \mu(I)\}$. We only have to show that $\mathcal{F}^*$ satisfies the two conditions in Theorem 7.20.

Take any $x, y \in \mu(I)$; thus, $x = p_a^{-1}(\xi)$, $y = p_b^{-1}(\xi)$ for some $a,b \in I$.

    1. $x \in C_x^* = C_a$, since $p_a(x) = \xi$; moreover, for any $z \in C_x^*$, $p_c(z) = \xi$ for some $c \in I$ by definition of an anchor; that is, $\mu(c) = z$, and $z \in \mu(I)$ yielding $C_x^* \subset \mu(I)$.
    2. Successively,

$$
\begin{array}{lll}
x \in C_y^* & \text{iff} & p_a^{-1}(\xi) \in C_b = C_y^* \\
& \text{iff} & p_b^{-1}(\xi) \in C_a \text{ (by hypothesis)} \\
& \text{iff} & y \in C_x^*. \quad \blacksquare
\end{array}
$$

In the language of homomorphism of psychometric families, some of the results obtained in Chapter 6 concerning the relation between parallel and subtractive families can be reformulated or generalized. For example:

7.22. Theorem. *Any subtractive psychometric family has a homomorphic image which is a parallel psychometric family. In particular, any Fechnerian discrimination family is 1-isomorphic to a parallel discrimination family.*

This theorem has a partial converse (see 7.23(i)).

Proof. Let $\mathscr{F} = \{p_a | a \in I\}$ be a subtractive psychometric family, say,

$$p_a(x) = F[u(x) - g(a)]$$

for some real valued, continuous functions g, u and F, with u, F strictly increasing. By Theorem 7.17,

$$\mathscr{F} \overset{(g,u)}{\longmapsto} \mathscr{F}^*$$

defines a homomorphic image $\mathscr{F}^* = \{p_s^* | s \in g(I)\}$ of $\mathscr{F}$. For any $s \in g(I)$ and $t \in C_s^*$, we have $s = g(a)$, $t = u(x)$ for some $a \in I$ and $x \in C_a$, with

$$p_s^*(t) = p_a(x) = F[u(x) - g(a)]$$
$$= F(t - s),$$

yielding if $p_s^*(t) = \pi$,

$$p_s^{*-1}(\pi) = t = F^{-1}(\pi) + s.$$

Consequently,

$$p_s^{*-1}(\pi) - p_s^{*-1}(\pi') = F^{-1}(\pi) - F^{-1}(\pi')$$

independent of s, whenever π, π' are in the range of p_s^*. From Theorem 6.5 we conclude that $\mathscr{F}^*$ is a parallel psychometric family. If $\mathscr{F}$ is a Fechnerian psychometric family, then $u = g$, and the above construction yields a parallel discrimination family $\mathscr{F}^*$ which is 1-isomorphic to $\mathscr{F}$. ∎

7.23. Theorem. (i) *If an anchored psychometric family has an homomorphic image that is a parallel discrimination family, then it is subtractive.*
(ii) *A discrimination family is Fechnerian iff it is isomorphic to a parallel discrimination family.*

The proofs are easy, and we omit them (see Exercise 10).

REPRESENTATION AND UNIQUENESS THEOREMS FOR SUBTRACTIVE FAMILIES

In Chapter 6, we encountered two conditions, called double and triple cancellation (cf. 6.14, 6.13), which were necessary for the existence of a subtractive representation (u,g,F) of a psychometric family $\mathscr{F} = \{p_a | a \in I\}$. Thus, if (u,g,F) is a subtractive representation, we have by definition

$$p_a(x) = F[u(x) - g(a)],$$

with u and F, two strictly increasing and continuous functions. Obviously, another necessary condition is the uncrossing property of Definition 7.8.

Obtaining a set of conditions that is both sufficient and not unduly strong is a more delicate matter. From a heuristic viewpoint, the following approach has some appeal. Notice that if (u,g,F) is a subtractive representation of $\mathscr{F}$, then with

$$g(a) = t,$$

$$p_t^*(s) = p_a[u^{-1}(s)] = F(s - t)$$

defines a subtractive psychometric family $\mathscr{F}^*$ homomorphic to $\mathscr{F}$ (cf. Theorem 7.17). Moreover, it is clear from the last equation that if $\mathscr{F}^*$ happens to be a discrimination family, then it is Fechnerian (Definition 6.8). Since we know a great deal regarding Fechnerian discrimination families, this remark suggests a relatively easy route for attacking the representation problem, the main steps of which are outlined below.

Starting from a psychometric family $\mathscr{F}$, we first construct a discrimination family $\mathscr{F}^*$ homomorphic to $\mathscr{F}$. Next, a balanced family $\mathscr{F}^{*\dagger}$ will be obtained from $\mathscr{F}^*$, and we require that $\mathscr{F}^{*\dagger}$ is Fechnerian. It will turn out that $\mathscr{F}^{*\dagger}$ is Fechnerian iff $\mathscr{F}$ satisfies the triple cancellation condition. From the fact that $\mathscr{F}^{*\dagger}$ is Fechnerian, we derive that $\mathscr{F}$ is subtractive. We have the following result.

7.24. Theorem.   *Let* $\mathscr{F} = \{p_a | a \in I\}$ *be a psychometric family, with a continuous anchor ξ satisfying*

$$p_a^{-1}(\xi) \in C_b \qquad \text{iff} \qquad p_b^{-1}(\xi) \in C_a, \tag{15}$$

for all $a, b \in I$. *Then* $\mathscr{F}$ *is subtractive iff it satisfies triple cancellation.*

Similar results have been obtained by Levine (1975) and Narens & Luce (1976).

7.25. Proof.   The necessity of triple cancellation has been established (cf. 6.12, 6.13). Let $\mathscr{F} = \{p_a | a \in I\}$ be a psychometric family satisfying the hypothesis of the theorem, together with triple cancellation.

This implies that $\mathscr{F}$ is uncrossed (set $a = a'$, $x = x'$, $y = y'$ in Definition 6.13). By Theorem 7.21, we can assert that $\mathscr{F}$ has an homomorphic image $\mathscr{F}^*$, which is a discrimination family. More specifically:

$$\mathscr{F} \xrightarrow{\;(\mu,\,=)\;} \mathscr{F}^*,$$

where μ is defined by $\mu(a) = p_\xi^{-1}(a)$.

Lemma 1.   Whenever $p_y^*(x) \leqslant p_{y'}^*(x')$, $p_z^*(y) \leqslant p_z^*(y')$ then $p_z^*(x) \leqslant p_z^*(x')$.

This can easily be verified. In other words, $\mathscr{F}^*$ satisfies the bicancellation axiom (Definition 4.10).

Lemma 2.   For any $x, x', y, y' \in \mu(I)$, whenever the members of one inequality are defined in the equivalence

$$p_{x'}^*(y') \leqslant p_x^*(y) \qquad \text{iff} \qquad p_y^*(x) \leqslant p_{y'}^*(x'),$$

the members of the other inequality are also defined, and the equivalence holds.

Proof.   With $x = \mu(a)$, $x' = \mu(a')$, $y = \mu(b)$ and $y' = \mu(b')$, the equivalence can be rewritten

$$p_{a'}[\mu(b')] \leqslant p_a[\mu(b)] \qquad \text{iff} \qquad p_b[\mu(a)] \leqslant p_{b'}[\mu(a')] \tag{16}$$

and it is clear from (15) that the members of one inequality are defined iff the members of the other inequality are also defined. (Indeed, $\mu(a) \in C_b$ iff $\mu(b) \in C_a$, etc.) The left member of (16) gives

$$p_{a'}(y') \leqslant p_a(y); \tag{17}$$

moreover, by definition

$$p_a(x) = p_{a'}(x') = \xi = p_b(y) = p_{b'}(y'), \tag{18}$$

and (17), (18) together yield

$$p_b(x) = p_b[\mu(a)] \leqslant p_{b'}(x') = p_{b'}[\mu(a')]$$

by the triple cancellation condition. The converse implication follows by symmetry. ∎

Since $\mathscr{F}^*$ is a discrimination family, the background sets are connected. Consequently, (Theorem 7.6) the set $T = \bigcup_{x \in \mu(I)} \mathscr{R}(p_x^*)$ is an open interval. It follows from Lemma 2 that there exist a continuous, strictly decreasing function K mapping T onto itself, such that

$$p_y^*(x) = K[p_x^*(y)]. \tag{19}$$

Let H be a balancing function (cf. Definition 6.10), and let

$$\mathscr{F}^{*\dagger} = \{p_x^{*\dagger} \mid x \in \mu(I)\}$$

be the corresponding balanced family, generated from $\mathscr{F}^*$ by the function H. In view of (19), we can assume that H is a continuous, strictly increasing function in one variable only, defined on T. Notice that since the bicancellation axiom holds for $\mathscr{F}^*$, it also holds for $\mathscr{F}^{*\dagger}$. This follows easily from the fact that

$$p_y^{*\dagger}(x) \leqslant p_y^{*\dagger}(x') \qquad \text{iff} \qquad p_y^*(x) \leqslant p_y^*(x'),$$

which itself results from the definition of $\mathscr{F}^{*\dagger}$. Thus, $\mathscr{F}^{*\dagger}$ is a balanced discrimination family satisfying bicancellation. Using Theorem 4.13, it can be deduced that $\mathscr{F}^{*\dagger}$ is Fechnerian and there exist real-valued, strictly increasing, continuous functions u, G such that

$$p_y^{*\dagger}(x) = G[u(x) - u(y)]$$

for all $y \in \mu(I)$ and $x \in C_y^{*\dagger}$. Successively, for all $a \in I$ and $x \in C_a$,

$$\begin{aligned}
p_a(x) &= p_{\mu(a)}^*(x) \\
&= H^{-1}[p_{\mu(a)}^{*\dagger}(x)] \\
&= (H^{-1} \circ G)\{u(x) - u[\mu(a)]\} \\
&= F[u(x) - g(a)],
\end{aligned}$$

with $F = H^{-1} \circ G$ and $g = u \circ \mu$, two continuous functions. This establishes the fact that $\mathscr{F}$ is subtractive. ∎

The above result immediately raises the question of the uniqueness of a subtractive representation. We have the following theorem.

7.26. Theorem.   *Let $\mathscr{F} = \{p_a | a \in I\}$ be a subtractive psychometric family with an anchor. Suppose that (g,u,F) and (g^*,u^*,F^*) are two subtractive representations of $\mathscr{F}$. Then necessarily*

$$g(t) = \beta_0 g^*(t) + \beta_1,$$

$$u(t) = \beta_0 u^*(t) + \beta_1 + \beta_2,$$

$$F(t) = F^*\left(\frac{t - \beta_2}{\beta_0}\right)$$

for some constants $\beta_0 > 0$ and β_1, β_2.

For a related result see Levine (1975).

Proof.   The hypotheses of the theorem imply that

$$F[u(x) - g(a)] = F^*[u^*(x) - g^*(a)] \tag{20}$$

for all $a \in I$ and $x \in C_a$. Let ξ be an anchor of the family $\mathscr{F}$. For any $a,b \in I$, we have

$$\begin{array}{lll} g(a) \leqslant g(b) & \text{iff} & g(a) + F^{-1}(\xi) \leqslant g(b) + F^{-1}(\xi) \\ & \text{iff} & u[p_a^{-1}(\xi)] \leqslant u[p_b^{-1}(\xi)] \\ & \text{iff} & p_a^{-1}(\xi) \leqslant p_b^{-1}(\xi). \end{array}$$

Consequently,

$$g(a) \leqslant g(b) \qquad \text{iff} \qquad g^*(a) \leqslant g^*(b)$$

and there exists a continuous, strictly increasing function v satisfying

$$g(a) = v[g^*(a)]$$

for all $a \in I$. Notice that since g^* is continuous and I is connected, v is defined on a real interval. Applying F^{-1} on both sides of (20), defining

$$H = F^{-1} \circ F^*, \qquad h = u \circ u^{*-1}$$

and setting

$$u^*(x) = s, \qquad g^*(a) = t,$$

we obtain

$$h(s) - v(t) = H(s - t),$$

which we rewrite

$$h(t + r) = v(t) + H(r), \tag{21}$$

with $r = s - t$. Each of h, v and H is a continuous, strictly increasing function.

Functional equation techniques apply to Equation 21, (cf. 3.10(i)) but the domains of the functions have to be examined. Since ξ is an anchor, the equation

$$F^*[u^*(x) - g^*(a)] = \xi \tag{22}$$

has a solution in x for every fixed $a \in I$, and has also a solution in a for every fixed $x \in \bigcup_{a \in I} C_a$. Without loss of generality, we can assume that

$$F^{*-1}(\xi) = 0, \tag{23}$$

$$g^*(a_0) = 0, \qquad \text{for some } a_0 \in I, \tag{24}$$

$$u^*(x_0) = 0, \qquad \text{for some } x_0 \in C_{a_0}. \tag{25}$$

(We leave to the reader to check these facts.) For all $a \in I$, the set $u^*(C_a)$ is an open interval, since u^{*-1} is a continuous function. It follows that

$$\mathscr{D}(H) = \bigcup_{a \in I} \{u^*(x) - g^*(a) | x \in C_a\}$$

is an open set. Notice also that, as a consequence of (23), (24), and (25), each of

$$\mathscr{D}(h), \mathscr{D}(v) \text{ and } \mathscr{D}(H)$$

is an open set containing 0, and so, in particular, each contains an interval containing 0; we have in fact $\mathscr{D}(h) = \mathscr{D}(v)$ (ξ being an anchor, (22), (23) entail that the equation $u^*(x) = g^*(a)$ can be solved for both a and x). Let J be an open interval containing 0, and such that

$$J \subset \mathscr{D}(h) \cap \mathscr{D}(H).$$

Going back to the functional equation (21) and restricting consideration to the points $t, r \in J$, we obtain by standard arguments, for all $t \in J$ and some constants $\beta_0 > 0$ and β_1, β_2,

$$h(t) = \beta_0 t + \beta_1 + \beta_2, \tag{26}$$

$$v(t) = \beta_0 t + \beta_1, \tag{27}$$

$$H(t) = \beta_0 t + \beta_2. \tag{28}$$

This result is easily extended to all points t in the domains of the functions h, v, H. Notice that for all $t \in \mathscr{D}(h) = \mathscr{D}(v)$.

$$h(t) = v(t) + H(0)$$
$$= v(t) + \beta_2. \tag{29}$$

Thus, if (26) holds everywhere on $\mathscr{D}(h)$, then (27) holds everywhere on $\mathscr{D}(v)$. Since H is completely determined by h and v, this means that we only have to show that (26) holds on $\mathscr{D}(h)$. Suppose that $t \in \mathscr{D}(h) - J$. Take a positive integer n satisfying $t = ns$ for some s, and large enough to ensure that $s \in J$. (This is always possible, since J is an open interval containing 0.) Clearly using (21),

$$h(2s) = v(s) + H(s),$$
$$h(3s) = v(2s) + H(s)$$
$$= h(2s) - \beta_2 + H(s) \qquad \text{(by (29))}$$
$$= v(s) - \beta_2 + 2H(s). \tag{30}$$

By induction, we obtain for $n \geqslant 2$,

$$h(ns) = v(s) - (n-2)\beta_2 + (n-1)H(s).$$

Replacing $v(s)$ and $H(s)$ by their expressions from (27) and (28), we obtain

$$h(ns) = \beta_0 ns + \beta_1 + \beta_2.$$

This shows that (26), and hence (27), (28), hold for all relevant values of the variable t. Using

$$h = u \circ u^{*-1}, \qquad g = v \circ g^* \qquad \text{and} \qquad H = F^{-1} \circ F^*,$$

the theorem follows by substitution in (26), (27), and (28). ■

RANDOM VARIABLES REPRESENTATIONS

In a subtractive model, the psychophysical effects of stimuli and backgrounds are symbolized by scale values, for example, the numbers $u(x)$, $g(a)$ in the equation

$$p_a(x) = F[u(x) - g(a)]. \tag{31}$$

The chance factors involved in the detection of a stimulus x over a background a have only an implicit representation, in the function F in (31). A natural counterpart of such model is one in which the effects of stimuli and backgrounds are explicitly formalized in terms of random variables. We assume in this case that to each stimulus x and background a correspond some random variables, $\mathbf{U}_x$ and $\mathbf{V}_a$, respectively, such that

$$p_a(x) = \mathbb{P}\{\mathbf{U}_x \geqslant \mathbf{V}_a\}, \tag{32}$$

where $\mathbb{P}$ denotes the probability measure. This representation generalizes that defined in 5.1 for discrimination systems.

Obviously, (31) and (32) are not incompatible. In most instances, (31) can in fact be regarded as a special case of (32). The general theory of such representations is yet to be developed, however. The result given below is indicative of what can be expected in that direction.

7.27. Theorem. *Let $\{p_a | a \in I\}$ be a psychometric family. Suppose that there exist two collections $\mathscr{V} = \{\mathbf{V}_a | a \in I\}$ and $\mathscr{U} = \{\mathbf{U}_x | x \in \bigcup_{a \in I} C_a\}$ of jointly distributed, continuous random variables such that*

$$p_a(x) = \mathbb{P}\{\mathbf{U}_x \geqslant \mathbf{V}_a\}$$

for all $a \in I$ and $x \in C_a$. Then necessarily

$$|p_a(x) + p_b(y) - p_a(y) - p_b(x)| \leqslant 1$$

whenever $a,b \in I$ and $x,y \in C_a \cap C_b$.

Proof. Suppose that the two collections $\mathscr{V}, \mathscr{U}$ exist satisfying the conditions. Take any $a,b \in I$, with $x,y \in C_a \cap C_b$. In the sequel, we restrict consideration to the elements of the sets $\{a,b\}$ and $[x,y]$. It is important to distinguish the elements in these two sets. So if $\{a,b\} \cap [x,y] \neq \varnothing$, we relabel the elements in $\{a,b\}$ appropriately. With $S = \{a,b\} \cup [x,y]$, let $\{\mathbf{T}_s | s \in S\}$ be a collection of random variables such that $\mathbf{T}_s = V_s$ if $s = a,b$ and $\mathbf{T}_s = U_s$ if $x \leqslant s \leqslant y$. Define a function $(s,t) \mapsto P_{s,t}$ mapping $S \times S$ into $[0,1]$ by

$$P_{s,t} = \mathbb{P}\{\mathbf{T}_s \geqslant \mathbf{T}_t\}.$$

Notice that P coincides with p on the set $[x,y] \times \{a,b\}$ in the sense that

$$P_{s,t} = p_t(s) \qquad \text{for } t \in \{a,b\} \text{ and } x \leqslant s \leqslant y.$$

Moreover, it is easy to check that by the continuity of random variables, (S,P) is a binary random utility model.

The continuity of the random variables is used here, to ensure that $\mathbb{P}\{\mathbf{T}_s = \mathbf{T}_t\} = 0$, which yields

$$P_{s,t} + P_{t,s} = 1.$$

This implies that

$$P_{s,t} + P_{t,q} + P_{q,r} + P_{r,s} \leqslant 3,$$

by an application of 5.3(iv). In particular, with $s = x$, $t = a$, $q = y$ and $r = b$, we obtain

$$p_a(x) + [1 - p_a(y)] + p_b(y) + [1 - p_b(x)] \leqslant 3,$$

that is

$$p_a(x) + p_b(y) - p_a(y) - p_b(x) \leqslant 1,$$

and the theorem follows by symmetry. ∎

EXERCISES

1. Prove Theorem 7.5.
2. Show that Definitions 6.2 and 7.2 are consistent, by proving that a connected set in a metric space is uncountable.
3. Check in detail that the Automatic Gain Control Model of Example 7.7(b) defines a psychometric family, which is subtractive iff the functions v and h are linearly related.
4. Check in detail the derivations leading to Equation 7.
5. Provide an algebraic proof of the equivalence between (i), (ii), and (iii) in Theorem 7.9.
6. Prove Lemma 1 in 7.12.
7. Adapt Theorem 7.11 and its proof in the case where there is some number $\pi \in (0,1)$ such that for all $a \in I$, we have $p_a(x) = \pi$ for some $x \in C_a$. Do not assume that $\mathscr{F}$ is conditionally overlapping (cf. 7.13(1)).

8. What is the isomorphism of $\mathscr{F}'$ onto $\mathscr{F}^*$ in 7.15(c)?
9. Prove Theorem 7.20.
10. Prove Theorem 7.23.
11. Prove Lemma 1 in 7.25.
12. Check that triple cancellation implies double cancellation.
13. Under the hypothesis of Theorem 7.27, prove the following: if for $1 \leqslant i \leqslant n$, $a_i \in I$ and $x_i \in \bigcap_{1 \leqslant i \leqslant n} C_{a_i}$, then

$$[p_{a_1}(x_1) - p_{a_2}(x_1)] + \cdots + [p_{a_{n-1}}(x_{n-1}) - p_{a_n}(x_{n-1})]$$
$$+ [p_{a_n}(x_n) - p_{a_1}(x_n)] \leqslant n - 1.$$

14. Prove that if a discrimination family $\mathscr{F}$ is 1-isomorphic to a parallel, centered family $\mathscr{F}^*$ having a major element, then $\mathscr{F}$ is symmetric iff it is parallel.

8

Sensitivity Functions—
Weber's Law

What is the smallest increment on a stimulus continuum, which is just detectable by a subject? In other terms: given a stimulus intensity equal to a, what is the smallest increment $\Delta(a)$ such that $a + \Delta(a)$ "just noticeably" exceeds a? This was one of the earlier questions raised by psychophysicists. This minimal increment is often referred to as the *just noticeable difference*, or *Jnd* for short.[1] A variant—or rather, a special case—of this question is: What is the minimum value of a stimulus that is "just detectable" by a subject? This is called the *absolute threshold*.

Various experimental methods for the the determination of $\Delta(a)$ have been designed, described in Chapter 9. Such questions are by no means straightforward, however, since they are ambiguous. For example, what is meant by "just noticeably"? Suppose that $a + \Delta(a)$ is judged as exceeding a on 65% of the trials. Does that mean that $a + \Delta(a)$ "just noticeably" exceeds a? An empirical criterion is clearly involved here. In the so-called method of *constant stimuli* (see Chapter 9), $\Delta(a)$ is often taken as a correct determination if $a + \Delta(a)$ is judged as exceeding a on 75% of the trials. (We are ignoring statistical issues for the moment.) The arbitrariness of this choice is troubling.[2]

Certainly, one would not want the general pattern of experimental results to depend critically on the choice of the criterion. In fact, as Luce and Edwards (1958) pointed out, there are theoretical difficulties involved in adopting a unique, fixed criterion. Accordingly, there is a trend in contemporary psychophysical research toward varying the value of the criterion across experimental conditions. We return to this point later on.

A basic notion of this chapter is a function Δ of two variables,

$$(a,\pi) \mapsto \Delta_\pi(a)$$

with $\pi, 0 < \pi < 1$, representing the value of the criterion. Thus, in the particular case discussed above, $a + \Delta_{.75}(a)$ is judged as exceeding a on 75% of the trials. Notice that $\Delta_\pi(a)$ may be negative for some values of π: it is natural for example to expect that $a + \Delta_{.25}(a) < a$, at least in some experimental situations.

---

1. The expression *difference limen* is also used. A definition of this concept is given in 8.14.
2. This arbitrariness is less apparent, but just as critical, in the method "of limits" or in the method "of adjustments" (see Chapter 9). A criterion random variable is implicitly involved in these methods. The arbitrariness lies in the choice of an index of central location, and also in the details of the experimental procedure.

There is an obvious relation between the function of one variable $\pi \mapsto \Delta_\pi(a)$, and the psychometric function p_a analyzed in the two preceding chapters. For instance, suppose that p_a is a psychometric function in a discrimination family $\mathcal{F}$ (Definition 6.8), such that $p_a(a) = .5$. As illustrated in Figure 8.1, we have in such case

$$\Delta_\pi(a) = p_a^{-1}(\pi) - a. \tag{1}$$

The collection of all the functions Δ_π contains thus exactly the same information as the family $\mathcal{F}$ of psychometric functions. The emphasis on these functions here is justified, however. Psychophysicists have found out that experimental plots of the functions Δ_π provided very revealing summaries of their data, and use such plots routinely. Correspondingly, these functions are of a considerable theoretical interest, as we will see.

A difficulty with Δ_π, as defined by (1), is that the subtraction

$$p_a^{-1}(\pi) - a$$

does not necessarily make sense, since a and $p_a^{-1}(\pi)$ may denote two objects of different nature. Consider, for example, a situation in which $p_a^{-1}(\pi) = x$ specifies the intensity x of a stimulus detected with a probability π over a background of noise a, where a denotes a wave form or a spectral density function (i.e., a possibly infinite dimensional vector). For this reason, we focus our developments on the closely related class of functions

$$a \mapsto \xi_\pi(a) = p_a^{-1}(\pi)$$

(see Fig. 8.1). A more general definition of the functions Δ_π will also be given.

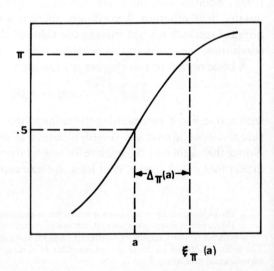

FIGURE 8.1. The functions Δ and ξ in a discrimination family $\mathcal{F} = \{p_a\}$ satisfying $p_a(a) = .5$. We have $\xi_\pi(a) = p_a^{-1}(\pi)$ and $\Delta_\pi(a) = \xi_\pi(a) - a$.

SENSITIVITY FUNCTIONS, WEBER FUNCTIONS

8.1. Definition. Let $\mathscr{F} = \{p_a | a \in I\}$ be a psychometric family (i.e., a family of psychometric functions satisfying certain hypotheses; cf. 6.1). The *sensitivity function* of $\mathscr{F}$ is a function ξ defined for all backgrounds (or standards) a, and all probabilities π in the range of a psychometric function p_a, by the equation

$$\xi_\pi(a) = p_a^{-1}(\pi).$$

(As usual, we write f^{-1} for the inverse of a one-to-one function f.) In words: $\xi_\pi(a)$ is the intensity of the stimulus yielding a response probability π, for the background a; that is,

$$p_a[\xi_\pi(a)] = \pi.$$

Let us assume that $\mathscr{F}$ is anchored at .5 (cf. 6.6; thus, .5 is a possible value for all the psychometric functions in the family). Then, the *Weber function* of $\mathscr{F}$ is a function Δ of two variables a and π, defined by

$$\Delta_\pi(a) = \xi_\pi(a) - \xi_{.5}(a).$$

This was illustrated in Figure 8.1 in the particular case where a denotes a real number (say, a physical intensity) and $\xi_{.5}(a) = a$.

It is important to distinguish in our notation the concept of Δ from that of Δ_π. The latter is a function of one variable, namely, the background or standard. In other words, in the notation $\Delta_{.75}$, the probability .75 is implicitly assumed to be fixed. Occasionally, it will nevertheless be convenient, by abuse of language, to refer to the functions Δ_π as the *Weber functions* of $\mathscr{F}$. A similar convention will apply to the functions ξ_π, which will be called the *sensitivity functions* of $\mathscr{F}$. Psychophysicists often analyze their data in terms of one or more functions

$$a \mapsto \Delta_\pi(a)/a,$$

in a situation in which division by a is legitimate. Such function will be called the *π-Weber fraction* of $\mathscr{F}$, or more simply, when no ambiguity can arise, a *Weber fraction*. Notice that since, in a case were $p_a(a) = .5$ for all intensities a, we have, by definition,

$$\frac{\Delta_\pi(a)}{a} = \frac{\xi_\pi(a)}{a} - 1,$$

any property of a Weber fraction will be almost exactly reflected in the corresponding function $\xi_\pi(a)/a$.

8.2. Remarks. The change of notation, from $p_a^{-1}(\pi)$ to $\xi_\pi(a)$, symbolizes an important shift of focus in our analysis. The quantity π, the probability of the response, ceases to be the variable of interest and becomes the parameter. Typically, at most a couple of values of π are considered in experimental plots of Weber functions or sensitivity functions. By contrast, the effect on $\Delta_\pi(a)$ or $\xi_\pi(a)$ of the variable *a* is investigated in minute detail. This is in line with a long tradition in psychophysical research in which the sensory scales uncovered by the analysis of the data are deemed of central importance. This point is a critical one and we pause for a while to discuss it in some detail.

Suppose, for example, that some psychometric family $\mathscr{F} = \{p_a\}$ is subtractive, in the sense of Definition 6.8. This means that the following representation holds for the response probabilities:

$$p_a(x) = F[u(x) - g(a)], \tag{2}$$

in which *u* and *F* are continuous and strictly increasing functions. The psychophysicist using such a model typically interprets the functions *u*, *g* as representing a rescaling of the physical variables by the sensory mechanisms. As such, these functions are far more important to him or her than the function *F* which, it is feared, may be plagued by nuisance variables of the "cognitive" type (response bias, motivation, etc).

Let us transform (2) in terms of the sensitivity function ξ. Setting $p_a(x) = \pi$ and $F^{-1} = h$, we obtain $\xi_\pi(a) = x$, which together with (2) yields

$$\xi_\pi(a) = u^{-1}[g(a) + h(\pi)] \tag{3}$$

Consequently, if the variable π in (3) is kept constant, the resulting equation in one variable only involves the functions *u*, *g* which for reasons given above, are the interesting ones.

Such is thus the strategy of the psychophysicist. It relies heavily on a couple of assumptions. One is that the sensitivity functions ξ_π can be determined empirically with enough accuracy. A number of methods have been designed for this purpose, which will be discussed in Chapter 9. Another, more critical, assumption is that the rescaling functions *u*, *g* in (2), (3) are unaffected by nuisance (i.e., nonsensory) variables. As far as I know, there is little experimental evidence suggesting that this assumption may be invalid.

As a by-product of our discussion, we have, in any event, the following result.

8.3. Theorem. *Let ξ be the sensitivity function of a psychometric family $\mathscr{F} = \{p_b | b \in I\}$. Then $\mathscr{F}$ is subtractive iff there exist three functions h, u, and g, with u and h strictly increasing and continuous, such that*

$$\xi_\pi(a) = u^{-1}[g(a) + h(\pi)].$$

Indeed, we have shown that (2) implies (3), and it is clear that the reverse implication also holds. As suggested by this theorem, all the results obtained in Chapters 6 and 7 regarding psychometric functions could be translated in terms of sensitivity functions or, when they are defined, in terms of Weber functions. A couple of additional examples are given below.

8.4. Theorem. *Let $\mathscr{F} = \{p_a | a \in I\}$ be a psychometric family, with sensitivity function ξ. Then, the following two conditions are equivalent.*

(i) $\mathscr{F}$ is a parallel family in the sense of Definition 6.4.

(ii) $\xi_\pi(a) - \xi_{\pi'}(a) = \xi_\pi(b) - \xi_{\pi'}(b)$,

for all π, π', and a, b such that both members are defined.

Moreover, each of (i), (ii) *is equivalent to the assumption that the Weber functions $a \mapsto \Delta_\pi(a)$ (assuming that they are defined, that is, $\mathscr{F}$ is anchored at .5) do not vary with the variable a.*

This result follows readily from the definitions and from Theorem 6.5.

8.5. Theorem. *If $\mathscr{F} = \{p_a | a \in I\}$ is an anchored psychometric family (in the sense of Definition 6.6) with a sensitivity function ξ, then $\mathscr{F}$ is parallel iff there exist two functions g, h with h strictly increasing and continuous, such that the equation*

$$\xi_\pi(a) = g(a) + h(\pi) \tag{4}$$

holds whenever $\xi_\pi(a)$ is defined. In particular, g is defined on I.

As suggested by a comparison of Theorems 8.4 and 8.5, the functions g, h do not necessarily exist if the assumption of anchoring is removed.

Proof. Suppose that $\mathscr{F}$ is an anchored, parallel psychometric family. By Theorem 6.7, it has a representation

$$p_a(x) = F[x - g(a)] \tag{5}$$

in which F, g are continuous functions. With $\xi_\pi(a) = p_a^{-1}(\pi) = x$, and $h = F^{-1}$, (5) is equivalent to (4). The converse proposition follows from Theorem 8.4. ■

Next we consider the effect of the balancing condition (Definition 6.8)

$$p_a(b) + p_b(a) = 1,$$

on the sensitivity function of a discrimination family.

8.6. Theorem. *A discrimination family $\mathscr{F} = \{p_b | b \in I\}$ is balanced iff its sensitivity function ξ satisfies*

$$\xi_{1-\pi}[\xi_\pi(a)] = a$$

whenever the left member of this equation is defined.

(See Exercise 4.)

These few results should suffice to familiarize the reader with the notions of Definition 8.1. Further results along these lines can be found in Falmagne (1982), or in the exercises.

LINEAR PSYCHOMETRIC FAMILIES—WEBER'S LAW

So far, no assumptions were made in this chapter regarding the structure of the set I of backgrounds of a psychometric family $\{p_a | a \in I\}$. Properties such as parallelism or subtractivity could be discussed while assuming that the elements

$a \in I$ were just labels for the psychometric functions p_a in the family. Of particular importance in this section will be the situation in which I is actually a (subset of *a*) vector space over the real numbers. For example, $a \in I$ may denote a spectral density function or, in the case of a discrimination family (cf. 6.8), a real number representing a physical intensity. What is critical here is that the multiplication

$$\lambda a$$

of a real vector a by a positive real number λ makes sense. From an empirical standpoint, the multiplication λa means that the intensity of the background has been multiplied by the factor λ. (In the case of a spectral density function, a denotes a real-valued function, and λa symbolizes the fact that all the intensities of the background have been multiplied by the same constant λ.) When such a situation arises, properties can be investigated in the data, which are both strong and of central interest for psychophysical research.

8.7. Definition.   A psychometric family $\mathscr{F} = \{p_b | b \in I\}$ is called *linear* iff the index set I is a (subset of *a*) vector space over the real numbers.

An important special case of a linear psychometric family arises when the indices of the psychometric function denote physical intensities. This case was referred to in 6.8 as a discrimination family.

We recall that in a psychometric family $\mathscr{F} = \{p_b | b \in I\}$, the notation C_b, for any $b \in I$, refers to the domain of the psychometric function p_b, which is an open interval (cf. Definition 6.2). The psychometric family $\mathscr{F}$ will be called *positive* iff each interval C_b is positive. (This is a typical case for physical intensities.) Most results in the remainder of this section will be obtained in the framework of linear, positive psychometric families.

The next definition will also be useful in connection with Weber's law, and more general forms of this law.

8.8. Definition.   Let V be a vector space over the real numbers. Let T be a subset of V. Let f be a real-valued function on T. Then f is said to be *homogeneous of degree* β *(on T)* iff for any real number $\lambda \neq 0$, whenever $a, \lambda a \in T$, then

$$f(\lambda a) = \lambda^\beta f(a).$$

8.9. Definition.   A linear, positive psychometric family $\mathscr{F} = \{p_b | b \in I\}$ satisfies *Weber's law* iff

$$p_a(x) = p_{\lambda a}(\lambda x) \tag{6}$$

whenever both members of (6) are defined, with $0 < \lambda < \infty$. In other words, $\mathscr{F}$ satisfies Weber's law iff the function $p, (a,x) \mapsto p_a(x)$, is homogeneous of degree 0. Occasionally, (6) will be referred to as *Weber's law*.

8.10. Remarks.   In two respects, this definition of Weber's law departs from tradition. Weber's law is usually stated in the special case in which the backgrounds are real numbers. For example, in the context of auditory detection of a stimulus embedded in noise, Weber's law would imply that the probability of a correct detection would not vary when both the stimulus and the noise are increased in intensity by the same number of decibels. The experimenter believes however that this prediction would apply for a fairly large set of spectral density functions specifying the noise. Such assumption is made explicit in Definition 8.9. Another difference is that Weber's law is most often expressed in terms of the Weber functions Δ_π. The equivalence is made clear in Theorem 8.12. We have two reasons for adopting Equation 6 as the defining condition of Weber's law, and not the more customary form

$$\Delta_\pi(\lambda a) = \lambda \Delta_\pi(a).$$

One reason is that (6) is more general: this equation makes sense in situations in which the Weber functions are not always defined. (The Weber function Δ_π was defined in 8.1 from the sensitivity function $\xi_{.5}$. There may be cases in which $\xi_{.5}$ is not obtainable.) Another reason is the fact that, in view of the binomial variability of the relative frequencies providing the basic data for (6), it is more readily amenable to statistical testing. In practice, however, evaluations of Weber's law are mostly based on investigating the empirical behavior of the Weber functions.

Some strengthening of our conditions will be useful for this and later results.

8.11. Definition. A linear psychometric family $\mathscr{F} = \{p_b | b \in I\}$ is called *solvable* iff for all $a \in I$ and all $x \in C_a$, the equation

$$p_{\lambda a}(\mu x) = p_a(x)$$

is solvable in μ for every λ, and is solvable in λ for every μ. We say that $\mathscr{F}$ has a *Weberian domain* iff for any $\lambda > 0$, $p_{\lambda a}(\lambda x)$ is defined whenever $p_a(x)$ is defined.

These strengthenings of our assumptions will occasionally be convenient, but are hardly innocuous. The reader is invited to reflect on the empirical impact of these two conditions. Both of them practically entail that neither of the two physical domains spanned by the function p is bounded, obviously not a realistic assumption. Neither of these conditions is essential, but they certainly render our developments much easier. In any event, they will be used sparingly in the sequel.

In Theorem 8.12, a central result of this chapter, we consider an important generalization of Weber's law, symbolized by the equation

$$p_{\lambda a}(\lambda^\beta x) = p_a(x),$$

and we establish the equivalence between this equation and some constraints on sensitivity function and Weber function data. In passing we show that our definition of Weber's law is equivalent to the traditional one. The interpretation of the exponent β is discussed in Remark 8.13(1).

8.12. Theorem. Let $\mathscr{F} = \{p_b | b \in I\}$ be a linear, positive, solvable psychometric family, with sensitivity function ξ. Then, the following three conditions are equivalent.

(i) *Every sensitivity function ξ_π is homogeneous of degree $\beta > 0$:*

$$\xi_\pi(\lambda a) = \lambda^\beta \xi_\pi(a).$$

(ii) *There is a constant $\beta > 0$ such that*

$$p_{\lambda a}(\lambda^\beta x) = p_a(x),$$

whenever both members of this equation are defined, with $0 < \lambda < \infty$.

(iii) *There exists a function F and a constant $\beta > 0$ such that*

$$p_a(x) = F(a/x^{1/\beta}).$$

Moreover, if $\mathcal{F}$ is anchored at .5, then each of (i) to (iii) is equivalent to the assumptions that any Weber function Δ_π is homogeneous of degree $\beta > 0$. In particular, Weber's law holds iff

$$\Delta_\pi(\lambda a) = \lambda \Delta_\pi(a), \tag{7}$$

that is, the Weber functions Δ_π are homogeneous of degree 1.

Proof. (i) *implies* (ii). Suppose that $p_a(x) = \pi$, $p_{\lambda a}(\lambda^\beta x) = \pi'$. Then $\xi_\pi(a) = x$, and successively

$$\xi_{\pi'}(\lambda a) = \lambda^\beta x = \lambda^\beta \xi_\pi(a) = \xi_\pi(\lambda a),$$

since $\mathcal{F}$ is solvable, and $\pi = \pi'$ follows by the strict monotonicity of $\xi_\pi(\lambda a)$ in the variable π.

(ii) *implies* (iii). Condition (ii) is equivalent to

$$p_{\lambda a}(\lambda^\beta x) = p_{\gamma a}(\gamma^\beta x)$$

whenever both members are defined with λ, $\gamma \in (0, \infty)$. Setting $z = \lambda^\beta x$ and $w = \gamma^\beta x$, we obtain $\lambda = (zx^{-1})^{1/\beta}$, $\gamma = (wx^{-1})^{1/\beta}$ yielding

$$p_{z^{1/\beta}(x^{-1/\beta}a)}(z) = p_{w^{1/\beta}(x^{-1/\beta}a)}(w).$$

This shows that the value of $p_{z^{1/\beta_s}}(z)$ does not depend on the choice of z. Fixing $z = K$, a constant, we obtain for any $a \in I$, $x \in C_a$, and $\lambda = (K/x)^{1/\beta}$

$$p_a(x) = p_{\lambda a}(\lambda^\beta x) = p_{(K/x)^{1/\beta}a}(K) = F(a/x^{1/\beta}),$$

with the function F defined by $F(s) = p_{K^{1/\beta_s}}(K)$. In fact, (ii) and (iii) are equivalent since, obviously,

$$F(a/x^{1/\beta}) = F[\lambda a/(\lambda^\beta x)^{1/\beta}].$$

(ii) *implies* (i). This is clear since, with

$$\pi = p_{\lambda a}(\lambda^\beta x) = p_a(x),$$

we have

$$\xi_\pi(\lambda a) = \lambda^\beta x = \lambda^\beta \xi_\pi(a).$$

If the Weber function is defined, it follows by substitution that the sensitivity functions are homogeneous of degree $\beta > 0$ iff the Weber functions Δ_π also satisfy this condition. Finally, the equivalence between Weber's law and Equation 7 is obtained from the case $\beta = 1$ of the equivalence between (i) and (ii). ∎

8.13. Remarks. (1) We will see that the homogeneity equation

$$\xi_\pi(\lambda a) = \lambda^\beta \xi_\pi(a)$$

plays an important role in the analysis of data, as a substitute to Weber's law. (This equation is often referred to as the *near-miss-to-Weber's-law*, cf. McGill & Goldberg, 1968.) The interpretation of the exponent β in this equation must be considered carefully. There seems to be a tendency in the psychophysical community to take this exponent as representing an critical aspect of neural coding of physical intensity. For a number of reasons, this position is open to challenge. One difficulty is indicated below. Suppose that $\mathscr{F}$ is a discrimination family satisfying this condition, together with $\xi_{.5}(a) = a$, for all intensities a. This implies that the Weber functions are also homogeneous of degree β:

$$\Delta_\pi(\lambda a) = \lambda^\beta \Delta_\pi(a). \tag{8}$$

But we also have

$$\Delta_\pi(\lambda a) = \xi_\pi(\lambda a) - \xi_{.5}(\lambda a) = \lambda^\beta \xi_\pi(a) - \lambda a = \lambda^\beta[\Delta_\pi(a) + a] - \lambda a,$$

which together with (8), implies

$$\lambda^\beta \Delta_\pi(a) = \lambda^\beta[\Delta_\pi(a) + a] - \lambda a,$$

that is,

$$a(\lambda^\beta - \lambda) = 0.$$

Since $a > 0$, we must conclude that $\beta = 1$. Thus, in the case of a discrimination family satisfying $p_a(a) = .5$, the assumption that the Weber functions are homogeneous of degree β in fact implies Weber's law.

The crux of the argument here is that the condition

$$p_a(a) = .5$$

or the balance condition

$$p_a(b) + p_b(a) = 1$$

which implies it, may result from a symmetry of the experimental paradigm that is not necessarily of a sensory nature. We return to this point later in this section.

(2) A special case of Theorem 8.12 is of historical interest. If Weber's law holds, then $\beta = 1$, and by virtue of Condition (iii) in Theorem 8.12, the choice probabilities take the form

$$p_a(x) = F(a/x) = F[e^{-(\log x - \log a)}],$$

yielding

$$p_a(x) = G(\log x - \log a), \tag{9}$$

with $G(s) = F(e^{-s})$, a strictly increasing, continuous function. Equation 9 has sometimes been given the interpretation that "the sensation grows as the logarithm of the excitation," a statement which has been christened "Fechner's law." Such interpretation has been at the center of a long controversy, and should not be dismissed or accepted casually. It relies, in part, on some empirical evidence—Weber's law. (How well Weber's law is supported by the data is considered in the next paragraph.) It also results on the somewhat arbitrary choice of a particular mathematical representation of such data, that is, Equation 9. Finally, it involves using a philosophically charged label such as "sensation." Each of these factors has contributed its share to the polemical aspects of the debate, an account of which can be found in Chapter 13 of this book.

8.14. Applications.   As an empirical prediction, Weber's law holds reasonably well for sensory continua such as, for example, loudness discrimination of Gaussian noises, loudness discrimination of pure tones, lifted weights, and visual brightness. As mentioned in the last section, the analysis of the data is sometimes based on the *just-noticeable-difference* (or Jnd) function, which can be computed from the sensitivity functions by the equation

$$\mathrm{Jnd}(a) = [\xi_{.75}(a) - \xi_{.25}(a)]/2. \tag{10}$$

The experimenter checks whether the ratio

$$\mathrm{Jnd}(a)/a \tag{11}$$

remains constant, while a varies on a chosen subset of the physical scale. (Thus, a takes values in the positive reals.) We have elected to base our developments on the sensitivity function rather than on the Jnd function. For various reasons, the sensitivity function is the appropriate notion to use as the cornerstone of the theory. Notice in this connection that the ratio (11) is constant if the functions

$$a \mapsto \xi_\pi(a)/a$$

are constant. More generally, the Jnd function is homogeneous of degree β if the sensitivity functions ξ_π are homogeneous of degree β. It is clear that the reverse implication does not necessarily hold.

A number of methods are used for the empirical determination of the sensitivity function. (These methods are described in Chapter 9.) Even though these methods differ drastically from an experimental viewpoint, many researchers seem to believe that the overall pattern of empirical results is not seriously affected by the method used. This opinion is not universal, however. (Luce and Green (1974) for example, analyze the data of six studies of the Weber fraction $\Delta_\pi(a)/a$ for tone intensities, with considerable discrepancies in the results.)

The experimental evidence favoring Weber's law is exemplified in Figure 8.2. For some sensory continua, the Weber fraction $\Delta_\pi(a)/a$, with $a > 0$, indeed remains constant over a substantial portion of the domain (2 to 3 log units, for audition and vision), thus supporting Weber's law. A more comprehensive description of the data would emphasize the fact that the Weber fraction is initially

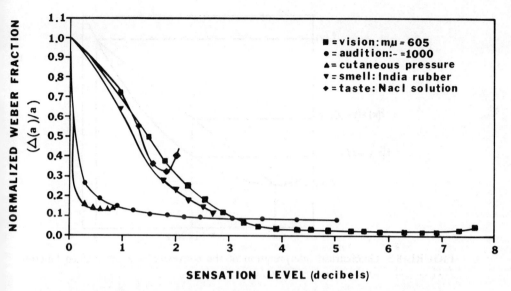

FIGURE 8.2. Weber fraction data for various sensory continua. The abscissa is in dB, sensation level. The Weber fractions have been normalized so as to be unity at threshold. From "Discrimination" by R. D. Luce and E. Galanter, 1963, in *Handbook of Mathematical Psychology, Vol. 1* by R. D. Luce, R. R. Bush, and E. Galanter (Eds.). New York: Wiley. Adapted with permission of authors. Copyright © 1963 by Duncan Luce.

decreasing. In fact, for audition and smell, it never increases. Finally, a conjecture that is validated by the data for all five continua in Figure 8.2 is that the Weber fraction is "convex." (That is, it never "curves downward." A precise definition of the convexity of a function is given below.) The reader should remember these aspects of the data, which will lead to a theoretical analysis in the next section.

The initial decrease of the Weber fraction is sometimes attributed to an absolute threshold of perception, while the late rise of the fraction in some cases is attributed to the sensory mechanisms reaching the limit of their operational range. However legitimate such interpretations might be, they do not necessarily justify an analysis of an empirical Weber fraction into fragments, each requiring a separate model. In this chapter, only models attempting a comprehensive description of the data are considered.

8.15. Definition. Let f be a real-valued function defined on a real interval (s,t). Then f is called *convex* iff

$$f[\lambda x + (1 - \lambda)y] \leqslant \lambda f(x) + (1 - \lambda)f(y) \tag{12}$$

whenever $s < x < t, s < y < t$, and $0 < \lambda < 1$. The function f is *strictly convex* iff the inequality in (12) is strict. If $-f$ is convex (respectively, strictly convex) then f is said to be *concave* (respectively, *strictly concave*).

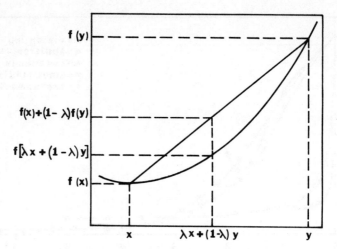

FIGURE 8.3. Geometrical interpretation of the convexity of a real valued function $f: f[\lambda x + (1 - \lambda)y] \leq \lambda f(x) + (1 - \lambda)f(y)$.

Any linear function is both convex and concave. Examples of strictly convex functions are $x \mapsto e^x, x \mapsto x^2$, for $-\infty < x < \infty$. The following results are easy consequences of the definition. Any convex function is continuous; if g is an increasing, convex function, and f is convex, then the composition $s \mapsto g[f(s)]$ is convex, (in particular, e^f is convex, in fact, strictly convex); if the second derivative f'' of f exists, then f is convex iff $f'' \geq 0$. A geometrical interpretation of convexity is that any segment of a straight line joining two points of the graph of a convex function f lies above or on the graph of f (see Fig. 8.3).

It is clear that the Weber fractions depicted in Figure 8.2 are convex in the sense of Definition 8.15. A case can be made that these functions are actually strictly convex. The failures of Weber's law illustrated in Figure 8.2 prompted psychophysicists to propose various alternatives.

ALTERNATIVES TO WEBER'S LAW

8.16. The near-miss-to-Weber's-law.   One generalization of Weber's law has been encountered earlier which, in terms of the sensitivity function, is symbolized by the equation

$$\xi_\pi(\lambda a) = \lambda^\beta \xi_\pi(a) \tag{13}$$

for $0 < \lambda < \infty$ and with $\beta > 0$, a constant independent of π. When the Weber function is defined, this is equivalent to

$$\Delta_\pi(\lambda a) = \lambda^\beta \Delta_\pi(a). \tag{14}$$

This prediction, which is often referred to as the "near-miss-to-Weber's-law" (McGill & Goldberg, 1968), has been supported experimentally in some situa-

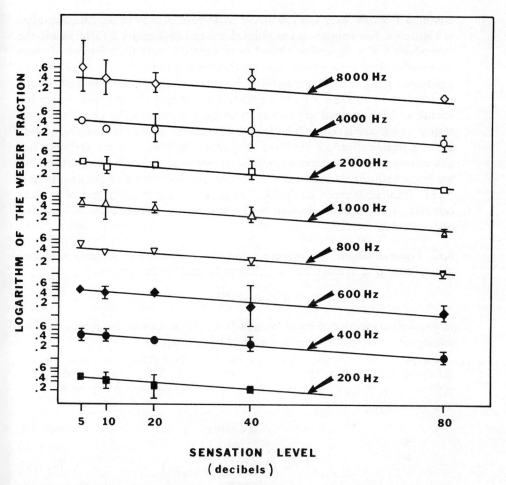

FIGURE 8.4. Values of the logarithm of the Weber fraction, averaged across subjects and replications, for various intensities and frequencies of pure tones. The abscissa is in dB, sensation level. The vertical bars indicate ±3 standard errors. A bar is omitted when its size is exceeded by that of the symbol. The same linear function has been fitted to the eight sets of data. From "Intensity Discrimination as a Function of Frequency and Sensation Level by W. Jesteadt, C. C. Wier, and D. M. Green, 1977, in *Journal of the Acoustical Society of America, 61*, pp. 169–177. Figure is reprinted with permission of authors and publisher.

tions (Jesteadt, Weir, & Green, 1977; cf. Fig. 8.4). Notice that the data in Figure 8.4 requires the exponent β in (14) to be smaller than 1: the Weber fraction

$$\Delta_\pi(\lambda)/\lambda = \lambda^{\beta-1}\Delta_\pi(1)$$

must be decreasing. It cannot be assumed however that the near-miss-to-Weber's-law holds generally, across experimental paradigms and sensory continua. For one thing, this law would fail to explain most of the data displayed in Figure 8.2. For another, it was pointed out earlier (Remark 8.13(1)) that in the case where $\beta \neq 1$, Equations 13 and 14 necessarily imply the existence of some asymmetry in the paradigm: the psychometric functions cannot satisfy the condition, $p_a(a) = .5$. This condition however, is sometimes inherent to the experimental paradigm (e.g., in a situation in visual psychophysics, where the stimuli to be compared are two spots of light symmetrically positioned with respect to a fixation point). It is also possible to ensure that this condition holds by a "normalization" of the data. As argued in 6.9(3), we are certainly not advocating such data tampering. The fact is, however, that such "normalizations" are fairly frequent. In such cases, it is clear that (14) describes the data only if $\beta = 1$—that is, Weber's law holds—or possibly, if β is a function of π. This, however, is not what is intended by the near-miss-to-Weber's-law, at least as I understand it.

8.17. Generalization.   In any event, the above discussion suggests a further generalization of Webers' law, which is embodied in the equation

$$\xi_\pi(\lambda a) = \lambda^{\beta(\pi)} \xi_\pi(a), \tag{15}$$

in which β is a function of π satisfying $\beta(.5) = 1$. (This ensures that $p_a(a) = .5$.) The consequences of that assumption deserve some attention.

Suppose that $\mathscr{F} = \{p_a | a \in I\}$ is a balanced, positive discrimination family satisfying (15), with $p_c(b) = \pi$ for some $c, b \in I$. This implies that $c \in C_b$, $p_b(c) = 1 - \pi$. Since C_b is an open interval, it contains some $a \neq c$, with $\lambda a = c$, and, successively,

$$
\begin{aligned}
\lambda a &= \xi_{1-\pi}[\xi_\pi(\lambda a)] &&\text{(by Theorem 8.6)} \\
&= \xi_{1-\pi}[\lambda^{\beta(\pi)} \xi_\pi(a)] &&\text{(by (15))} \\
&= \lambda^{\beta(1-\pi)\beta(\pi)} \xi_{1-\pi}[\xi_\pi(a)] &&\text{(by (15))} \\
&= \lambda^{\beta(1-\pi)\beta(\pi)} a &&\text{(by Theorem 8.6)}
\end{aligned}
$$

which gives

$$\lambda^{\beta(1-\pi)\beta(\pi)} = \lambda,$$

and thus

$$\beta(1 - \pi)\beta(\pi) = 1,$$

since we can assume that $a \neq 0$ and $\lambda \neq 0, 1$.

Theorem 8.18 summarizes this discussion.

8.18. Theorem.   *Let $\mathscr{F}$ be a balanced discrimination family with sensitivity function ξ satisfying* (15) *for some real valued function β; then, necessarily,*

$$\beta(\pi)\beta(1 - \pi) = 1 \tag{16}$$

for all π in the domain of β.

We point out that, somewhat unexpectedly, the available data would prevent β to be an increasing function of the probability. To see this, suppose that the near-miss-to-Weber's-law holds for a particular probability $\pi > \frac{1}{2}$. As indicated in 8.16, this is possible only if $\beta(\pi) < 1$, since the Weber fraction

$$\Delta_\pi(\lambda a)/\lambda = \lambda^{\beta(\pi)-1}\Delta_\pi(a)$$

must be decreasing. This fact together with (16), leads to

$$\beta(\pi) < \beta(1 - \pi).$$

But $1 - \pi < \pi$; we conclude that β cannot be an everywhere increasing function. By continuity, β has to decrease on part of its domain; it may of course be nonmonotonic.

As an illustration of the situation described in this theorem, suppose that the choice probabilities satisfy the equation

$$p_a(b) = \frac{[\log(\tau/a)]^\gamma}{[\log(\tau/a)]^\gamma + [\log(\tau/b)]^\gamma}$$

where τ and γ are constants, and $a,b < \tau$. Indeed, with $p_a(b) = \pi$, we easily obtain

$$\xi_\pi(a) = \tau(a/\tau)^{[(1-\pi)/\pi]^{1/\gamma}}$$

yielding

$$\xi_\pi(\lambda a) = \lambda^{[(1-\pi)/\pi]^{1/\gamma}}\xi_\pi(a).$$

This is a particular case of (15), in which

$$\beta(\pi) = [(1 - \pi)/\pi]^{1/\gamma}.$$

As far as I know, the effect of the choice probability π on the estimated value of the exponent β in (15) has never been investigated from an experimental viewpoint.

8.19. Other examples. A couple of other substitutes to Weber's law are of interest. As in the case of the near-miss-to-Weber's-law, each of the following examples is a special case of the representation

$$\xi_\pi(a) = u^{-1}[g(a) + h(\pi)],$$

as can be checked without difficulty.

(a) Let the sensitivity function ξ of a discrimination family be defined by the equation

$$\xi_\pi(\lambda a) = \lambda^\beta[\xi_\pi(a) - K] + K, \tag{17}$$

where K is a positive constant. In the style of Theorem 8.12, this is equivalent to the representation

$$p_a(x) = F[a(x - K)^{-1/\beta}] \tag{18}$$

for the choice probabilities (we assume $x > K$). Provided that $\beta > 1$ and

$\xi_\pi(a) > K$, the function

$$\lambda \mapsto \xi_\pi(\lambda a)/\lambda$$

is convex on the positive real numbers, with a minimum at the point

$$\lambda = [K/(\beta - 1)(\xi_\pi(a) - K)]^{1/\beta}.$$

Thus, the Weber fractions are also convex in the same conditions, a fact worth noticing in connection with our discussion of the data displayed in Figure 8.2. It is clear that this model generalizes the near-miss-to-Weber's-law. The constant K may be interpreted as a measure of a threshold value.

(b) In the case where $\mathscr{F}$ is a discrimination family, we also consider the representation

$$\xi_\pi(a) = [h(\pi) + \delta a^{\beta'}]^{1/\beta} \tag{19}$$

for the sensitivity functions, involving a strictly increasing, continuous function h and three positive constants β, β', and δ. This leads immediately to the representation

$$p_a(x) = F[x^\beta - \delta a^{\beta'}], \tag{20}$$

with $F = h^{-1}$, for the choice probabilities. This model has been discussed by several authors (see, for example, Parker & Schneider, 1980). It is not consistent with Weber's law. However, for appropriately chosen values of the parameters, it would predict the main features (monotonicity, convexity) of data such as that pictured in Figure 8.2.[3]

(c) The late increase of the Weber fraction is often interpreted as resulting from a saturation of the sensory or neuronal mechanisms. In turn, this leads us to postulate that the sensory scale—e.g., the function u in (2)—is bounded. An example along these lines is given below. It is assumed that the sensitivity functions satisfy the equation

$$\xi_\pi(a) = K\{h(\pi)f(a)/[1 - h(\pi)f(a)]\}^{1/\beta}, \tag{21}$$

with

$$f(a) = a^{\beta'} + K',$$

and $\beta, \beta', K, K' > 0$, constants. Using simple algebra, we obtain for the response probabilities, the form

$$p_a(\pi) = G[x^\beta/(x^\beta + K^\beta)f(a)],$$

or equivalently, as a difference model,

$$p_a(x) = F\{\ln[x^\beta/(x^\beta + K^\beta)] - \ln f(a)\},$$

with $F(\ln s) = G(s)$. Thus,

$$u(x) = \ln[x^\beta/(x^b + K)] < 0.$$

3. It is shown in Chapter 14 that this model is not "meaningful" if $\delta = 1$ and $\beta \neq \beta'$.

Again, such model is capable of accommodating typical Weber fraction data (cf. Alpern, Rushton, & Tori 1970a, 1970b, 1970c).

Other models have been proposed, which differ only in details from one or the other of those discussed in this section. They will not be reviewed here. Our purpose in this subsection is not to single out one particular mathematical expression as the appropriate model for the sensitivity function. In fact, it is quite conceivable that the choice of a suitable model (a model that would provide a good fit to the data, from a statistical viewpoint) may depend not only on the sensory continuum envisaged, but also on rather specific details of the experimental paradigm.

Accordingly it makes sense to investigate, from a theoretical viewpoint, aspects of the data that may perhaps be robust to minor changes of the experimental procedure. A couple of examples are given in the next section.

8.20. Some references.   Weber fraction data are compiled for example in Boring, Langfeld, and Weld (1948, p. 268) and Holway and Pratt (1936, p. 337), for various sensory continua. Luce and Green (1974; see also Green, 1978, p. 257) review a number of experimental studies of the discrimination of the difference in the amplitudes of a sinusoidal tone. The data are plotted in terms of the Weber fraction. Laming (1982; see also his monograph, 1983) examines a collection of models and data for the Weber fraction. In a particular theoretical framework, he obtains results that narrow down the possible forms of the distribution of the random representation (in the sense of 5.1).

INEQUALITIES

In 8.14, we pointed out that, in a number of empirical cases, the Weber fractions were decreasing, or at least nonincreasing. The following simple result is worth noticing in this connection.

8.21. Theorem.   Let $\mathscr{F} = \{p_b | b \in I\}$ be a linear, positive psychometric family, with Weberian domain and sensitivity function ξ. Let $0 < \pi_0 < 1$ be fixed. Then the two following conditions are equivalent.

(i) Whenever $p_a(x) \geqslant \pi_0$ the function $\lambda \mapsto p_{\lambda a}(\lambda x)$ is increasing (respectively, strictly increasing).

(ii) Whenever $\pi \geqslant \pi_0$ the function $\lambda \mapsto \xi_\pi(\lambda a)/\lambda$ is decreasing (respectively, strictly decreasing).

If the Weber functions Δ_π are defined, and $p_a(a) = .5$ (thus, in a case of a discrimination system), we have

$$\frac{\Delta_\pi(a)}{a} = \frac{\xi_\pi(a)}{a} - 1,$$

and each of (i), (ii) is equivalent to

(iii) for $\pi \geqslant \pi_0$, the function $\lambda \mapsto \Delta_\pi(\lambda a)/\lambda$ is decreasing (respectively strictly decreasing).

Proof.   Suppose that $\pi \geqslant \pi_0$ and $\lambda' \geqslant \lambda$. Let

$$x = \xi_\pi(\lambda a)/\lambda, \qquad y = \xi_\pi(\lambda'a)/\lambda'.$$

(i) *implies* (ii). Successively,

$$\pi_0 \leqslant p_{\lambda a}(\lambda x) = \pi = p_{\lambda'a}(\lambda'y) \leqslant p_{\lambda'a}(\lambda'x)$$

yielding, $y \leqslant x$.
(ii) *implies* (i). If

$$y = \xi_\pi(\lambda'a)/\lambda' \leqslant \xi_\pi(\lambda a)/\lambda = x$$

then,

$$\pi = p_{\lambda'a}(\lambda'y) = p_{\lambda a}(\lambda x) \geqslant p_{\lambda a}(\lambda y). \qquad \blacksquare$$

8.22. Remarks.   The connections between Weber's law and the weaker conditions (i) or (ii) in Theorem 8.21 must be appreciated. Suppose, for example, that Condition (i) holds for some psychometric family $\{p_b | b \in I\}$ satisfying the conditions of the theorem. Thus, the function $\lambda \mapsto p_{\lambda a}(\lambda x)$ is increasing whenever $p_a(x) \geqslant \pi_0$. Since p is bounded, we must have

$$\lim_{\lambda \to \infty} p_{\lambda a}(\lambda x) = p_a^*(x) \qquad (22)$$

for some number $p_a^*(x)$ depending on $a \in I$ and $x \in C_a$. From (22), it follows that

$$p_{\lambda a}^*(\lambda x) = p_a^*(x) \qquad (23)$$

$p_a^*(x) \geqslant \pi_0$ and $\lambda \geqslant 1$. It is tempting to translate (23) by saying that "Weber's law holds asymptotically." Such careless phrasing should be avoided however since it may elicit erroneous conclusions. In particular, as demonstrated by Example 8.23, the functions p_a^* are not necessarily psychometric functions.

8.23. Example.   Let $\{p_a | a > 0\}$ be a positive discrimination family defined by

$$p_a(x) = \frac{e^x}{e^x + e^a}.$$

Notice that $p_a(x) \geqslant \frac{1}{2}$ iff $x \geqslant a$. For $p_a(x) > \frac{1}{2}$, we have, successively,

$$\lambda > \lambda' \qquad \text{iff} \qquad \lambda(x - a) > \lambda'(x - a)$$
$$\text{iff} \qquad [1 + e^{-\lambda(x-a)}]^{-1} > [1 + e^{-\lambda'(x-a)}]^{-1}$$
$$\text{iff} \qquad p_{\lambda a}(\lambda x) > p_{\lambda'a}(\lambda'x).$$

On the other hand, we have

$$\lim_{\lambda \to \infty} p_{\lambda a}(\lambda x) = p_a^*(x) = \begin{cases} 1 & \text{if} & x > a; \\ .5 & \text{if} & x = a; \\ 0 & \text{if} & x < a. \end{cases}$$

The limit functions p_a^* are not continuous and thus are not psychometric functions. Some strengthening of our conditions is required. The features of this example are suggestive of the developments below.

After Inverson (1983; see also Falmagne, 1977), we have the following variation of Theorem 8.21.

8.24. Theorem. *Let $\mathcal{F} = \{p_b | b \in I\}$ and ξ be as in Theorem 8.21. Then, the two following conditions are equivalent:*

(i) $\lim_{\lambda \to \infty} p_{\lambda a}(\lambda x) = p_a^*(x)$, *for all $a \in I$ and $x \in C_a$, where the functions p_a^* are strictly increasing and continuous;*

(ii) $\lim_{\lambda \to \infty} \xi_\pi(\lambda a)/\lambda = \xi_\pi^*(a)$ *for all sensitivity functions ξ_π, where the function ξ^* is strictly increasing and continuous in π.*

Moreover, when these conditions hold, then

$$\xi_\pi^*(a) = p_a^{*-1}(\pi).$$

In other words, ξ^* is the sensitivity function of the asymptotic psychometric family $\{p_a^* | a \in I\}$.

Proof. Define

$$L_{\lambda a}(x) = p_{\lambda a}(\lambda x).$$

Notice that $L_{\lambda a}$ is strictly increasing and continuous. We obtain $L_{\lambda a}^{-1}(\pi) = \xi_\pi(\lambda a)/\lambda$. Suppose that (i) holds, that is, $L_{\lambda a}$ converges as $\lambda \to \infty$ to a continuous, strictly increasing function p_a^*. This implies that $L_{\lambda a}^{-1}$ also converges to a continuous, strictly increasing function $\pi \mapsto \xi_\pi^*(a)$ and (ii) follows from the definition of $L_{\lambda a}^{-1}$. The converse case, that (ii) implies (i), is similar. The fact that $p_a^*[\xi_\pi^*(a)] = \pi$ results from the assumption of continuity. We leave the details to the reader. ∎

FECHNER'S PROBLEM REVISITED

As illustrated by the material covered in this chapter, psychophysicists often collect their data to yield estimates of the sensitivity function or the Weber function. Theories or laws then naturally take the form of constraints on ξ_π or Δ_π, rather than on the choice probabilities $P_{a,b}$. This suggests that we reconsider Fechner's problem from the viewpoint of ξ_π.

8.25. Problem. Let $\mathcal{F} = \{p_b | b \in I\}$ be a discrimination family. Under which condition on the sensitivity function ξ of $\mathcal{F}$ does there exist two continuous, strictly increasing functions u and h satisfying

$$\xi_\pi(a) = u^{-1}[u(a) + h(\pi)]? \tag{24}$$

With $\xi_\pi(a) = b$, $p_a(b) = \pi$ and $F = h^{-1}$, (24) immediately yields

$$p_a(b) = F[u(b) - u(a)].$$

Problem 8.25 is thus equivalent to Representation Problem 4.5. Here, however, conditions are sought that directly constrain the sensitivity function, and only indirectly the choice probabilities. We give an example of such a condition.

Take two probabilities π, π' and suppose that both $\xi_\pi[\xi_{\pi'}(a)]$ and $\xi_{\pi'}[\xi_\pi(a)]$ are defined for some $a \in I$. We obtain, assuming that (24) holds,

$$
\begin{aligned}
\xi_\pi[\xi_{\pi'}(a)] &= u^{-1}\{u[\xi_{\pi'}(a)] + h(\pi)\} \\
&= u^{-1}\{(u \circ u^{-1})[u(a) + h(\pi) + h(\pi')]\} \\
&= \xi_{\pi'}[\xi_\pi(a)].
\end{aligned}
$$

8.26. Definition.   The sensitivity function ξ of a discrimination family

$$
\mathcal{F} = \{p_b | b \in I\}
$$

is called *commutative* iff for any two probabilities π, π' and any $a \in I$, whenever one member of the equation

$$
(\xi_\pi \circ \xi_{\pi'})(a) = (\xi_{\pi'} \circ \xi_\pi)(a) \tag{25}
$$

is defined, the other member is also defined, and the equation holds. Occasionally, when this condition is satisfied we will say for short that $\mathcal{F}$ is *commutative*. We have the following result.

8.27. Theorem.   *A commutative discrimination family $\mathcal{F} = \{p_b | b \in I\}$ satisfies the quadruple condition. Consequently, its sensitivity function ξ has a representation*

$$
\xi_\pi(a) = u^{-1}[u(a) + h(\pi)]
$$

where u and h are strictly increasing continuous function.

Proof.   We show first that $\mathcal{F}$ satisfies the weak quadruple condition. (In view of 4.11, the weak quadruple condition implies the quadruple condition. Note that we can assume that $\mathcal{F}$ is balanced. See the comments after 4.13 in this connection.) We recall that $p_a(b) = P_{b,a}$, the choice probability. Suppose that

$$
p_b(a) = p_{b'}(a') = \pi, \tag{26}
$$

and

$$
p_{a'}(a) = \pi', \qquad p_{b'}(b) = \pi''. \tag{27}
$$

We have to show that $\pi' = \pi''$. In terms of the sensitivity function, (26), (27) translate into

$$
\xi_\pi(b) = a, \qquad \xi_\pi(b') = a',
$$

$$
\xi_{\pi'}(a') = a, \qquad \xi_{\pi''}(b') = b.
$$

We obtain

$$
\begin{aligned}
a = \xi_{\pi'}[\xi_\pi(b')] &= \xi_\pi[\xi_{\pi''}(b')] \\
&= \xi_\pi[\xi_{\pi'}(b')],
\end{aligned}
$$

by commutativity. Using strict monotonicity, the last equation yields

$$
\xi_{\pi''}(b') = \xi_{\pi'}(b')
$$

and thus $\pi' = \pi''$. We conclude that $\mathcal{F}$ satisfies the weak quadruple condition.

Since $\mathcal{F}$ may be assumed to be balanced, we can apply Theorem 4.13 and assert the existence of two strictly increasing, continuous functions u and F such that

$$p_a(b) = F[u(b) - u(a)],$$

or equivalently, with $p_a(b) = \pi$, $F^{-1} = h$, and $\xi_\pi(a) = b$

$$\xi_\pi(a) = u^{-1}[u(a) + h(\pi)]. \quad \blacksquare$$

It is plausible that the hypothesis of Theorem 8.27 can be weakened. In particular, we venture the following.

8.28. Conjecture. *A discrimination family $\mathcal{F} = \{p_b\}$ with sensitivity function ξ satisfies the quadruple condition iff Equation 25 holds whenever both members are defined, for any two probabilities π, π'.*

EXERCISES

1. In 8.1, the sensitivity function ξ and the Weber function Δ were defined starting from the psychometric functions p_b in some family $\mathcal{F}$. Provide direct definitions of ξ and Δ, and prove the equivalence between these concepts and those defined in 8.1.

2. Suppose that the psychometric functions in some discrimination family $\mathcal{F} = \{p_b | b \in I\}$ satisfy Case III of Thurstone's law of comparitive judgments (cf. 5.5), that is, assume that

$$p_b(a) = \Phi\left\{\frac{\mu(a) - \mu(b)}{[\sigma(a)^2 + \sigma(b)^2]^{1/2}}\right\}$$

in which u and σ are real values or functions. Suppose also that Weber's law holds. Infer from these assumptions the possible analytic forms of the functions u and σ.

3. Prove Theorem 8.4.

4. Prove Theorem 8.6.

*5. Suppose that in Theorem 8.5, the background sets are assumed to be connected (cf. Chapter 7). What is the impact of this assumption on the domain of the function h in (4)?

6. In the proof of Theorem 8.24, prove in detail that the function $\pi \mapsto \xi_\pi^*(a) = b$ is the inverse of the function $b \mapsto p_a^*(b) = \pi$, a being the parameter.

7. Let ξ be a commutative sensitivity function in the sense of 8.26. Prove that for any finite sequence of probabilities $\pi_1, \pi_2, \ldots, \pi_n$, and any permutation ρ on the set $\{1, 2, \ldots, n\}$ whenever one member of the equation

$$(\xi_{\pi_1} \circ \xi_{\pi_2} \circ \cdots \circ \xi_{\pi_n})(a) = (\xi_{\pi_{\rho(1)}} \circ \xi_{\pi_{\rho(2)}} \circ \cdots \circ \xi_{\pi_{\rho(n)}})(a)$$

is defined, the other member is also defined, and the equation holds.

*8. In 8.26 and 8.27, a condition of the sensitivity function ξ was investigated, which was shown to be closely related to the quadruple condition of a discrimination system (cf. 4.10). Find by similar methods a condition on ξ which corresponds to bicancellation. Formulate and prove a representation theorem in the style of 8.27.

*9. Analyze the more general representation

$$\xi_\pi(a) = u^{-1}[g(a) + h(\pi)]$$

(cf. Theorem 8.3). Find conditions on ξ corresponding to double and triple cancellation. Formulate and prove appropriate representation theorems.

10. Prove that the discrimination model

$$p_a(b) = \frac{[\log(\tau/a)]^\gamma}{[\log(\tau/a)]^\gamma + [\log(\tau/b)]^\gamma}$$

where τ and γ are constants, $0 < a$ and $b < \tau$, leads to the sensitivity function having the form

$$\xi_\pi(a) = \tau(a/\tau)^{[(1-\pi)/\pi]^{1/\gamma}}$$

which gives

$$\xi_\pi(\lambda a) = \lambda^{[(1-\pi)/\pi]^{1/\gamma}} \xi_\pi(a)$$

thus, a particular case of (15) in which

$$\beta(\pi) = [(1-\pi)/\pi]^{1/\gamma}$$

(cf. 8.18).

9

Psychophysical Methods

In Chapter 8, we introduced the concept of the sensitivity function ξ, which we defined from a family $\{p_a\}$ of psychometric functions by the formula

$$(a,\pi) \mapsto \xi_\pi(a) = p_a^{-1}(\pi)$$

(cf. Fig. 8.1 and Definition 8.1). Thus $\xi_\pi(a)$ is the stimulus intensity judged by the subject as exceeding a with a probability π,

$$p_a[\xi_\pi(a)] = \pi.$$

The Weber function was then obtained from the expression

$$\Delta_\pi(a) = \xi_\pi(a) - \xi_{.5}(a) \tag{1}$$

From a theoretical viewpoint, the sensitivity function contains exactly the same information as the family of psychometric function. There is a consensus, however, that, at least for some purposes, the sensitivity function is a more useful measure of the subject performance, a position that was argued in detail in Chapter 8.

The problem discussed here is that of the empirical determination of the sensitivity function or the Weber function. Various methods have been employed. We begin by reviewing those introduced by the early psychophysicists.

TRADITIONAL PSYCHOPHYSICAL METHODS

Since to many people, the interest of the *method of limits* and of the *method of adjustments* is mostly historical, only a brief description will be given. For more details, the reader is referred, for example, to Engen (1971) or Fechner (1966). Each method involves a subject making successive comparisons of a stimulus with a standard or background. In the determination of the absolute threshold, the value of the background is considered to be negligible.

9.1. The method of limits. In a discrimination situation, the experimenter varies at each trial the value of the stimulus, in small ascending or descending steps. At each step, the subject reports whether the stimulus appears smaller or larger than the standard. For example, the experimenter may start with a stimulus value quite noticeably smaller than the standard, and increase this value by successive steps until the subject reports "larger."[1] The experimenter records

1. In some situations, an "equal" category is also used.

the values of the stimulus at which the subject's response shift from one category to another. This method is used in applied situations, such as audiology, to provide, by averaging the observed values, a quick estimate of the *point of subjective equality* $p_a^{-1}(.50)$. The procedure is similar in a detection situation. The subject reports at each trial whether the stimulus is perceptible or not, and the threshold is estimated by averaging the stimulus values at those trials where a shift in response took place. As Levitt (1970) pointed out, this method has serious defects from the viewpoint of efficiency (the observations may be poorly placed), and validity (the estimates may be substantially biased) (see Anderson, McCarthy, & Tukey, 1946; Brown & Cane, 1959).

9.2. The method of adjustments.   This method resembles the previous one. The subject adjusts the value of the stimulus, which can be varied continuously (e.g., by turning a dial), and sets it to apparent equality with the standard. Repeated applications of this procedure yields an empirical distribution of stimulus values that is used to compute—or estimate—the Jnd.

9.3. The method of constant stimuli.   This method, which has been encountered earlier (6.1), purports to estimate experimentally a number of suitably located points of some psychometric function p_a. If a particular mathematical expression is assumed for the psychometric functions (derived for instance from a mathematical model), then this expression is fitted to the experimental points. (Typically, the mathematical expression of p_a is only specified up to the values of some parameters, which have to be estimated from the data.) Finally, an estimate of the Jnd is provided for example by

$$\Delta_{.75}(a) = \xi_{.75}(a) - \xi_{.5}(a),$$

a special case of Equation 1.

As an illustration, suppose that the logistic distribution is assumed as a model for a psychometric family $\{p_a | a \in I\}$. Say we assume that for all $a \in I$ and $b \in C_a$ we have

$$p_a(b) = \{1 + \exp[-(b - \alpha(a))/\beta(a)]\}^{-1}, \tag{2}$$

(cf. Johnson & Kotz, 1970). The quantities $\alpha(a)$ and $\beta(a)$ are real parameters, which have to be estimated from the relative frequencies of the choices in the data (using, for instance, a minimum chi-square procedure. We assume, of course, that $\beta(a) > 0$.) Equation 2 yields

$$\xi_\pi(a) = \alpha(a) - \beta(a)\ln\left(\frac{1 - \pi}{\pi}\right), \tag{3}$$

and thus

$$\Delta_\pi(a) = -\beta(a)\ln\left(\frac{1 - \pi}{\pi}\right) \tag{4}$$

$$\geqslant 0$$

if $\pi \geqslant .5$.

If no specific mathematical model is assumed, but the psychometric function appears to be approximately linear say, between values .20 and .80, then a straight line can be fitted to the experimental points in that interval, replacing the mathematical form used above, to estimate critical values of the sensitivity function or the Weber function.

In general, each of these three methods suffers from one or more of the following defects.

(i) Absence of control of the criterion (9.1, 9.2).
(ii) No theoretical justification for important aspects of the procedure (9.1, 9.2).
(iii) The estimates may be biased (9.1, 9.2).
(iv) Costs; a large amount of data is often wasted (all three methods).

In computerized laboratories, sophisticated versions of Method 9.3 are used routinely, which we now describe. These methods are applicable when the exact mathematical form of the psychometric functions are unknown. In our discussion of the adaptive methods, we assume that the reader is familiar with the basic notions and the terminology of the theory of stochastic processes (cf. e.g., Parzen, 1962).

ADAPTIVE METHODS

Consider the problem of finding a point ξ in the domain of a psychometric function p_a, such that $p_a(\xi) = \pi$, where π is chosen arbitrarily in the range of p_a. Notice that the location of ξ depends on both a and π; ξ is thus a function of the two variables a and π. Actually, ξ is the sensitivity function introduced earlier, with $\xi_\pi(a) = p_a^{-1}(\pi)$ (Fig. 8.1). In the rest of this section, we assume that the background a is fixed. We will thus occasionally simplify our notation and write $\xi_\pi = p^{-1}(\pi)$.

It must be realized that the problem of estimating ξ_π with an acceptable degree of accuracy from the data is not trivial, since the exact mathematical form of the psychometric function may be unknown. A couple of practical methods are described below. They differ from the methods described in the preceding section in that the course of the experiment depends critically on the data: the stimulus presented on trial n depends on the subject's responses on one or more of the preceding trials. At present, none of these methods taken by itself is completely free of defects. As indicated in 9.8, however, a suitable combination of methods provides an estimation procedure that seems to be reasonable for empirical applications.

From a theoretical standpoint, the sequence of stimulus-response pairs will be regarded as a stochastic process (Parzen, 1962). For the time being, we assume that the process is stationary. The following notations are used. The stimulus presented at trial n will be denoted by X_n, a random variable. The subject's responses will be coded

1   if a is not judged as exceeding X_n; and

0   otherwise.

Thus, 0,1 are the values of a random variable, which we denote by Z_n. We have, by definition,

$$\mathbb{P}\{Z_n = 1|X_n\} = p_a(X_n).$$

In the following methods, the succession of stimuli is governed by an equation of the form

$$X_{n+1} = X_n + \theta(\pi, n, Z_n, Z_{n-1}, X_{n-1}, \ldots),\tag{5}$$

in which θ is a function that may vary with the probability π assigned to the target value $\xi_\pi(a)$, the trial number n, the subject's response on that trial, and possibly some stimulus-response pairs on earlier trials.

9.4. Stochastic approximation. Fix π, $0 < \pi < 1$ and choose a point x_1 arbitrarily, somewhere in the neighborhood of $\xi_\pi(a)$, the point to be estimated. (Since $\xi_\pi(a)$ is unknown, an educated guess has to made. The accuracy of this guess is not crucial.) Present the pair (x_1, a) to the subject. Determine a second point x_2 by the following rule:

$$x_2 = \begin{cases} x_1 + c\pi & \text{if } Z_1 = 0, \\ x_1 - c(1 - \pi) & \text{if } Z_1 = 1, \end{cases}$$

where $c > 0$ is some constant, the choice of which is of importance, as we will see. Thus, x_2 is a value of the random variable X_2. We have $X_1 = x_1$ by convention. The above rule can be rewritten compactly as

$$X_2 = X_1 - c[Z_1 - \pi].$$

Next, we determine successively $x_3, x_4, \ldots, x_n, \ldots$, using the rule

$$X_{n+1} = X_n - \frac{c}{n}(Z_n - \pi).\tag{6}$$

This yields

$$\theta(\pi, n, Z_n) = \frac{c}{n}(\pi - Z_n),$$

in the notation of Equation 5. The sequence of pairs of random variables (X_n, Z_n) is known as a *Robbins-Monro process*. It can be shown that, as n gets large, X_n tends to a normal random variable, with expectation equal to ξ_π, and a vanishing variance. This results holds under general differentiability assumptions regarding the psychometric function p_a (which seem quite reasonable in the present context), and provided that the constant c is chosen appropriately. For details refer to Robbins and Monro (1951) or Wasan (1969). In practice, an estimate of ξ_π is provided by a sample value of X_n for some large n. This method constitutes a substantial improvement over the preceding ones. It is not very economical, however, since a large number of trials is needed, only the last one of which is actually used. Moreover, if the number of trials is not large, the estimate of ξ_π is biased, the size and direction of the bias depending on the curvature of the psychometric function at the point to be estimated. One difficulty is that the convergence of c/n is slow, from the viewpoint of the scale of a psychophysical experiment.

As suggested by Kesten (1958) and Pavel (personal communication), the convergence of the estimation process can be speeded up significantly by modifying the constant c in (6) as a function of the subject's responses on trials preceding trial n. For example, the value of c/n in (6) could fail to decrease in the case of a succession of identical responses. (We refer to this modification of the method as *accelerated stochastic approximation*.) Finally, it must be remembered that there are often practical limitations to the resolution of the apparatus used to generate the stimuli. In psychoacoustics, for instance, the minimum difference between distinct stimuli is often of the order of $\frac{1}{4}$ dB and sometimes more.

Even assuming that an accelerated stochastic approximation method is used, these limitations may suffice to render the estimate unacceptable. Stochastic approximation nevertheless has its use as an early component of an adaptive estimation procedure (see 9.8).

9.5. Up-down or staircase method.   This method is probably the most popular one. The essential difference with the stochastic approximation method is that on each trial, the value of the stimulus is changed by a constant amount, either positively or negatively. In other terms in (5),

$$|\theta(\pi, Z_n, Z_{n-1}, X_{n-1}, \ldots)| = |X_{n+1} - X_n|$$

is constant for all trials n, the direction of the change depending on the probability π, on the subject's responses, etc. The increments by which the stimulus is either increased or decreased are referred to as *steps*. A sequence of steps in one direction, in a realization of this process, is called a *run*.

The staircase method is illustrated in Figure 9.1, in which the value of the stimulus presented at the first trial is set arbitrarily equal to 0 and the step size is equal to 1. There are eight runs, corresponding to trials 1–2, 2–5, 5–7, etc. Three variants of the method are described as follows.

9.6. Variants.   (1) In the *simple* up-down method, the problem is to estimate $\xi_{.5}$. As in 9.4, an educated guess is made for the initial value X_1 of the stimulus. The successive remaining values are then obtained by the rule

$$X_{n+1} = X_n + \delta(1 - 2Z_n). \tag{7}$$

In words: δ is the step size, and the stimulus is increased by δ in the case of a

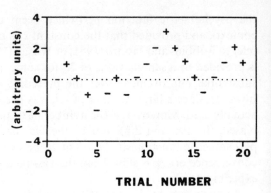

FIGURE 9.1. Exemplary data for the simple up-down method. The initial value is arbitrarily set at 0. The step size is equal to 1. There are eight runs, corresponding to trial 1–2, 2–5, 5–7, etc.

negative response ($\mathbf{Z}_n = 0$), and decreased by δ in the case of a positive one ($\mathbf{Z}_n = 1$). In Figure 9.1, the succession of responses is "no, yes, yes, yes, no, ... " etc. The choice of the step size is obviously important, and will be commented on in a moment. Since

$$\mathbb{P}\{\mathbf{Z}_n = 1 | \mathbf{X}_n\} = p_a(\mathbf{X}_n),$$

it is apparent that (7) defines a discrete parameter Markov chain $\{\mathbf{X}_n\}$ with state space $\{x_1 \pm n\delta | n = 1,2,...\}$. The states are recurrent, with a finite mean recurrent time, which implies (see e.g., Parzen, 1962, p. 252) that the distribution of $\mathbf{X}_n$ converges as $n \to \infty$. In particular, taking expectations and limits in (7), and denoting as customary the expectations by E, we obtain, after rearranging,

$$0 = \lim_{n \to \infty} E(\mathbf{X}_{n+1}) - \lim_{n \to \infty} E(\mathbf{X}_n) = \delta[1 - 2 \lim_{n \to \infty} E(\mathbf{Z}_n)].$$

Using the fact that p_a is a bounded, continuous function, this gives successively, with obvious notation,

$$.5 = \lim_{n \to \infty} E(\mathbf{Z}_n) = \lim_{n \to \infty} \mathbb{P}\{\mathbf{Z}_n = 1\}$$

$$= \lim_{n \to \infty} E[\mathbb{P}\{\mathbf{Z}_n = 1 | \mathbf{X}_n\}] = \lim_{n \to \infty} E[p_a(\mathbf{X}_n)]$$

$$= E[p_a(\mathbf{X}_\infty)] \approx p_a[E(\mathbf{X}_\infty)], \tag{8}$$

in which the approximation holds if we assume either that the psychometric function p_a is approximately linear in the region of concentration of the mass of $\mathbf{X}_\infty$, or that the distribution of $\mathbf{X}_\infty$ is approximately symmetric. (Indeed, in this last case, the expectation of $\mathbf{X}_\infty$ is confounded with its median $M(\mathbf{X}_\infty)$, and for any strictly increasing function f, we have $M[f(\mathbf{X}_\infty)] = f[M(\mathbf{X}_\infty)]$. See also Exercise 4.) In principle, the value $\xi_{.5} \approx E(\mathbf{X}_\infty)$ can be estimated by the statistic

$$\frac{1}{k} \sum_{i=1}^{k} \mathbf{X}_{n+i},$$

for n sufficiently large. As Wetherill (1963) pointed out, a practical estimate of $\xi_{.5}$ is provided by averaging the peaks and the valleys in all the runs. As an illustration, the data of Figure 9.1 would yield for this estimate, the value

$$\tfrac{1}{8}(0 + 1 - 2 + 0 - 1 + 3 - 1 + 2 + 1) = \tfrac{3}{8}.$$

It is easy to verify that this method amounts to considering the midpoint of every second run as an estimate of $\xi_{.5}$, and then computing the average of these midpoints. Thus, in Figure 9.1

$$\tfrac{1}{4}(-.5 - .5 + 1 + 1.5) = \tfrac{3}{8}.$$

These estimates are sometimes referred to as the *midrun estimates*. A even number of runs should be used, in order to reduce a bias in the estimation. The bias is then small provided that to a reasonable approximation, the psychometric function or the distribution of X_n satisfy the conditions indicated above. This procedure based on the midrun estimates is known to be fairly efficient. In fact, for a small number of trials ($n < 30$), it is more efficient than a maximum likelihood estimate (Wetherill, Chen, & Vasudeva, 1966). There are various problems with this procedure, only some of which will be mentioned here (see Levitt, 1970.)

One problem concerns the choice of the step size δ, the value of which should be small as compared to the "spread" of the psychometric function. As a rule of thumb, a good choice is to get δ equal to the slope of the psychometric function at the point to be estimated. (If we assume that the psychometric function is approximately linear in some neighborhood of the target value, then this value of δ can be shown to minimize the variance of the asymptotic distribution of the stimuli presented, cf. Wetherill, 1963.) Since both locations and spread are typically unknown at the early stage of experimentation, this recommendation is only of heuristic use. A frequently employed, reasonable procedure is to start the first few (say, 10) trials of each experimental session with a large step size, which is then decreased for the useful part of the data.

Another source of difficulty is that the subject may become aware of the systematic character of the stimulus changes. In turn, this may induce a strategy of anticipation of these changes, which may be responsible for a bias in the responses. This is easily taken care of by "interleaving" two or more staircase processes (involving different estimates) within each experimental session. This remark also applies, obviously, to the stochastic approximation procedure.

It is clear that, as described here, the staircase procedure is only of limited use, since it only permits the estimation of the point $\xi_{.5}$.

(2) Following Derman (1957), the simple up-down procedure can be adapted to provide, at least in principle, an estimate of ξ_π for any choice of π. The idea is simple enough. From a given psychometric function p_a, let us define a new psychometric function p_a^* by

$$p_a^*(x) = \alpha p_a(x),$$

where α is a multiplicative constant, $.5 \leqslant \alpha \leqslant 1$, the role of which will be made clear in a moment. Applying the simple up-down method to p_a^* will yield a stimulus value ξ satisfying

$$\alpha p_a(\xi) = p_a^*(\xi) \approx .5.$$

Thus,

$$p_a(\xi) \approx \frac{1}{2\alpha},$$

and for any $\pi, .5 \leqslant \pi < 1$, an appropriate choice of α will yield an estimate of ξ_π. In the style of Equations 5 and 7, this amounts to set

$$X_{n+1} = X_n + \delta(1 - 2Z_n Y_\pi), \tag{9}$$

where Y_π is a random variable taking value 1 with probability $1/2\pi$ and value 0 with probability $1 - (1/2\pi)$, and independent of the random variables X_n's. We have thus, clearly,

$$\alpha p_a(X_n) = p_a^*(X_n) = \mathbb{P}\{Z_n Y_\pi = 1\}. \tag{10}$$

A similar method is used in the case of the determination of a point ξ_π with $0 < \pi < .5$. For example, we define a psychometric function

$$p_a^*(x) = (1 - \alpha)p_a(x) + \alpha,$$

with

$$0 < \alpha = \frac{.5 - \pi}{1 - \pi} < .5.$$

Again, applying the simple up-down procedure to p_a^* yields the required estimate of ξ_π. An objection to Derman's method is that the slope of p_a^* is smaller that the slope of p_a, a fact that may reduce the efficiency of the procedure.

(3) The impact of this objection is less critical in the so-called *transformed up-down* method, where the function p_a^* is defined differently, for example, by one of the following expressions:

$$p_a^*(x) = p_a(x)^n; \qquad\qquad n = 2,3,4,\ldots \tag{11}$$

$$p_a^*(x) = 1 - [1 - p_a(x)]^n; \qquad\qquad n = 2,3,4,\ldots \tag{12}$$

$$p_a^*(x) = [1 - p_a(x)]p_a(x) + p_a(x). \tag{13}$$

Such transformations have been used by a number of authors (see Levitt, 1970, for some references). As an illustration, we discuss the case $n = 2$ in (11). We consider the psychometric function $p_a^*(x) = p_a(x)^2$. As in the simple up-down procedure, we search for an estimate of a point ξ satisfying

$$.5 = p_a^*(\xi) = p_a(\xi)^2,$$

that is,

$$p_a(\xi) = \sqrt{.5} \approx .707.$$

The case $n = 2$ in (11) is thus useful when this particular point of the psychometric function is of interest. The relevant stochastic process is defined as follows. Pick x_1 as usual. Set $x_2 = x_1$ if $Z_1 = 1$, and $x_2 = x_1 - \delta$ if $Z_n = 0$. For $n = 3,4,\ldots$, we use the rule

$$X_{n+1} = X_n + \theta(Z_n, Z_{n-1}, X_{n-1}),$$

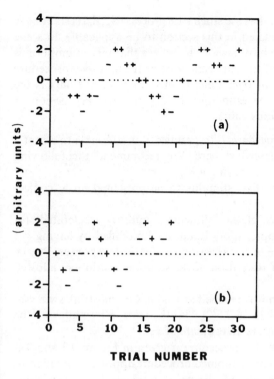

FIGURE 9.2. (a) Exemplary data for the transformed up-down method, Equation 11. The conventions regarding initial value and step size are as in Figure 9.1: $x_1 = 0$ and $\delta = 1$. (b) Recoding of the data of Figure 9.2a, eliminating consecutive repetitions of identical stimulus values. Six runs are obtained, corresponding to trials 1–3, 3–7, 7–10, etc.

in which the function θ is defined by

$$\theta(\mathbf{Z}_n, \mathbf{Z}_{n-1}, \mathbf{X}_{n-1}) = \begin{cases} \delta & \text{if } \mathbf{Z}_n = 0; \\ -\delta & \text{if } \mathbf{Z}_n = \mathbf{Z}_{n-1} = 1 \text{ and } \mathbf{X}_n = \mathbf{X}_{n-1}; \\ 0 & \text{in all other cases.} \end{cases}$$

An example of realization of such process is pictured in Figure 9.2a. The point $\xi_{.5}$ of p_a^*, which is also the point $\xi_{\sqrt{.5}}$ of p_a can be estimated by the midrun procedure. A slight adaptation of our definition of a run must be introduced however. For the data of Figure 9.2a, a strict application of this definition leads to a count of four runs between trials 1 and 10, while we mean to have only two runs: 1–5, 5–10, with respective midpoints -1 and 0. The clearest approach is to begin by recoding the data, to eliminate the repetitions of a stimulus on consecutive trials. The function of this recoding is made transparent by a comparison of Figure 9.2a and 9.2b. The exact definition given below is somewhat involved, however. Let $\{x_n\}$ be a realization of the process $\{\mathbf{X}_n\}$. Consider the largest subsequence $\{x_{n_i}\}$ of $\{x_n\}$, such that $x_{n_i} \neq x_{n_{i+1}}$ for $i = 1, 2, \ldots$. Define $x_i^* = x_{n_i}$, for $i = 1, 2, \ldots$. The sequence $\{x_i^*\}$ will be called the *recoding* of $\{x_n\}$. An illustration of such recoding is given in Figure 9.2b, starting from the data of Figure 9.2a. By eliminating the repetitions, the number of trials has been reduced to 19. There are 6 runs: 1–3, 3–7, 11–15, etc., with respective midpoints $-1, 0, 0$, etc.

9.7. Remarks.   The assumption that the stochastic process (X_n, Z_n) is stationary is critical for the procedure discussed in this section to be applicable. In some situations, the experimenter may have reasons to believe that this assumption is not warranted. An examination of the data generated by the up-down procedure may then reveal a systematic drift over time. If this happens, not only is the adaptive procedure useless for the estimation of ξ_π, but the very notion of psychometric function is of dubious value.

9.8. A recommended adaptive procedure.   In practice, it is advisable to adopt a combination of the methods described here. We recommend the following procedure. To estimate a point ξ_π satisfying $p_a(\xi_\pi) = \pi$.

Step 1.   Choose $X_1 = x_1$, the first stimulus to be presented, in a (conjectured) neighborhood of ξ_π.

Step 2.   Determine the values of the following stimuli by accelerated stochastic approximation; for example, apply Equation 6 modified by having c/n remaining constant in the course of a succession of identical responses. Pursue this procedure up to the limit of resolution of the stimulus continuum allowed by the apparatus.

Step 3.   Suppose that this limit is reached at trial n. On that trial, switch to a suitable up-down procedure such as 9.6(2). Use the midrun estimates on the data from trial n onward to compute an estimate of ξ_π.

An example of application of this procedure is given in Figure 9.3 and Table 9.1 for some simulated data. This combined procedure appears to avoid most of the criticisms elicited by other methods discussed in this section. So far, how-

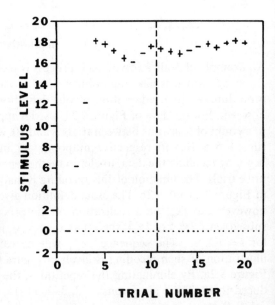

FIGURE 9.3. Simulated application of the adaptive procedure recommended in 9.8 to estimate $\xi_{.75}$. The vertical dotted line separates the two modes of the procedure. See the legend of Table 9.1 for details.

TABLE 9.1. *Simulation of the adaptive procedure recommended in 9.8, to estimate $\xi_{.75}$. From trial 1 to 10, accelerated stochastic approximation is used, with $x_1 = 0$ and $c = 8$. [The successive values of the stimulus are obtained from Eq. (6) except that c/n does not vary in the course of repetitions of a response.] From trial 11 on, method 9.6(2) is used, with $\alpha = .5/.75$. The values of $Y_{.75}$ are obtained by random sampling with $\mathbb{P}\{Y_{.75} = 1\} = \alpha$. Starting at trial 11, the peak and valley estimate of $\xi_{.75}$ would be obtained by averaging 17, 16.75, 17.5, etc.*

Trial number	Stimulus value	Response (Z_n)	$Y_{.75}$	Computation of x_{n+1}
1	0	0	—	$0 - 8(0 - .75) = 6$
2	6	0	—	$6 - 8(0 - .75) = 12$
3	12	0	—	$12 - 8(0 - .75) = 18$
4	18	1	—	$18 - (8/4)(1 - .75) = 17.5$
5	17.5	1	—	$17.5 - (8/4)(1 - .75) = 17$
6	17	1	—	$17 - (8/4)(1 - .75) = 16.5$
7	16.5	1	—	$16.5 - (8/4)(1 - .75) = 16$
8	16	0	—	$16 - (8/8)(0 - .75) = 16.75$
9	16.75	0	—	$16.75 - (8/8)(0 - .75) = 17.5$
10	17.5	1	—	$17.5 - (8/10)(1 - .75) = 17.3*$
11	17.25	1	—	$17.25 + .25(1 - 2) = 17$
12	17	1	—	$17 + .25(1 - 2) = 16.75$
13	16.75	1	0	$16.75 + .25(1 - 0) = 17$
14	17	0	1	$17 + .25(1 - 0) = 17.25$
15	17.25	0	1	$17.25 + .25(1 - 0) = 17.5$
16	17.5	1	1	$17.5 + .25(1 - 2) = 17.25$
17	17.25	1	0	$17.25 + .25(1 - 0) = 17.5$
18	17.5	1	0	$17.5 + .25(1 - 0) = 17.75$
19	17.75	1	1	$17.75 + .25(1 - 2) = 17.5$
20	17.50	1	1	$17.5 + .25(1 - 2) = 17.25$

* We suppose that the limit of resolution of the apparatus is .25. Thus the starred value of 17.3 computed at trial 10 is replaced by the stimulus value of 17.25 at trial 11.

ever, no serious test of this procedure has been made, and its theoretical properties are largely unknown. The last word is by no means said on the question of designing an optimal adaptive procedure, as indicated by recent activity in this field (Pavel, Note 1; Vorberg, Note 3).

REFERENCE NOTES

A basic paper is Levitt (1970), which contains a discussion of adaptive procedures geared toward psychophysical applications. A fairly complete mathematical treatment is available in the monograph by Wasan (1969). In general, the adaptive procedures are based on a class of stochastic learning models, a discussion of which is contained in Norman (1972).

EXERCISES

1. Sometimes, the just noticable difference $\text{Jnd}(a)$ is estimated empirically from the equation

$$\text{Jnd}(a) = \frac{\xi_{.75}(a) - \xi_{.25}(a)}{2} \tag{14}$$

Compare this procedure with that based on Equation 1, which leads us to estimate

$$\Delta_{.75}(a) = \xi_{.75}(a) - \xi_{.5}(a),$$

and discuss the possible objections to (14), if any. Do $\text{Jnd}(a)$ and $\Delta_{.75}(a)$ provide exactly the same information in all cases?

2. Give the derivations of Equation 3 and 4.

3. Adapt the derivations leading to (3) and (4), but starting from different models. Consider in particular the two models

$$p_a(b) = \Phi[b^{\beta(a)} - \alpha(a)] \tag{15}$$

$$p_a(b) = \Phi\{[b - \alpha(a)]^{\beta(a)}\} \tag{16}$$

in which Φ is the standard normal distribution function, and $\alpha(a)$, and $\beta(a)$ are real parameters. What is the essential difference between (15) and (16) as far as the form $\Delta_{.75}(a)$ is concerned?

4. Give an example where, using the approximation (8), $E[p_a(\mathbf{X}_\infty)] \approx p_a[E(\mathbf{X}_\infty)]$ leads to a positive (respectively negative) bias, that is,

$$E[p_a(\mathbf{X}_\infty)] < p_a[E(\mathbf{X}_\infty)], \qquad (\text{resp.} >).$$

5. Justify in detail the derivation of (8).

6. Justify Equations 9 and 10.

7. Discuss in detail the case $0 < \pi < .5$ in Variant 9.6(2).

8. Which value of n in (12) leads to a good estimate of $\xi_{.80}(a)$? Give the details of the derivation in this case.

10

Signal Detection Theory

Any psychophysical task has cognitive components, this term covering a variety of such factors as response bias, guessing strategy, motivation, etc. So far in our approach to psychophysical theory, we have implicitly assumed that such factors could be bypassed or controlled by careful experimental design. In fact, we have ignored them. This position is not without its weaknesses; an example will make this clear.

Consider a task in which a subject is required to detect a stimulus embedded in noise. On some proportion of the trials, the noise is presented alone. Across conditions, the intensity of the stimulus is varied, providing the basic data for a psychometric function. Two kinds of errors can be made in such a task which, as mentioned earlier, is often referred to as the yes/no paradigm: the subject may fail to report a stimulus presented; this is called a *miss*; the subject may report a detection on a "noise alone" trial; this is called a *false alarm*, or a *false positive*. A correct detection will be referred to as a *hit*. The remaining case is a *correct rejection*.

A guessing strategy is available to the subject in this situation: When he or she is not quite sure that the stimulus was presented on a trial, the subject may nevertheless claim to have detected it. Such a strategy would succeed in a situation in which a miss is much more heavily penalized than a false alarm. For example, suppose that the system of rewards and penalties is the one displayed in the following table, in which the numbers represent monetary values.

		Responses	
		Yes	No
Stimulus	Yes	3 Hit	−3 Miss
	No	−1 False alarm	3 Correct rejection

Thus, each correct detection brings 3 monetary units (mus), each miss costs 3 mus, etc. Such a table is often referred to as a *payoff matrix*. It is reasonable to suppose that, if the two types of trials are equiprobable, the particular payoff matrix displayed above would favor a guessing strategy over a conservative one. (For instance, if the subject reports a detection at every trial, whether or not the stimulus was presented, the average gain per trial is 2 mus, while the opposite strategy of responding "No Detection" at every trial results in an average gain of 0 mus.) Obviously, another payoff matrix may evoke a completely different strategy. A naive experimenter may be tempted to believe that if a constant payoff matrix is used across conditions varying stimulus intensity, the subject strategy will not change, a fact that can be tested by checking that the proportion of false alarms remain constant. Unfortunately, a subject's interpretation of a payoff matrix is largely his or her own affair, and this interpretation may change drastically from one condition to another. Needless to say, these remarks also apply when no explicit payoff matrix is used, but the subject strategy is induced by verbal instructions. The problem at hand is thus that of disentangling the purely sensory aspects of the task from those resulting from the subject strategy.

This chapter discusses a particular solution to this problem, usually referred to as "signal detection theory," even though its applicability extends far beyond the detection of signals. Our presentation is far from exhaustive. It should, however, be sufficient to acquaint the reader with the most commonly used notions and techniques of signal detection theory. For an extensive treatment of this topic, see Green and Swets (1974).

ROC GRAPHS AND CURVES

For simplicity, we will ignore statistical variability for the moment, and identify response frequencies and probabilities.

Let us suppose that, for a given stimulus intensity, three payoff matrices have been used—θ_1, θ_2, and θ_3—inducing three different guessing strategies. Let s and n denote the stimulus and the noise, respectively. Let $p_s(\theta_i)$ and $p_n(\theta_i)$, $i = 1, 2, 3$, be the hit and false alarm probabilities. For concreteness, some hypothetical data is displayed as follows.

	$p_n(\theta_i)$	$p_s(\theta_i)$
θ_1	.10	.35
θ_2	.40	.75
θ_3	.65	.90

A useful graphic representation of such data is often used by psychophysicists, in which each pair of response probabilities $[p_n(\theta_i), p_s(\theta_i)]$ is pictured as a point in the unit square (see Figure 10.1, but ignore the three curves for the moment).

There is a large consensus in psychophysics that, by appropriately choosing the payoff matrix, any type of strategy can be induced in the subject, ranging from

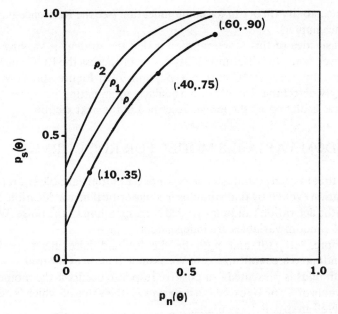

FIGURE 10.1   Three ROC curves and one ROC graph containing three points.

the most conservative one (if the slightest doubt arise, say "No Detection"), to the most daring guessing. It is also reasonable to suppose that any change in a payoff matrix that would increase the probability of a false alarm would also increase (continuously) the probability of a hit. (This assumption is supported by many data.) In other words, this means that the three points in Figure 10.1 belong to the graph of a continuous function ρ mapping the closed interval $[0,1]$ into itself. We have thus

$$\rho[p_n(\theta)] = p_s(\theta),$$

in which θ ranges in a large set Θ of payoff matrices θ.

10.1. Definition.   Let Θ be a set (of payoff matrices); for each $\theta \in \Theta$, let $p_n(\theta)$ and $p_s(\theta)$ be the probabilities of a false alarm and of a hit, respectively. Then the set of points

$$\{[p_n(\theta), p_s(\theta)] \mid \theta \in \Theta\},$$

in the unit square is called an *ROC graph*. When an ROC graph is the graph of a continuous function ρ mapping the closed interval $[0,1]$ into itself, it will be called an *ROC curve*. The function ρ will be referred to as the *ROC function*. As mentioned, ROC functions are generally assumed to be increasing.

Three examples of ROC curves are displayed in Figure 10.1. The acronym "ROC" stands for "receiver-operating-characteristic", and is borrowed from signal detectability theory in telecommunication (see the Reference Notes at the end of the chapter).

The basic idea of this representation is that the strategy is varying along the ROC curves, while the discriminability is varying across the ROC curves. In this framework, the three ROC curves ρ, ρ_1, and ρ_2 in Figure 10.1 correspond to increasingly detectable stimuli. A particularly illuminating interpretation of an ROC curve is offered by the model described in the next section.

A RANDOM VARIABLE MODEL FOR ROC CURVES

Suppose that to each stimulus s corresponds a random variable $\mathbf{U}_s$, representing the activation evoked by that stimulus in some critical neural location. Similarly, let $\mathbf{U}_n$ be the activation random variable corresponding to the noise. We assume that these random variables are independent.

As before, let $p_s(\theta)$ and $p_n(\theta)$ be the hit and false alarm probabilities, corresponding to a payoff matrix θ. We assume that on every trial—whether or not the stimulus is presented—a positive response occurs if the momentary (or sample) value of $\mathbf{U}_s$ or $\mathbf{U}_n$ exceeds a criterion λ_θ, the value of which is determined by the payoff matrix θ. In symbols:

$$p_s(\theta) = \mathbb{P}\{\mathbf{U}_s > \lambda_\theta\} \tag{1}$$

and

$$p_n(\theta) = \mathbb{P}\{\mathbf{U}_n > \lambda_\theta\}. \tag{2}$$

Such a model is in the spirit of the random utility, or Thurstone-type models discussed in Chapter 5.

In the context of ROC curves, it entails a couple of interesting simple results. Suppose that

$$p_n(\theta) > p_n(\theta')$$

For some payoff matrices θ and θ'. Using (2) and (1) successively, this implies that

$$\lambda_\theta < \lambda_{\theta'},$$

yielding

$$p_s(\theta) \geqslant p_s(\theta').$$

This means that the ROC function $p_n(\theta) \mapsto p_s(\theta)$ must be nondecreasing, a prediction which, as indicated earlier, is consistent with many data. Another, basic result is that the area under the ROC curve (the integral of the ROC function from 0 to 1) is equal to the probability that $\mathbf{U}_s$ exceeds $\mathbf{U}_n$:

$$\mathbb{P}\{\mathbf{U}_s > \mathbf{U}_n\}.$$

The argument is spelled out as follows. Using the independence of random variables in question, we have

$$\mathbb{P}\{\mathbf{U}_s > \mathbf{U}_n\} = \int_{-\infty}^{\infty} \mathbb{P}\{\mathbf{U}_s > \lambda | \mathbf{U}_n = \lambda\} \, d\mathbb{P}\{\mathbf{U}_n \leqslant \lambda\}$$

$$= \int_{-\infty}^{\infty} \mathbb{P}\{\mathbf{U}_s > \lambda\} \, d\mathbb{P}\{\mathbf{U}_n \leqslant \lambda\}. \tag{3}$$

According to this model, the response probabilities $p_s(\theta) = \mathbb{P}\{\mathbf{U}_s > \lambda_\theta\}$ and $p_n(\theta) = \mathbb{P}\{\mathbf{U}_n > \lambda_\theta\}$ depend on the payoff matrix θ only through the number λ_θ. There is thus no ambiguity in writing $p_s(\lambda)$ for $p_s(\theta)$ and $p_n(\lambda)$ for $p_n(\theta)$, with $\lambda = \lambda_\theta$. Consequently, using ρ to denote the ROC function, and assuming that λ varies in $(-\infty, +\infty)$ (this assumption will be weakened in a moment), (3) yields

$$\mathbb{P}\{\mathbf{U}_s > \mathbf{U}_n\} = \int_{-\infty}^{\infty} p_s(\lambda) \, d[1 - p_n(\lambda)]$$

$$= -\int_{-\infty}^{\infty} \rho[p_n(\lambda)] \, dp_n(\lambda)$$

$$= \int_{\infty}^{-\infty} \rho[p_n(\lambda)] \, dp_n(\lambda).$$

Changing variables, from λ to $p_n(\lambda) = p$, we obtain, finally,

$$\mathbb{P}\{\mathbf{U}_s > \mathbf{U}_n\} = \int_0^1 \rho(p) \, dp, \tag{4}$$

as asserted. In the framework of this model, the area below the ROC curve appears thus as a reasonable measure of the detectability of the stimulus. The next definition and theorem summarize this discussion.

10.2. Definition. Let $\rho = \{[p_n(\theta), p_s(\theta)] | \theta \in \Theta\}$ be an ROC curve. (Thus ρ is an increasing, continuous function mapping $[0,1]$ into itself.) Let $\theta \mapsto \lambda_\theta$ be a mapping of Θ onto some open interval J. Let $\mathbf{U}_s$ and $\mathbf{U}_n$ be two independent random variables with a mass concentrated in J, that is, $\mathbb{P}\{\mathbf{U}_s \in J\} = \mathbb{P}\{\mathbf{U}_n \in J\} = 1$. We say then that the pair $(\mathbf{U}_s, \mathbf{U}_n)$ is a *random representation of ρ with criterion λ* iff for any payoff matrix $\theta \in \Theta$ the hit and false alarm probabilities satisfy the equation

$$p_\mathbf{S}(\theta) = \mathbb{P}\{\mathbf{U}_\mathbf{S} > \lambda_\theta\}$$

for $\mathbf{S} = s, n$.

Since the integration leading to (4) can obviously be carried over J, we have the following theorem.

10.3. Theorem. *If $(\mathbf{U}_s, \mathbf{U}_n)$ is a random representation of an ROC curve ρ then*

$$\mathbb{P}\{\mathbf{U}_s > \mathbf{U}_n\} = \int_0^1 \rho(p) \, dp,$$

thus a measure of the area under the ROC curve ρ.

This result suggests thus evaluating the detectability of the stimulus by estimating empirically the area under the ROC curve. Such a measure is appealing in that, at least in principle, it is not affected by nonsensory factors (represented here by the payoff matrices), which have been integrated out.

In practice however, it will typically be the case that only a few scattered points of some hypothetical ROC curve have been sampled empirically. This means that an interpolation procedure must take place. A way out of this difficulty is to make specific assumptions concerning the distributions of the random variables $\mathbf{U}_s$ and $\mathbf{U}_n$. Such assumptions would determine—up to the values of a couple of parameters—the exact analytic form of the ROC curve. If the assumptions are valid, a couple of suitably placed points of the ROC curve will suffice to estimate the parameters of the ROC curve experimentally, and the area under the ROC curve can then be evaluated by integration.

10.4. Remarks.   (1) One may be suspicious of such a method and object that the estimated value of the area will be model bound. This objection is not as strong as it may appear. Notice in this connection that Equation 4 was obtained without making any assumption regarding the distribution of the random variables $\mathbf{U}_s$ and $\mathbf{U}_n$. In fact, the shape of these distributions is arbitrary to some extent. For instance, let us assume that (1), (2) and (4) hold for some random variables $\mathbf{U}_s, \mathbf{U}_n$. For any strictly increasing continuous function g, we have

$$p_s(\theta) = \mathbb{P}\{g(\mathbf{U}_s) > g(\lambda_\theta)\} = \mathbb{P}\{\mathbf{U}'_s > \lambda'_\theta\}$$

and

$$p_n(\theta) = \mathbb{P}\{g(\mathbf{U}_n) > g(\lambda_\theta)\} = \mathbb{P}\{\mathbf{U}'_n > \lambda'_\theta\},$$

with $\mathbf{U}'_s = g(\mathbf{U}_s)$, $\mathbf{U}'_n = g(\mathbf{U}_n)$ and $\lambda'_\theta = g(\lambda_\theta)$. It is clear that the representation of the response probabilities provided by the random variables $\mathbf{U}'_s$ and $\mathbf{U}'_n$ is equivalent to that obtained with $\mathbf{U}_s$ and $\mathbf{U}_n$. In particular, the predicted ROC curve is not changed by the transformation. Later on in this chapter, we make precise hypotheses regarding the distributions of random variables entering into equations (1), (2), and (4). When evaluating these hypotheses, the reader should keep in mind the above remark pointing out to the relative arbitrariness of the distributions of $\mathbf{U}_s$ and $\mathbf{U}_n$.

(2) It must be realized that the random variable model discussed here does not necessarily describe a rational strategy. Depending on how optimality is defined, and on more specific assumptions on the random variables $\mathbf{U}_s$ and $\mathbf{U}_n$, the decision rule embodied in (1) and (2) may or may not be optimal.

To illustrate this point, let π be the probability of a stimulus trial, and suppose that for some criterion value λ_0

$$\mathbb{P}\{\mathbf{U}_n > \lambda_0\}(1 - \pi) > \mathbb{P}\{\mathbf{U}_s > \lambda_0\}\pi. \tag{5}$$

A special case of this assumption is seen in Figure 10.2, which is by no means unrealistic.

Nevertheless, (5) leads to a somewhat undesirable conclusion. When reacting to an activation value exceeding λ_0, the subject reports a detection, even though

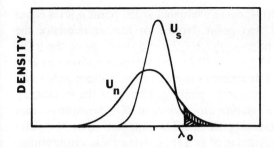

FIGURE 10.2. Two normal densities of U_s and U_n for which Equation 5 holds, with $\pi = 1 - \pi = .5$.

the likelihood of a stimulus trial is then smaller than that of a noise trial. Such a conclusion easily follows from the above inequality. Indeed, denoting by S, as before, the stimulation at a given trial (thus $S = s$ or $S = n$), (5) holds if and only if, successively,

$$\mathbb{P}\{U_s > \lambda_0 | S = n\}\, \mathbb{P}\{S = n\} > \mathbb{P}\{U_s > \lambda_0 | S = s\}\, \mathbb{P}\{S = s\}$$

iff

$$\mathbb{P}\{S = n, U_s > \lambda_0\}/\mathbb{P}\{U_s > \lambda_0\} > \mathbb{P}(S = s, U_s > \lambda_0)/\mathbb{P}\{U_s > \lambda_0\}$$

iff

$$\mathbb{P}\{S = n | U_s > \lambda_0\} > \mathbb{P}\{S = s | U_s > \lambda_0\}.$$

In words, this last inequality means that the conditional probability of a noise trial, when observing the event $U_s > \lambda_0$, is greater than that of a stimulus trial. However, according to the model, the subject will report a detection. A definition of optimality suggested by that argument would require that such situation does not arise; that is,

$$\mathbb{P}\{U_s > \lambda\}\pi > \mathbb{P}\{U_n > \lambda\}(1 - \pi),$$

for all criterion values λ. This definition does not take into account the monetary gains or losses resulting from the strategy. Other definitions of optimality are conceivable, one of which will be considered shortly.

ROC ANALYSIS AND LIKELIHOOD RATIOS

The slope of the ROC curve is susceptible of an interesting interpretation. Let us assume that the random variables U_s and U_n have densities, f_s and f_n, respectively with $f_n > 0$. Writing as before ρ for the ROC function, we have, successively,

$$d\rho[p_n(\theta)]/dp_n(\theta) = d\mathbb{P}\{U_s > \lambda_\theta\}/d\,\mathbb{P}\{U_n > \lambda_\theta\}$$
$$= d[1 - \mathbb{P}\{U_s \leqslant \lambda_\theta\}]/d[1 - \mathbb{P}\{U_n \leqslant \lambda_\theta\}]$$
$$= \frac{-f_s(\lambda_\theta)}{-f_n(\lambda_\theta)}$$
$$= \frac{f_s(\lambda_\theta)}{f_n(\lambda_\theta)}.$$

In other terms, the slope of the ROC curve evaluated at the point $p_n(\theta)$ is equal to the ratio of the densities at that point. Notice for further reference the monotonicity relation between the ratio $f_s(\lambda_\theta)/f_n(\lambda_\theta)$ and the slope of the ROC curve. Since, as a consequence of Definition 10.2, λ_θ decreases as $p_n(\theta)$ increases, a decrease in the slope of the ROC function in some interval corresponds to an increase in the ratio $f_s(\lambda_\theta)/f_n(\lambda_\theta)$, in the corresponding interval of the variable λ_θ. Typical data strongly support the assumption of concave ROC functions—that is, ROC functions with nonincreasing slopes. This suggests that the ratio $f_s(\lambda)/f_n(\lambda)$ should be an increasing function of λ.[1] Let us review these assumptions.

10.5. Definition. A random representation (U_s, U_n) of some ROC curve is called *differentiable* iff the random variables have densities f_s, f_n, respectively, with $f_n > 0$. The random representation is called *rational* iff the ratio

$$\ell(x) = f_s(x)/f_n(x) \tag{6}$$

is a continuous strictly increasing function of x. In statistics, a ratio such as that appearing in (6) is often referred to as a *likelihood ratio*. The assumption that a random representation is rational suggests a drastically different interpretation of the model, in which the strategy of the subject is consistent with that of a statistician engaged in a decision task and applying an optimal decision procedure. Let us elaborate this. Since ℓ is strictly increasing, we have (cf. remark 10.4(1))

$$\begin{aligned}
p_s(\theta) &= \mathbb{P}\{U_s > \lambda_\theta\} \\
&= \mathbb{P}\{\ell(U_s) > \ell(\lambda_\theta)\} \\
&= \mathbb{P}\{f_s(U_s)/f_n(U_s) > \ell(\lambda_\theta)\}.
\end{aligned} \tag{7}$$

By a similar argument, we also obtain

$$p_n(\theta) = \mathbb{P}\{f_s(U_n)/f_n(U_n) > \ell(\lambda_\theta)\}. \tag{8}$$

Notice that two new random variables appear in (7) and (8):

$$U_s' = f_s(U_s)/f_n(U_s)$$

$$U_n' = f_s(U_n)/f_n(U_n)$$

We have thus a random representation (U_s', U_n') with criterion $\ell(\lambda_\theta)$.

The successive steps of the procedure described by (7) and (8) are reviewed in Figure 10.3, which is self-explanatory. Thus, if an ROC curve has a rational random representation, the subject decision strategy may be reinterpreted as relying on a computation of a likelihood ratio. When perceiving a neural signal of

---

1. We recall that a function g mapping a subset of $\mathbb{R}$ into $\mathbb{R}$ is called *increasing* iff $x \leq y$ implies $g(x) \leq g(y)$, for all x,y in the domain of g. It is called *strictly increasing* iff the two inequalities are replaced by the strict inequality $<$. A similar convention applies to the terms decreasing, convex, and concave.

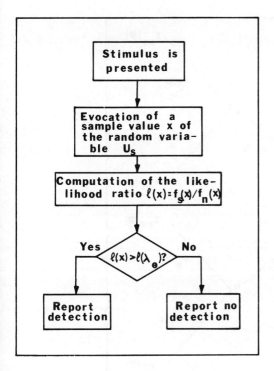

FIGURE 10.3. Successive stages of the decision process, elicited by the presentation of the stimulus s, in the case of the likelihood ratio model. The diagram is identical in the case of the presentation of the noise n, except that $\mathbf{U}_s$ is replaced by $\mathbf{U}_n$.

subjective intensity x, the subject somehow "computes" $f_s(x)/f_n(x)$ and reports a detection if his or her likelihood ratio exceeds the criterion value $\ell(\lambda_\theta)$. The comparison with the behavior of a statistician can be pursued a step further, however.

We assume that the subject's procedure maximizes the expected value of his or her gain, as determined by the payoff matrix θ. Let $\gamma(\theta)_{ss}$ and $\gamma(\theta)_{nn}$ be the gains resulting from a hit and a correct rejection, respectively; let $\gamma(\theta)_{ns}$ and $\gamma(\theta)_{sn}$ be the the costs attached to a false alarm and a miss. Let π be the probability that a stimulus is presented on any trial. The expected value $G(\theta,\pi)$ of the gain is easily computed from the tree diagram of Figure 10.4, which displays the possible paths and their probabilities.

We obtain

$$G(\theta,\pi) = \pi\{p_s(\theta)\gamma_{ss}(\theta) - [1 - p_s(\theta)]\gamma_{ns}(\theta)\}$$
$$+ (1 - \pi)\{[1 - p_n(\theta)]\gamma_{nn}(\theta) - p_n(\theta)\gamma_{sn}(\theta)\},$$

which we rewrite

$$G(\theta,\pi) = \pi[\gamma_{ss}(\theta) + \gamma_{ns}(\theta)][p_s(\theta) - p_n(\theta)\beta_\theta], \qquad (9)$$

with

$$\beta_\theta = (1 - \pi)[\gamma_{sn}(\theta) + \gamma_{nn}(\theta)]/\pi[\gamma_{ss}(\theta) + \gamma_{ns}(\theta)]. \qquad (10)$$

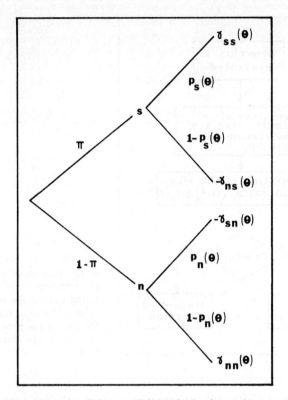

FIGURE 10.4. Tree diagram of the possible paths in the yes/no paradigm with their probabilities and their outcomes.

The statistician's decision procedure concerns the response probabilities $p_s(\theta)$ and $p_n(\theta)$, which can be manipulated via the quantity λ_θ in the equations

$$p_s(\theta) = \mathbb{P}\{\mathbf{U}_s > \lambda_\theta\}$$

and

$$p_n(\theta) = \mathbb{P}\{\mathbf{U}_n > \lambda_\theta\}.$$

Since $\pi[\gamma_{ss}(\theta) + \gamma_{ns}(\theta)]$ is constant, a value of λ_θ maximizes the expected gains $G(\theta,\pi)$ in (9) if and only if it maximizes

$$\mathbb{P}\{\mathbf{U}_s > \lambda_\theta\} - \mathbb{P}\{\mathbf{U}_n > \lambda_\theta\}\beta_\theta.$$

It follows that the required value of λ_θ must satisfy

$$f_s(\lambda_\theta) - f_n(\lambda_\theta)\beta_\theta = 0,$$

that is,

$$\ell(\lambda_\theta) = \frac{f_s(\lambda_\theta)}{f_n(\lambda_\theta)} = \beta_\theta.$$

We conclude that the subject strategy is optimal in the sense of a maximisation of the expected gain, if the response probabilities satisfy the two equations

$$p_s(\theta) = \mathbb{P}\{\mathbf{U}_s > \ell^{-1}(\beta_\theta)\}, \tag{11}$$

$$p_n(\theta) = \mathbb{P}\{\mathbf{U}_n > \ell^{-1}(\beta_\theta)\}, \tag{12}$$

with β_θ defined by (10). The next definition and theorem summarize the results of this section.

10.6. Definition. Let $\rho = \{[p_n(\theta), p_s(\theta)] | \theta \in \Theta\}$ be an ROC curve, with a *gain function* defined by the matrix

Responses

		Yes	No
S		$\gamma_{ss}(\theta)$	$\gamma_{sn}(\theta)$
Stimulus			
n		$\gamma_{ns}(\theta)$	$\gamma_{nn}(\theta)$

Let $\mathcal{U} = (\mathbf{U}_s, \mathbf{U}_n)$ be a rational random representation of ρ with criterion λ and density functions f_s, f_n. Then the criterion λ is *optimal for some* $\theta \in \Theta$ *and some stimulus probability* π (*in the sense of a maximization of the expected gain*) iff the value λ_θ maximizes the function $G(\theta, \pi)$ in (9), with $p_s(\theta) = \mathbb{P}\{\mathbf{U}_s > \lambda_\theta\}$ and $p_n(\theta) = \mathbb{P}\{\mathbf{U}_n > \lambda_\theta\}$.

This definition of optimality is consistent with the notion that only the criterion λ is under the subject's control. (In this definition, the choice of the criterion implicitly depends on the probability π of the stimulus. A more exact notation for the criterion would be $\lambda_{\theta,\pi}$.)

10.7. Theorem. Let $\mathcal{U} = (\mathbf{U}_s, \mathbf{U}_n)$ be a random representation with criterion λ, of an ROC curve $\rho = \{[p_n(\theta), p_s(\theta)] | \theta \in \Theta\}$. Suppose that $\mathcal{U}$ is differentiable, with density functions f_s, f_n then:

(i) ρ is differentiable and for every $\theta \in \Theta$, its slope at the point $[p_n(\theta), p_s(\theta)]$ is equal to the likelihood ratio

$$\ell(\lambda_\theta) = f_s(\lambda_\theta)/f_n(\lambda_\theta);$$

(ii) $\mathcal{U}$ is rational iff ρ is strictly concave, in which case

$$p_n(\theta) = \mathbb{P}\{f_s(\mathbf{U}_n)/f_n(\mathbf{U}_n) > \ell(\lambda_\theta)\},$$

$$p_s(\theta) = \mathbb{P}\{f_s(\mathbf{U}_s)/f_n(\mathbf{U}_s) > \ell(\lambda_\theta)\}.$$

(iii) *Moreover, if* $\mathcal{U}$ *is rational, then the criterion* λ *is optimal for some payoff matrix* θ *and stimulus probability* π *iff*

$$\lambda_\theta = \ell^{-1}(\beta_\theta),$$

with β_θ defined by (10), in which case the ROC curve is described by Equations 11 and 12.

Further developments along these lines can be found in the exercises. If precise assumptions are made concerning the distributions of the random variables U_s and U_n, it can then be checked whether the subject's strategy is optimal in the above sense, by evaluating the fit of the above equation to the data. This comparison of the subject's strategy with that of a statistician engaged in a decision-making task was discussed in some detail since it is an inherent part of the common wisdom in this field. It must be clear, however, that the analysis of the data in terms of ROC curves is a useful device to disentangle sensory from cognitive components of the task, whether or not the subject strategy happens to be optimal.

This analysis is also valuable, or at least relevant, in cases of experimental procedures or paradigms somewhat different from that envisaged so far in this section. Two examples are discussed in the next two sections.

ROC ANALYSIS AND THE FORCED CHOICE PARADIGM

In the two-alternative-forced-choice paradigm (often abbreviated 2AFC), the subject's task is to decide on every trial which of two locations, or two intervals of time, contains the stimulus. Even though the effect on performance of guessing strategies is minimized in such paradigm, an ROC analysis will be useful. In particular, the connections between the predictions in the yes/no and the 2AFC paradigms are of interest.

For concreteness, we consider as before an auditory detection situation. On every trial, the subject is presented with two successive intervals of time, of equal duration, one of which containing the stimulus (a click, say) embedded in noise, the other one containing only the noise. There are thus two types of trials, depending on whether the stimulus was in the first or in the second interval. We denote these two cases by (s,n) and (n,s), respectively. Let $p_{1,sn}$ and $p_{2,ns}$ be the corresponding probabilities of a correct response, and let $p_{2,sn}$ and $p_{1,ns}$ be the error probabilities. By design, we must have

$$p_{1,sn} + p_{2,sn} = 1$$

and

$$p_{1,ns} + p_{2,ns} = 1,$$

since the subject is forced to choose one of the two intervals on every trial. For the time being, let us suppose that the two probabilities of a correct response are equal,

$$p_{1,sn} = p_{2,ns}. \tag{13}$$

This assumption, which is not always realistic and can be rejected for some data, will be relaxed in a moment. From a purely sensory viewpoint, the 2AFC paradigm differs only a little from the yes/no paradigm, and it makes sense to apply the same theoretical analysis. Let us assume that

$$p_{1,sn} = \mathbb{P}\{\mathbf{U}_s > \mathbf{U}_n\} = p_{2,ns}, \tag{14}$$

in which $\mathbf{U}_s$ and $\mathbf{U}_n$ are independent random variables with the same interpretation as before. If we assume that $\mathbf{U}_s$ and $\mathbf{U}_n$ are continuous, we have

$$\mathbb{P}\{\mathbf{U}_s = \mathbf{U}_n\} = 0,$$

which implies, for the probabilities of errors,

$$p_{2,sn} = 1 - p_{1,sn} = \mathbb{P}\{\mathbf{U}_n > \mathbf{U}_s\} = p_{1,ns}.$$

The idea is that each of the two intervals provides a sample of one of the random variables $\mathbf{U}_s$ and $\mathbf{U}_n$, and the subject's response is based on a comparison of these samples. In the case of an (s,n) trial, for instance, if x_1 and x_2 are sample values of $\mathbf{U}_s$ and $\mathbf{U}_n$ respectively, the subject will choose interval 1 (the correct one) if $x_1 > x_2$.

Notice that, under the assumption of rationality (cf. Definition 10.5: $\mathbf{U}_s$ and $\mathbf{U}_n$ have densities f_s, f_n with $f_n > 0$, and the ratio $\ell(x) = f_s(x)/f_n(x)$ is a strictly increasing function of x), we have

$$\mathbb{P}\{\mathbf{U}_s > \mathbf{U}_n\} = \mathbb{P}\{f_s(\mathbf{U}_s)/f_n(\mathbf{U}_s) > f_s(\mathbf{U}_n)/f_n(\mathbf{U}_n)\}.$$

This means that the above interpretation of the subject's decision process as based on a comparison of samples of $\mathbf{U}_s$ and $\mathbf{U}_n$ is equivalent to another, in which he or she would behave as a statistician and compare likelihood ratios.

In any event, the conclusion to be derived from (14) is that the probability of a correct response in the 2AFC paradigm, under the assumption that $p_{1,sn} = p_{2,ns}$, is equal to the area under the ROC curve in the corresponding yes/no paradigm.

As indicated, the assumption that $p_{1,sn} = p_{2,sn}$ may be unrealistic. We briefly examine here the possibility that the subject may be biased toward one of the two intervals. A systematic way of inducing such a bias would be to assign different probabilities to the events (s,n) and (n,s). Our random variable model for the 2AFC paradigm can be generalized as follows. Let Θ be a set of bias-inducing conditions; let $p_{1,sn}(\theta)$ and $p_{1,ns}(\theta)$ be the two probabilities of choosing the first interval, in condition θ, for the two cases (s,n) and (n,s). We assume that the effect of a given condition $\theta \in \Theta$ is to transform the distribution of the random variable corresponding to the second interval. Specifically, we assume that the following two equations hold:

$$p_{1,sn}(\theta) = \mathbb{P}\{\mathbf{U}_s > g_\theta(\mathbf{U}_n)\}$$

$$p_{1,ns}(\theta) = \mathbb{P}\{\mathbf{U}_n > g_\theta(\mathbf{U}_s)\},$$

where g_θ is a strictly increasing, continuous function. With obvious notation, the two remaining probabilities are computed from the equations

$$p_{1,sn}(\theta) + p_{2,sn}(\theta) = 1,$$

$$p_{1,ns}(\theta) + p_{2,ns}(\theta) = 1,$$

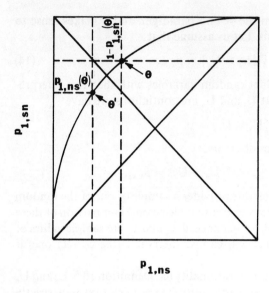

FIGURE 10.5. Hypothetical ROC curve symmetric with respect to the negative diagonal of the unit square, in the 2AFC paradigm. We have $p_{1,ns}(\theta') = 1 - p_{1,sn}(\theta)$, and $p_{1,sn}(\theta') = 1 - p_{1,ns}(\theta)$.

which are inherent to the 2AFC paradigm. Let us suppose for a moment that the set of points

$$[p_{1,ns}(\theta), p_{1,sn}(\theta)],$$

generated by varying $\theta \in \Theta$, is an ROC curve. Under fairly general properties on the set of transformations $(g_\theta | \theta \in \Theta)$, it follows then that this ROC curve must be symmetric with respect to the negative diagonal of the unit square (see Fig. 10.5). One such property is that if g_θ is a strictly increasing transformation, then there must be some condition $\theta' \in \Theta$ corresponding to the "opposite" transformation, $g_\theta^{-1} = g_{\theta'}$. Indeed, we have then

$$
\begin{aligned}
1 - p_{1,sn}(\theta) &= \mathbb{P}\{g_\theta(\mathbf{U}_n) > \mathbf{U}_s\} \\
&= \mathbb{P}\{\mathbf{U}_n > g_\theta^{-1}(\mathbf{U}_s)\} \\
&= \mathbb{P}\{\mathbf{U}_n > g_{\theta'}(\mathbf{U}_s)\} \\
&= p_{1,ns}(\theta').
\end{aligned}
$$

and

$$
\begin{aligned}
p_{1,sn}(\theta') &= \mathbb{P}\{\mathbf{U}_s > g_{\theta'}(\mathbf{U}_n)\} \\
&= \mathbb{P}\{\mathbf{U}_s > g_\theta^{-1}(\mathbf{U}_n)\} \\
&= \mathbb{P}\{g_\theta(\mathbf{U}_s) > \mathbf{U}_n\} \\
&= 1 - p_{1,ns}(\theta).
\end{aligned}
$$

The two equations,

$$1 - p_{1,sn}(\theta) = p_{1,ns}(\theta'),$$

$$p_{1,sn}(\theta') = 1 - p_{1,ns}(\theta)$$

express the symmetry property of the ROC curve mentioned above. This situation is illustrated in Figure 10.5.

ROC ANALYSIS OF RATING SCALE DATA

In the same experimental situation, consider a procedure in which, rather that giving a yes/no detection response at every trial, the subject is required to quantify his or her certainty that the stimulus was presented. Suppose for example that a six-category rating scale is used, ranging from 0 (certainty that the stimulus was not presented) to 5 (certainty that the stimulus was presented). Some hypothetical, but plausible data is given in Table (15), which displays the relative frequencies of the ratings in the two types of trials.

Rating Value

	0	1	2	3	4	5
Noise trials	.10	.15	.35	.20	.15	.05
Stimulus trials	.05	.10	.30	.20	.25	.10

(15)

Let R_s and R_n be two random variables corresponding to the ratings in the two types of trials. (For example, $\mathbb{P}\{R_s = 3\}$ is the probability of observing a rating of 3, on a trial when the stimulus was presented). Since the experimental situation is unchanged except for the subject's responses, it makes sense to suppose that the same underlying activation random variables U_s and U_n are responsible for the ratings. The following model seems reasonable: an observed rating will exceed a value i ($i = 0,\ldots,4$) only if the activation random variable exceeds a criterion λ_i, the value of which depends on the rating considered.

In symbols:

$$\mathbb{P}\{R_s > i\} = \mathbb{P}\{U_s > \lambda_i\},$$
$$\mathbb{P}\{R_n > i\} = \mathbb{P}\{U_n > \lambda_i\}.$$

Observe that the right members of these two equations strongly resemble those of Equations 1 and 2, defining a random representation of an ROC curve (cf. Definition 10.2). This suggests an ROC analysis of the data. It is as if each possible value of the rating (with the exception of the maximal one) would implicitly define a particular payoff matrix, and a recoding of the rating data into two yes/no classes. In the example of Table (15), the value $i = 3$ leads to the recoding

write *yes*   if $i = 4,5$

write *no*   if $i = 1,2,3,$

with

Proportion of "False alarms": $.05 + .15 = .20$

Proportion of "Hits": $.10 + .25 = .35.$

The results of this recoding, the proportion of ratings exceeding i, are displayed in Table (16).

Rating Value

i	0	1	2	3	4	
n	.90	.75	.40	.20	.05	(16)
s	.95	.85	.55	.35	.10	

The corresponding ROC graph is displayed in Figure 10.6. In general, the probabilities of "hits" and "false alarms" corresponding to each rating value i up to (but not including) the maximal one are given by the equations

$$p_s(i) = \mathbb{P}\{\mathbf{R}_s > i\},$$

$$p_n(i) = \mathbb{P}\{\mathbf{R}_n > i\}$$

with the ROC graph $\{[p_n(i), p_s(i)] | i = 0, 1, \ldots, m - 1\}$, m denoting the maximal rating value.

An obvious advantage of this method is its efficiency. The subject is required to make more sophisticated responses than in the yes/no procedure, which results in a substantial economy in the collection of the data. This was illustrated in our example, in which only one condition, rather than five, had to be run to obtain a five-points ROC graph. On the negative side, it must be remarked that the points

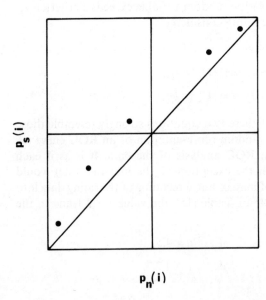

FIGURE 10.6. ROC graph obtained for the rating scale data displayed in Table (16).

of an experimental ROC graph are not independent, which may create difficulties in fitting and evaluating a model.

Finally, we mention that data collected by the rating scale procedure, but analyzed by methods different from those discussed here, may provide a sharp test of some models. We will return to this point later on in this chapter.

THE GAUSSIAN ASSUMPTION

In principle, an ROC analysis is feasible without making any assumptions on the distributions of the random variables U_s and U_n (cf. Bamber, 1975). However, the application is greatly facilitated if such assumptions are made. We discuss in this section the case of Gaussian distributions.

10.8. Definition. Let $\mathscr{U} = (U_s, U_n)$ be a random representation of an ROC curve $\rho = \{[(p_n(\theta), p_s(\theta)] \,|\, \theta \in \Theta\}$ with criterion λ. Then $\mathscr{U}$ is called *Gaussian (with parameters $\mu_s, \sigma_s, \mu_n, \sigma_n$)* iff U_s and U_n are normally distributed random variables and $\mu_s, \sigma_s, \mu_n, \sigma_n$ denote their expectations and standard deviations, respectively. In such case we have clearly

$$p_s(\theta) = \mathbb{P}\{U_s > \lambda_\theta\} = \Phi\left(\frac{\mu_s - \lambda_\theta}{\sigma_s}\right), \tag{17}$$

$$p_n(\theta) = \mathbb{P}\{U_n > \lambda_\theta\} = \Phi\left(\frac{\mu_n - \lambda_\theta}{\sigma_n}\right), \tag{18}$$

in which Φ denotes, as usual, the distribution function of a standard normal random variable.

From Equations 17 and 18, it is apparent that the ROC curve is determined by four parameters at most: the means and the standard deviations of the random variables U_s and U_n. (In fact, we will see that only two parameters are necessary.) From a practical viewpoint, it will be convenient to rewrite (17) and (18) in terms of the so-called "z scores." With

$$z_s(\theta) = \Phi^{-1}[p_s(\theta)]$$

$$z_s(\theta) = \Phi^{-1}[p_n(\theta)]$$

and dropping θ in the notations, we obtain

$$z_s = \frac{\mu_s - \lambda}{\sigma_s}$$

$$z_n = \frac{\mu_n - \lambda}{\sigma_n}$$

Eliminating λ in these equations and solving for z_s, yields

$$z_s = z_n \frac{\sigma_n}{\sigma_s} + \frac{\mu_s - \mu_n}{\sigma_s}. \tag{19}$$

In other terms: when the hit and false alarm probabilities are transformed into z scores, the ROC curve is transformed into a straight line with slope σ_n/σ_s and intercept $(\mu_s - \mu_n)/\sigma_s$. Using linear regression, these two parameters can be estimated from the response frequencies of the data. Notice that the ROC curve only specifies two of the four parameters μ_s, μ_n, σ_s, and σ_n.

For example, we can assume, without loss of generality, that $\mu_n = 0$ and $\sigma_n = 1$. The area under the ROC curve can be computed from the equations

$$\mathbb{P}\{U_s > U_n\} = \mathbb{P}\{U_s - U_n > 0\}$$

$$= \Phi\left[\frac{\mu_s - \mu_n}{(\sigma_s^2 + \sigma_n^2)^{1/2}}\right]. \tag{20}$$

It is easy to show that this Gaussian representation is rational if, and only if, $\sigma_s = \sigma_n$ and $\mu_s > \mu_n$ (Exercise 5). By Theorem 10.7, the ROC function ρ is strictly concave iff the random representation is rational. Thus, ρ is strictly concave iff $\sigma_s = \sigma_n$ and $\mu_s > \mu_n$. As pointed out, typical ROC data are consistent with the assumption that the underlying ROC functions are concave. The above argument suggests that the special case $\sigma_s = \sigma_n$ deserves a serious consideration.

10.9. Theorem. *Let $\mathcal{U} = (U_s, U_n)$ be a Gaussian random representation of an ROC curve $\rho = \{[p_n(\theta), p_s(\theta)] \mid \theta \in \Theta\}$ with parameters μ_s, σ_s, μ_n, and σ_n. Then,*

$$\int_0^1 \rho(p)dp = \mathbb{P}\{U_s > U_n\} = \Phi\left[\frac{\mu_s - \mu_n}{(\sigma_s^2 + \sigma_n^2)^{1/2}}\right],$$

expressing the area under the ROC curve. Also, with

$$z_s(\theta) = \Phi^{-1}[p_s(\theta)] \tag{21}$$

and

$$z_n(\theta) = \Phi^{-1}[p_n(\theta)], \tag{22}$$

we have

$$z_s(\theta) = z_n(\theta)\frac{\sigma_n}{\sigma_s} + \frac{\mu_s - \mu_n}{\sigma_s}.$$

Moreover, the four following conditions are equivalent:

(i) *$\mathcal{U}$ is rational.*
(ii) *ρ is strictly concave.*
(iii) *$\sigma_s = \sigma_n$ and $\mu_s > \mu_n$.*
(iv) *$z_s(\theta) = z_n(\theta) + [(\mu_s - \mu_n)/\sigma_s]$, with $\mu_s > \mu_n$.*

In (iv), we can always choose to set $\sigma_s = 1$, which yields

$$\mathbb{P}\{U_s > U_n\} = \Phi\left(\frac{\mu_s - \mu_n}{\sqrt{2}}\right). \tag{23}$$

In the special case where U_s and U_n are independent Gaussian random variables with equal variances, the ROC curves, replotted in the units of the z scores, are thus parallel straight lines with a slope equal to 1. The only parameter remaining in the model is the difference $\mu_s - \mu_n > 0$.

10.10. Definition. When this model is used, $\sigma_s = \sigma_n = 1$, a standard measure of the detectability of the stimulus is

$$d'(s,n) = \mu_s - \mu_n.$$

Notice that d' is closely related to the other measure, the area under the ROC curve. Indeed from Equation 23, we have

$$\mathbb{P}\{\mathbf{U}_s > \mathbf{U}_n\} = \Phi[d'(s,n)/\sqrt{2}].$$

Obviously, the use of d' as a measure of discriminability is justified only if the underlying assumptions are supported by the data. Thus, it must be checked that the empirical ROC graphs, transformed by Equations 21 and 22, are predicted reasonably well by a set of parallel straight lines with slope 1.

Occasionally, it is convenient to plot the empirical ROC graphs and the theoretical ROC curves on "double probability" paper (a two-dimensional Cartesian representation in which the coordinates are in units of the normal integral).

THE THRESHOLD THEORY

A rather different interpretation of an ROC analysis of yes/no detection data is possible, in which the basic, underlying notions are not activation random variables, but detection states. A number of such models have been proposed, which differ in particular by the number of (unobservable) states postulated, or by the exact relation linking the states to the responsible probabilities or other observable quantities (e.g., response latencies, ratings). We now discuss a simple example, due to Luce (1960, 1963a, 1963b).

10.11. Basic notions. We assume that the presentation of the stimulus or noise elicit one of two sensory states in the subject: either a neural threshold has been exceeded, or it has not. The event that the threshold is exceeded may lead to a "yes" response (the subject reports a detection), but not necessarily so. We also assume that a payoff matrix Θ may induce one of two opposite response strategies: (i) a *conservative strategy*, in which the subject never says "yes" when the threshold has not been exceeded; when the threshold has been exceeded, the subject only says "yes" with a probability β_θ depending on the payoff matrix; (ii) a *guessing strategy*, in which the subject always says "yes" when the threshold has been exceeded; when the threshold has not been exceeded, the subject says yes with a probability α_θ, depending on the payoff matrix. This means that the collection Θ of payoff matrices is partitioned into two classes: Θ_c, the set of payoff matrices inducing a conservative strategy and Θ_g, the set of payoff matrices inducing a guessing strategy. The event that the threshold has been exceeded will be denoted by $\mathbf{D} = 1$; the complementary event will be denoted by $\mathbf{D} = 0$. Thus, in the framework of a probabilistic model, $\mathbf{D}$ is a random variable taking values 0,1. As before, the letter $\mathbf{S}$ denotes the stimulation; we have two cases: $\mathbf{S} = s$ (the stimulus is presented) and $\mathbf{S} = n$ (only the noise is presented). The probability that the stimulation determines a neural event exceeding the threshold ($\mathbf{D} = 1$) only depends on $\mathbf{S}$, and will be denoted $q(\mathbf{S})$. Notice that we have introduced four numerical parameters: two for the response probabilities, β_θ and α_θ; and two for the probabilities of the states, $q(s)$ and $q(n)$. In the framework of an ROC analysis, however, two of these parameters will be eliminated in the equations, leaving only $q(s)$ and $q(n)$ to be estimated from the data. Finally, we denote by Y_θ and N_θ the two events of a "yes" and a "no" response, respectively.

10.12. Axioms for the threshold theory.   We provide a summary of these assumptions in the form of two axioms.

State Axiom T1.

$$\mathbb{P}\{\mathbf{D} = 1|\mathbf{S}\} = q(\mathbf{S}), \qquad \text{for } \mathbf{S} = s,n.$$

(The probability that stimulation exceeds the threshold is equal to $q(s)$ if the stimulus is presented, and to $q(n)$ if the noise is presented, these probabilities being independent of the payoff matrix.)

Response Axiom T2.   For any payoff matrix $\theta \in \Theta = \Theta_c + \Theta_g$

$$\mathbb{P}\{Y_\theta|\mathbf{S}, \mathbf{D}\} = \begin{cases} (1 - \mathbf{D})\alpha_\theta + \mathbf{D}, & \text{if } \theta \in \Theta_g, \\ \beta_\theta \mathbf{D}, & \text{if } \theta \in \Theta_c, \end{cases}$$

independent of $\mathbf{S}$.

(The probability of a "yes" response to a stimulation only depends on the payoff matrix θ, and whether the threshold has been exceeded or not. If θ is in Θ_g, it is equal to 1 or α_θ, depending on whether $\mathbf{D} = 1$ or $\mathbf{D} = 0$, respectively. If θ is in Θ_c, this probability is equal to β_θ or 0, again depending on whether $\mathbf{D} = 1$ or $\mathbf{D} = 0$.)

10.13. Remarks.   The form of these axioms deserves perhaps some comments. In general, the task of the theoretician in signal detection is to predict, for a payoff matrix $\theta \in \Theta$, the corresponding point of the ROC curve, that is, the two conditional probabilities of observable events

$$p_\mathbf{S}(\theta) = \mathbb{P}\{Y_\theta|\mathbf{S}\}, \qquad \text{for } \mathbf{S} = s, n.$$

In the threshold theory, this is accomplished by postulating the existence of two unobservable detection events $\mathbf{D} = 0$ and $\mathbf{D} = 1$. By a standard rule of elementary probability, we have, for $\mathbf{S} = s, n$,

$$\mathbb{P}\{Y_\theta|\mathbf{S}\} = \mathbb{P}\{Y_\theta|\mathbf{D} = 1, \mathbf{S}\}\mathbb{P}\{\mathbf{D} = 1|\mathbf{S}\} + \mathbb{P}\{Y_\theta|\mathbf{D} = 0, \mathbf{S}\}\mathbb{P}\{\mathbf{D} = 0|\mathbf{S}\}. \quad (24)$$

Thus, the point of the ROC curve—the left member of the above equation—can be obtained by specifying all the probabilities in the right member, which is achieved by T1 and T2.

10.14. Form of the ROC curve. As shown by a simple calculation, these axioms predict an ROC curve made of two segments of a straight line (see Fig. 10.7). The upper portion describes the guessing strategy and contains the corner (1,1) of the unit square. The points of that segment are generated by varying θ in Θ_g. The lower portion describes the conservative strategy, contains the point (0,0), and is generated by varying θ in Θ_c. Let us demonstrate this.

Applying Axiom T1 to (24) yields

$$p_\mathbf{S}(\theta) = \mathbb{P}\{Y_\theta | \mathbf{D} = 1, \mathbf{S}\}q(\mathbf{S}) + \mathbb{P}\{Y_\theta | \mathbf{D} = 0, \mathbf{S}\}[1 - q(\mathbf{S})] \qquad (25)$$

Case $\theta \in \Theta_g$.   Using Axiom T2, (25) specializes into

$$p_s(\theta) = q(s) + \alpha_\theta[1 - q(s)]$$
$$p_n(\theta) = q(n) + \alpha_\theta[1 - q(n)].$$

Eliminating α_θ in these two equations and solving for $p_s(\theta)$, we obtain

$$p_s(\theta) = p_n(\theta)[1 - q(s)]/[1 - q(n)] + [q(s) - q(n)]/[1 - q(n)], \qquad (26)$$

a linear function containing the point (1,1). Thus, as θ varies in Θ_g, the points of the ROC curve moves along a segment of a straight line specified by Equation 26. Notice that in this case we have $q(n) \leqslant p_n(\theta)$.

Case $\theta \in \Theta_c$.   From (25) and Axiom T2, we obtain

$$p_s(\theta) = \beta_\theta q(s),$$
$$p_n(\theta) = \beta_\theta q(n).$$

Eliminating β_θ yields

$$p_s(\theta) = p_n(\theta)q(s)/q(n), \qquad (27)$$

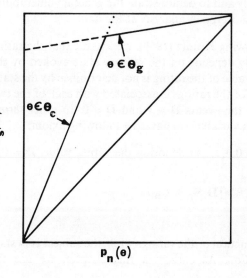

FIGURE 10.7. An example of an ROC curve in the 2-state threshold model. The upper limb of the curve corresponds to Equation 26, $\theta \in \Theta_g$; the lower limb corresponds to Equation 27, $\theta \in \Theta_c$.

the equation of a straight line going through the origin. Here, we have $p_n(\theta) \leqslant q(n)$.

Equations 26 and 27 together specify the class of ROC curves predicted by Luce's two-state-threshold theory. This prediction has been shown to hold reasonably well for some data (cf. Luce 1963a). In other cases, however, the theory is not so successful. For example, Nachmias and Steinman (1963) have shown that, in some empirical situations, the probability $q(n)$ that the threshold is exceeded on noise trials (as estimated from the data) has to vary with signal strength. Such a fact is obviously difficult to accommodate in the framework of the two-state-threshold theory.

RATING DATA AND THE THRESHOLD THEORY

It is natural to inquire about the predictions of the threshold theory concerning data obtained by the rating scale procedures. Some authors have pointed out that rating scale data characteristically favor an ROC function with smooth curvature, a fact that may appear to be inconsistent with the two segments of straight lines predicted by the threshold theory (Broadbent & Gregory, 1963; Nachmias & Steinman, 1963; Swets, 1961; Watson, Rilling, & Bourbon, 1964). Actually, as stated above and in the cited papers of Luce, the theory is not relevant to rating data, and no inferences can legitimately be made in this respect. (The only "response axiom" is T2, which concerns itself specifically with the response probabilities in the yes/no paradigm.) If rating scale data are to be predicted by the theory, a new axiom is required. There are various candidates, one of which is briefly considered in 10.15. There are two reasons for including such a discussion in this chapter: to show by a counterexample that the argument against the two-state theory based on the curvature of the ROC curve implied by the data does not apply and to demonstrate the general vulnerability of two-state theories to a particular type of analysis of the data.

10.15. Additional axiom.   Following Krantz (1969), we assume that the rating given by a subject on a trial only depends on the sensory state evoked by the stimulation. However, the exact value of the rating is not determined by the state. Instead, a particular distribution of the ratings is associated with each of the two sensory states corresponding to the events $\mathbf{D} = 1$ and $\mathbf{D} = 0$. In other terms, denoting by $\mathbf{R}$ the rating random variable, we have the following axiom:

Rating Axiom T3.   With $i = 0, 1, \ldots, m$ denoting the rating value, $\mathbf{D} = 0, 1$ and $\mathbf{S} = s, n$

$$\mathbb{P}\{\mathbf{R} \leqslant i \,|\, \mathbf{D}, \mathbf{S}\} = G_{\mathbf{D}}(i),$$

independent of $\mathbf{S}$.

Thus, $G_{\mathbf{D}}$ is the distribution function of the ratings while the subject is in state $\mathbf{D}$, irrespective of the stimulation. As earlier in this chapter, we use the abbreviation

$$\mathbb{P}\{\mathbf{R_S} \leqslant i\} = \mathbb{P}\{\mathbf{R} \leqslant i | \mathbf{S}\}$$

and we derive the prediction for the ROC curve. For $\mathbf{S} = s, n$ we have

$$\mathbb{P}\{\mathbf{R_S} \leqslant i\} = \mathbb{P}\{\mathbf{R_S} \leqslant i | \mathbf{D} = 1\} \mathbb{P}\{\mathbf{D} = 1 | \mathbf{S}\}$$
$$+ \mathbb{P}\{\mathbf{R_S} \leqslant i | \mathbf{D} = 0\} \mathbb{P}\{\mathbf{D} = 0 | \mathbf{S}\}$$
$$= G_1(i)q(\mathbf{S}) + G_0(i)[1 - q(\mathbf{S})],$$

by T1 and T3. For the two cases $\mathbf{S} = s$ and $\mathbf{S} = n$, we obtain thus

$$\mathbb{P}\{\mathbf{R}_s \leqslant i\} = q(s)G_1(i) + [1 - q(s)]G_0(i), \tag{28}$$

$$\mathbb{P}\{\mathbf{R}_n \leqslant i\} = q(n)G_1(i) + [1 - q(n)]G_0(i). \tag{29}$$

Eliminating $G_1(i)$ in these two equations and solving for $\mathbb{P}\{\mathbf{R}_s > i\}$, with $i = 1, 2, \ldots, m - 1$, yields the following prediction for the ROC curve:

$$\mathbb{P}\{\mathbf{R}_s > i\} = \mathbb{P}\{\mathbf{R}_n > i\}q(s)/q(n) - [1 - G_0(i)][q(s) - q(n)]/q(n). \tag{30}$$

Notice that the ROC function defined by (30) depends on G_0, and need not yield an ROC curve made of two segments of straight lines. The model is, in fact, quite flexible as far as the ROC rating data are concerned (Exercise 8).

10.16. A critical test of the threshold theory.   On the other hand, it is doubtful that this particular version of the two-state theory is viable, since it makes extremely strong predictions concerning some other aspect of the rating data. Using an argument of Falmagne (1968), Vorberg (Note 3) points out that the observed distributions of the ratings should satisfy a very constraining fixed point property. This property stems from the fact that, as indicated by (28) and (29), the distribution of ratings for $\mathbf{S} = s$ or $\mathbf{S} = n$ is a "mixture" of the two latent distributions G_1 and G_0, in proportion $q(\mathbf{S})$ and $1 - q(\mathbf{S})$, respectively. This property is easily stated in words. Consider the empirical histograms of ratings obtained for s and n in some situation (e.g, for some payoff matrix θ). Suppose that the histograms "cross" at some rating value j (say the proportions of ratings are not significantly different). Then the histogram of the ratings obtained for any other stimulus s' should have—except for statistical errors—the same proportion of ratings j (see Fig. 10.8). The argument is as follows. Let k_s, k_n, g_0, and g_1 be the probability distributions of $\mathbf{R}_s, \mathbf{R}_n, G_0$, and G_1, respectively. Thus, k_s and k_n idealize the histograms mentioned above. Taking finite differences in (28) and (29) gives

$$k_s(i) = q(s)g_1(i) + [1 - q(s)]g_0(i) \tag{31}$$

and

$$k_n(i) = q(n)g_1(i) + [1 - q(n)]g_0(i). \tag{32}$$

Suppose that $k_s(j) = k_n(j)$ for some rating value j. From (31) and (32), it follows

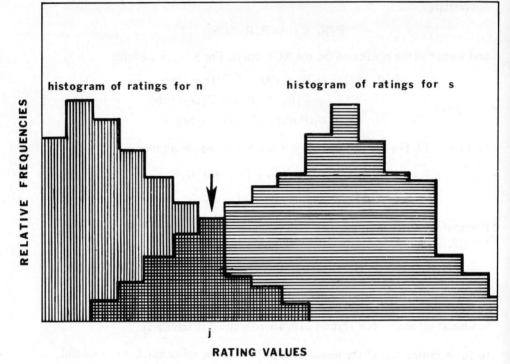

RATING VALUES

FIGURE 10.8. The fixed point property of the 2-state threshold model applied to hypothetical rating scale data. The two histograms have relative frequencies which do not differ significantly at the rating value j. Any other histogram of ratings (say of stimulus s') should have approximately the same relative frequency at the value j.

necessarily that

$$g_1(j) = g_0(j) = k_s(j) = k_n(j).$$

(We assume that $q(n) \neq q(s)$.)

Consequently, if s' is some other stimulus, it must be the case that

$$k_{s'}(j) = q(s')g_1(j) + [1 - q(s')]g_0(j)$$
$$= g_1(j)$$
$$= k_s(j) = k_n(j),$$

as asserted.

A GENERAL SIGNAL DETECTION MODEL

The models discussed in this chapter are special cases of a general signal detection model. This model has no predictive power, but is nevertheless of some interest for classification purposes, and also because its consideration may suggest other special cases.

As usual, we start from a payoff matrix $\{[p_n(\theta), p_s(\theta)]|\theta \in \Theta\}$. The symbols $\mathbf{S}$, $\mathbf{U_S}$, and λ_θ have the same meaning as earlier in this chapter. Let

$$\theta \mapsto \alpha_\theta, \qquad \theta \mapsto \beta_\theta$$

be two functions mapping the set Θ of payoff matrices into the closed interval $[0,1]$.

10.17. Axiom. For $\mathbf{S} = s, n$ and any $\theta \in \Theta$, we have

$$p_\mathbf{S}(\theta) = \mathbb{P}\{\mathbf{U_S} > \lambda_\theta\}\beta_\theta + \mathbb{P}\{\mathbf{U_S} \leqslant \lambda_\theta\}\alpha_\theta.$$

A tree diagram displaying the stages of the detection/decision process symbolized by this axiom is given in Figure 10.9.

A tempting interpretation of this model is as follows. The number λ_θ denotes a neural threshold, the value of which may be affected by the payoff matrix. For example, it is conceivable that the subject might lower λ_θ by decreasing the intensity of the noise in some neural location, a process that may be stressing. Under another name, such a process would be called "selective attention." If $\mathbf{U_S} > \lambda_\theta$, a detection occurs, but this event involves no certainty that a stimulus was actually presented. The subject then gives a "yes" response with a probability β_θ, also depending on the payoff matrix. A similar interpretation can be given of the lower branch of the tree diagram of Figure 10.9.

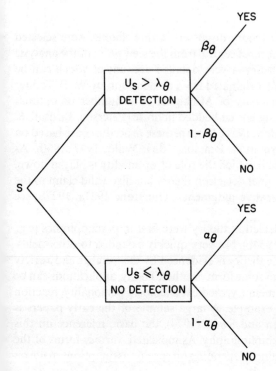

FIGURE 10.9. Tree diagram of the decision process elicited by the stimulation $\mathbf{S} = s,n$ in the general model defined by 10.17.

If it is assumed that $\beta_\theta = 1$ and $\alpha_\theta = 0$, this model reduces to the random variable model of Definition 10.2.

Suppose, on the other hand, that λ is constant. With $S = s, n$, we then write

$$q(S) = \mathbb{P}\{U_s > \lambda\},$$

which yields, by the above axiom

$$p_S(\theta) = q(S)\beta_\theta + [1 - q(S)]\alpha_\theta. \tag{33}$$

Let $\{\Theta_g, \Theta_c\}$ be a partition of the collection Θ of payoff matrices, and assume that

$$\beta_\theta = 1 \qquad \text{iff} \qquad \theta \in \Theta_g,$$

and

$$\alpha_\theta = 0 \qquad \text{iff} \qquad \theta \in \Theta_c.$$

Equation 33 then gives the two cases

$$p_S(\theta) = \begin{cases} q(S) + [1 - q(S)]\alpha_\theta & \text{if } \theta \in \Theta_g, \\ q(S)\beta_\theta & \text{if } \theta \in \Theta_c, \end{cases}$$

a result that is easily shown to be equivalent to the threshold model defined in 10.12.

Other special cases are considered in the exercises.

REFERENCE NOTES

The notions of signal detection theory discussed in this chapter were selected from a vast literature, as being the most central from the view point of the analysis of psychophysical data. This theory, a very detailed account of which can be found in Green and Swets (1974), originated from an adaption by W. P. Tanner and his co-workers at the University of Michigan, of a number of optimal procedures for the detection of signals embedded in noise (Peterson, Birdsall, & Fox, 1954; van Meter & Middleton, 1954). In turn, these procedures are based on statistical decision theory (Neyman & Pearson, 1933; Wald, 1947, 1950). As emphasized by our presentation, in which the role of optimality is played down, the random variable model of signal detection theory has also valid claim to the parentage of the law of comparative judgments (Thurstone 1927a, 1927b; see Chapter 5).

The applications of signal detection theory were first in psychophysics (e.g., Tanner & Swets, 1953, 1954a, 1954b), but very quickly extended to other fields. The extraordinary success of the theory is evidenced by the number and variety of the papers in which it is used in some form or other. Today, applications can be found, for instance, in learning, memory, medical diagnosis, personality, reaction time, and skills (vigilance), for example. A large sample of the early papers is collected in Swets (1964). Green and Swets (1974), the basic reference on this topic, contains a very extensive bibliography. As indicated, various forms of the random variable model are obtained depending on specific assumptions made on the distributions of the random variables U_s and U_n. A discussion of these special cases is provided in Egan (1975). Difficulties of the threshold theory are reviewed by Krantz (1969) who also discusses a three-state version of this theory.

EXERCISES

1. Ponder the role of the assumption of independence of the random variables U_s and U_n in Theorem 10.3. Show by a counterexample that this assumption cannot be dropped.
2. Suppose that $\mathscr{U} = (U_s, U_n)$ is a rational random representation of some ROC curve ρ. Let g be a strictly increasing, continuous function mapping $\mathbb{R}$ into $\mathbb{R}$. Under which additional conditions on g is $\mathscr{U}^* = [g(U_s), g(U_n)]$ a differentiable (rational) random representation of ρ?
3. (*Continuation.*) Apply the results of Exercise 2 to the situation in which $g(x) = f_s(x)/f_n(x) = \ell(x)$, the likelihood ratio. What is the criterion of $\mathscr{U}^*$ in such case? Consider in particular the situation in which $\mathscr{U}$ is Gaussian.
4. (*Continuation.*) Let $\mathscr{U}$ and $\mathscr{U}^*$ be as in Exercise 2, and $g = \ell$. Let the stimulus probability π be fixed. Show that if λ is optimal for all payoff matrices θ, then β (as defined by Equation 10) is the criterion of $\mathscr{U}^*$.
5. Show that a Gaussian random representation $\mathscr{U}$ of an ROC curve with parameters μ_s, σ_s, μ_n, and σ_n is rational iff $\sigma_s = \sigma_n$ and $\mu_s > \mu_n$ (cf. Theorem 10.9).
6. Check the derivation of Equations 9 and 10 and of the result $\ell(\lambda_\theta) = \beta_\theta$.
7. Suppose that $\mathbb{P}\{S = s\} = .75$, and let a payoff matrix θ be defined by

$$\gamma_{ss}(\theta) = 3, \qquad \gamma_{sn}(\theta) = -2,$$

$$\gamma_{ns}(\theta) = -1 \qquad \gamma_{nn}(\theta) = 3.$$

   (i) Compute β_θ as defined by Equation 10.
   (ii) Assume that the ROC curve has a Gaussian random representation, with parameters $\mu_s = \sigma_s = \sigma_n = 1$ and $\mu_n = 0$, with a criterion λ, which is optimal for θ and $\pi = .75$. Compute λ_θ.
   (iii) Compute the coordinates of the point $[p_n(\theta), p_s(\theta)]$ of the ROC curve.

8. Check the derivation of Equation 30. Under which conditions on an ROC curve ρ, is a perfect fit of this equation feasible? Are these conditions satisfied by the data displayed in (16)? The parameters of this equation are the ratio $q(s)/q(n)$, and the values $G_0(i)$, $i = 0,\dots,m - 1$. Estimate these parameters in some optimal way with regard to the data of (16).
9. Is there a model for ROC data that is inconsistent with the general model defined by Axiom 10.17? In other words, does Axiom 10.17 put any constraint on the data?
10. Construct, in the style of 10.12, a signal detection model predicting a concave ROC curve made of three segments of straight lines.

11

Psychophysics with Several Variables or Channels

We consider here a number of paradigms and models designed to analyze how a subject integrates the information flowing from several sensory inputs. Examples of how this may arise have been encountered in earlier chapters. In the yes/no paradigm discussed in Chapter 10, for instance, the subject had to detect a stimulus s embedded in a "masking" noise n. The subject's responses were regarded as resulting from some operation combining, on the sensory side, the effect of both s and n on the organism, and on the cognitive side, factors affecting decision making.

Another example, which this chapter treats in some detail, is offered by an auditory detection situation in which a stimulus is presented binaurally. The intensities in the two auditory channels may be manipulated independently, and the resulting performance may be investigated. This chapter discusses this and various other cases.

The word "channel" is frequently used in psychophysics. As far as I know, however, no satisfying, generally accepted definition has been given for this term, even though several have been proposed. Depending on the context, "two channels" may mean that two sensory modalities are involved, or two neurophysiological locations, or two psychophysical variables, or even the same psychophysical variable but with different intensities. For the time being, we advise the reader to use the term "channel" intuitively, and to check any ambitious drive toward rigor or consistency.

A GENERAL MODEL FOR TWO-CHANNEL DETECTION

11.1. The detection of binaural stimuli. In a version of the yes/no paradigm, the stimulus is a binaural 1000 cps tone (a,x) embedded in a masking noise (n,n'). The letters a,x denote the intensities of the stimulus in the left and right auditory channels, respectively; n and n' stand for the intensities of the noise in the two channels. As in the standard yes/no paradigm, the binaural noise (n,n') is presented alone on some proportion of the trials. To evaluate a possible response bias, the experimenter varies the payoff matrix across conditions. (See Chapter 10 for a discussion of payoff matrices.) Let us denote by $p_{ax}(\theta)$ and $p_{nn'}(\theta)$ the probabilities of a correct detection and of a false alarm, respectively, with a payoff matrix θ.[1]

Monaural stimuli are also presented on some trials. Let $p_a(\theta)$ be the probability of detection of a stimulus of intensity a, embedded in a noise n, in the left auditory channel. Let $p_n(\theta)$ be the corresponding probability of a false alarm. With obvious notation, let $p_x(\theta)$ and $p_{n'}(\theta)$ be the probabilities of a "yes" response in the right auditory channel. The (idealized) data can be regarded as made of three ROC curves

$$\rho_{12} = \{[p_{ax}(\theta), p_{nn'}(\theta)] | \theta \in \Theta\} \tag{1}$$

$$\rho_1 = \{[p_a(\theta), p_n(\theta)] | \theta \in \Theta\} \tag{2}$$

$$\rho_2 = \{[p_x(\theta), p_{n'}(\theta)] | \theta \in \Theta\}. \tag{3}$$

This paradigm can easily be transposed to other experimental situations (e.g., binocular perception). An important theoretical problem concerns the relation between these three ROC curves. In particular, a model should provide an explanation for the typical data: the presentation of the stimulus through two channels often determines an improvement of detection performance. For reasons made clear in Chapter 10, this result may be symbolized by the inequality

$$\int_0^1 \rho_{12}(p) \, dp \geqslant \int_0^1 \rho_i(p) \, dp \qquad \text{for} \qquad i = 1, 2. \tag{4}$$

The data in many instances would suggest a strict inequality in (4).

11.2. A random variable model. Extending the random variable model for signal detection defined in 10.2, we assume that the presentation of a stimulus of intensity a in the left auditory channel evokes some activity in a specific neural location, the intensity of which is a sample of a random variable $\mathbf{U}_{1,a}$. Correspondingly, the presentation of x in the right channel generates a sample of a random variable $\mathbf{U}_{2,x}$. On noise-alone trials, samples are taken from two random variables $\mathbf{V}_{1,n}$ and $\mathbf{V}_{2,n'}$, representing the neural activity generated by the masking noises n and n'. We assume that these four random variables are independent. On a trial where the binaural stimulus (a,x) is presented, the information available to the organism is thus a sample of a pair of random variables $(\mathbf{U}_{1,a}, \mathbf{U}_{2,x})$. We suppose that $\mathbf{U}_{1,a}$ and $\mathbf{U}_{2,x}$ are combined or pooled in some way, resulting in a random variable

$$\mathbf{Q}_{ax} = F(\mathbf{U}_{1,a}, \mathbf{U}_{2,x}),$$

where F is a real-valued function of two real variables, which we suppose to be continuous and increasing in each of its variables. The subject reports a detection if $\mathbf{Q}_{ax}$ exceeds a criterion λ_θ, the value of which depends in general on the payoff

---

1. Our notation is consistent with that of Chapter 10. A more explicit, but heavier, notation for these probabilities would have been $p_{ax,nn'}(\theta)$ and $p_{00,nn'}(\theta)$. A similar remark also applies to the notation of the probabilities in the two monaural cases.

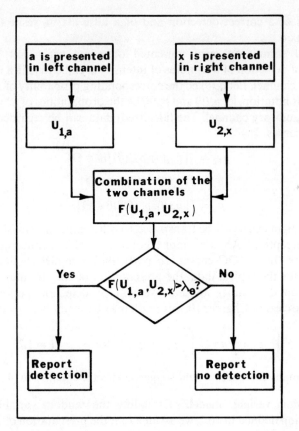

FIGURE 11.1. A general random variable model for the pooling of information from two sensory channels. The cases of the model are obtained by specifying the function F.

matrix θ. These assumptions are illustrated in Figure 11.1, and formalized by the equation

$$p_{ax}(\theta) = \mathbb{P}\{F(\mathbf{U}_{1,a},\mathbf{U}_{2,x}) > \lambda_\theta\} \tag{5}$$

Similar assumptions hold for the binaural noise trials, with the same function F operating on the pair of random variables $(\mathbf{V}_{1,n},\mathbf{V}_{2,n'})$. In the terminology of Definition 10.2, the pair of random variables

$$[F(\mathbf{U}_{1,a},\mathbf{U}_{2,x}), F(\mathbf{V}_{1,n},\mathbf{V}_{2,n'})]$$

is thus a random representation of the ROC curve ρ_{12}, with criterion λ. In the two monaural cases, it is tempting to assume that $(\mathbf{U}_{1,a},\mathbf{V}_{1,n})$ and $(\mathbf{U}_{2,x},\mathbf{V}_{2,n'})$ are random representations of ρ_1 and ρ_2, respectively, with the same criterion λ. These assumptions are summarized in Definition 11.3.

11.3. Definition. Let Θ be a collection of payoff matrices, and let ρ_{12}, ρ_1, and ρ_2 be the three ROC curves defined by (1), (2), and (3). We say then that

$(\mathbf{U}_{1,a},\mathbf{U}_{2,x},\mathbf{V}_{1,n},\mathbf{V}_{2,n'})$ is a *joint random representation of* $(\rho_{12},\rho_1,\rho_2)$, *with pooling function F and criterion* λ, iff the following axioms hold.

1. F is a real-valued, continuous function of two real variables, increasing in each variable and satisfying

$$F(s,t) \geqslant s,t;$$

2. $[F(\mathbf{U}_{1,a},\mathbf{U}_{2,x}), F(\mathbf{V}_{1,n},\mathbf{V}_{2,n'})]$ is a random representation of ρ_{12}.
3. $(\mathbf{U}_{1,a},\mathbf{V}_{1,n})$ is a random representation of ρ_1.
4. $(\mathbf{U}_{2,x},\mathbf{V}_{2,n'})$ is a random representation of ρ_2.
5. All three random representations have the same criterion λ.

Notice that, using successively Axioms 2, 5, 1, 3, and 5 again,

$$p_{ax}(\theta) = \mathbb{P}\{F(\mathbf{U}_{1,a},\mathbf{U}_{2,x}) > \lambda_\theta\} \geqslant \mathbb{P}\{\mathbf{U}_{1,a} > \lambda_\theta\} = p_a(\theta)$$

Clearly, similar inequalities holds for $p_x(\theta)$, and for the false alarm probabilities. We have thus the following simple result.

11.4. Theorem. *Let* ρ_{12}, ρ_1, *and* ρ_2 *be the three ROC curves of Definition 11.3. Suppose that a joint random representation exists. Then, for any payoff matrix*

$$\theta \in \Theta,$$

$$p_{ax}(\theta) \geqslant p_a(\theta), p_x(\theta) \tag{6}$$

and

$$p_{nn'}(\theta) \geqslant p_n(\theta), p_{n'}(\theta). \tag{7}$$

Equations 6 and 7 bear some superficial resemblance to Equation 4. It must be clear, however, that these equations do not necessarily signify an improvement in performance. Actually, the axioms defining a joint random representation are not sufficient to obtain Equation 4. The same remark applies to the "probability summation" model described in the next section (see Exercise 1).

Several particular cases of the random variable model will be discussed, corresponding to special forms of the pooling function F of Definition 11.3.

PROBABILITY SUMMATION

This heading covers a class of models in which the increase of the detection rate resulting from having the stimulation delivered to two or more channels is attributed to chance alone. For an analogy, consider a group of N observers watching the same visual display. Suppose that the probability p of detecting a faint stimulus is the same for all observers, and that the group reports a detection if at least one of the N observers claims to have detected the stimulus. Assuming that the observers responses are independent, the detection probability of the group is

$$1 - (1 - p)^N \geqslant p.$$

The application of that idea in psychophysics can be traced back to Pirenne (1943), and plays an important role in current theorizing, especially in visual perception. We limit our discussion to a two-channel situation. We hasten to say that, despite its intuitive appeal, this analogy will not necessarily lead to a model formalizing an improvement of performance (in the sense of Equation 4, for instance). Indeed, the proportion of false alarms resulting from having N observers pooling their observations as above will also increase.

In any event, in the random variable model, this notion leads to the assumption that the subject reports a detection if at least one of the two activation random variables exceeds the threshold λ_θ. (Sometimes different criteria are postulated for the two channels. This assumption seems more general. See Remark 11.8(1), however.)

11.5. Definition.   A joint random representation with pooling function F is a *probability summation model* iff

$$F(s,t) = \max \{s,t\},$$

in which "max" stands for the maximum in the set of numbers $\{s,t\}$. (Thus $\max \{s,t\} = s$ iff $s \geqslant t$.) Using the assumption of independence of the random variables, we obtain, for the hit probabilities, with familiar notation,

$$
\begin{aligned}
p_{ax}(\theta) &= \mathbb{P}\{\max \{\mathbf{U}_{1,a},\mathbf{U}_{2,x}\} > \lambda_\theta\} \\
&= 1 - \mathbb{P}\{\lambda_\theta \geqslant \max \{\mathbf{U}_{1,a},\mathbf{U}_{2,x}\}\} \\
&= 1 - \mathbb{P}\{\lambda_\theta \geqslant \mathbf{U}_{1,a}, \lambda_\theta \geqslant \mathbf{U}_{2,x}\} \\
&= 1 - \mathbb{P}\{\lambda_\theta \geqslant \mathbf{U}_{1,a}\}\mathbb{P}\{\lambda_\theta \geqslant \mathbf{U}_{2,x}\},
\end{aligned}
\tag{8}
$$

yielding

$$p_{ax}(\theta) = 1 - [1 - p_a(\theta)][1 - p_x(\theta)]. \tag{9}$$

This equation can also be written

$$p_{ax}(\theta) = p_a(\theta) + p_x(\theta)[1 - p_a(\theta)],$$

which shows that (9) is indeed a special case of (6). For the false alarm probabilities, a similar derivation gives

$$p_{nn'}(\theta) = 1 - \mathbb{P}\{\lambda_\theta \geqslant \mathbf{V}_{1,n}\}\mathbb{P}\{\lambda_\theta \geqslant \mathbf{V}_{2,n'}\}, \tag{10}$$

and thus

$$p_{nn'}(\theta) = 1 - [1 - p_n(\theta)][1 - p_{n'}(\theta)] \tag{11}$$

as a special case of (7).

11.6. Remarks on empirical testing.   Of the assumptions used in the above derivations, two are critical. One is that of the independence of the random variables. The other is that of the equality of the criterion, for a given payoff matrix, between the binaural case and the monaural cases. These assumptions render the model testable. Indeed, any stimulus pair (a,x) and noise pair (n,n')

yields four monaural probabilities and two binaural probabilities, to be explained by four parameters. This leads to a standard chi-square (or likelihood ratio) test with $6 - 4 = 2$ degrees of freedom. For (implicitly) fixed θ, (9) or (11) have, in fact, been tested by a number of authors, with mixed results. It is not clear that, at this level of generality, the predictions of the model are sufficiently constraining to be rejected convincingly by the available data. The negative evidence, some of which is reviewed by Blake and Fox (1973), is mostly circumstantial (by which I mean that it has no direct bearing on the predictions formally derivable from the assumptions).

We can also use a stronger version of the invariance assumption concerning the criterion: for a given payoff matrix θ, the criterion λ_θ is constant over conditions varying the intensities of the stimuli a and x, and of the noises n and n'. This assumption is frequently made (explicitly or not). It lends itself to an empirical test similar to the one we just described.

The standard measurement techniques of signal detection theory, such as the estimation of the area under the ROC curve, are not used here. In fact signal detection theory was introduced explicitly to deal with situations in which an assumption such as the strong criterion invariance does not hold.

To sum up, a rejection of this model could be attributed to a one of several possibilities, particularly (i) a failure of the invariance assumption on the criterion (ii) a failure of the independence assumption or (iii) a failure of the assumption concerning the form of the pooling function, $F(s,t) = \max\{s,t\}$.

11.7. Distributional assumptions: A special case. The model can be strengthened in a different way, by making specific assumptions concerning the distributions of the random variables. There are obviously numerous possibilities. The particular case discussed here is meant as an illustration, chosen in view of the relative simplicity of the developments. The analysis of the data will be in the framework of signal detection theory.

Our aim is to derive an explicit expression for the ROC curve in the binaural situation, involving parameters that also determine the ROC curves in the monaural situations. We begin by assuming that each of the four activation random variables has a logistic distribution, that is,

$$\mathbb{P}\{\mathbf{U}_{1,a} \leqslant \lambda_\theta\} = \left\{1 + \left[\exp\left(\frac{\lambda_\theta - \mu_{1,a}}{\beta_{1,a}}\right)\right]^{-1}\right\}^{-1}.$$

with a similar equation for the three other cases. We recall that $E(\mathbf{U}_{1,a}) = \mu_{1,a}$ and $\mathrm{Var}(\mathbf{U}_{1,a}) = \beta_{1,a}^2 \pi^2/3$ (Johnson & Kotz, 1970).

Assume that $\beta_{1,n} = \beta_{2,n'}$. Without loss of generality, we can set

$$\mu_{1,n} = 0 \quad \text{and} \quad \beta_{1,n} = \beta_{2,n'} = 1.$$

Dropping θ in the notation, Equation 10 becomes

$$p_{nn'} = 1 - [1 + \exp(-\lambda)]^{-1}\{1 + \exp[-(\lambda - \mu_{2,n'})]\}^{-1}$$

$$= 1 - \exp(2\lambda - \mu_{2,n'})[1 + \exp(\lambda) + \exp(\lambda - \mu_{2,n'}) + \exp(2\lambda - \mu_{2,n'})]^{-1}.$$

This is a quadratic equation in $t = e^{\lambda}$. Only one solution is acceptable however, yielding

$$t(p_{nn'}, \mu_{2,n'}) = [1 + e^{-\mu_{2,n'}} + D^{1/2}][2e^{-\mu_{2,n'}}p_{nn'}/(1 - p_{nn'})]^{-1},$$

$$D = (1 + e^{-\mu_{2,n'}})^2 + 4e^{-\mu_{2,n'}}p_{nn'}/(1 - p_{nn'}).$$

To obtain the equation of the ROC curve in the binaural situation (p_{ax} as a function of $p_{nn'}$), it suffices to replace $\lambda = \ln t$ in (8) by its expression above. We have, with $\mu = \ln \gamma$,

$$\mathbb{P}\{\mathbf{U}_{1,a} \leqslant \lambda\} = \{1 + \exp[-(\lambda - \mu_{1,a})/\beta_{1,a}]\}^{-1}$$
$$= \{1 + \exp[-(\ln t(p_{nn'}, \mu_{2,n'}) - \ln \gamma_{1,a})/\beta_{1,a}]\}^{-1}$$
$$= \{1 + [\gamma_{1,a}/t(p_{nn'}, \mu_{2,n'})]^{1/\beta_{1,a}}\}^{-1}.$$
$$= G(p_{nn'}, \mu_{2,n'}, \gamma_{1,a}, \beta_{1,a}),$$

the last equation defining the function G. Similarly,

$$\mathbb{P}\{\mathbf{U}_{2,x} \leqslant \lambda\} = \{1 + [\gamma_{2,x}/t(p_{nn'}, \mu_{2,n'})]^{1/\beta_{2,x}}\}^{-1}$$
$$= G(p_{nn'}, \mu_{2,n'}, \gamma_{2,x}, \beta_{2,x}).$$

We obtain thus, for the equation of the ROC curve,

$$p_{ax} = 1 - G(p_{nn'}, \mu_{2,n'}, \gamma_{1,a}, \beta_{1,a})G(p_{nn'}, \mu_{2,n'}, \gamma_{2,x}, \beta_{2,x}),$$

a function depending on five parameters $\gamma_{1,a}$, $\gamma_{2,x}$, $\beta_{1,a}$, $\beta_{2,x}$, and $\mu_{2,n}$. These parameters also explain the two ROC curves in the two monaural cases. It can, of course, be checked whether $\beta_{1,a} = \beta_{2,x} = 1$ fits the data, which would reduce to three the number of parameters used to predict the three ROC curves.

11.8. Remarks. (1) As exemplified above, the probability summation model defined by Equations 8 to 11 takes different forms depending on specific assumptions regarding the distributions of the random variables. The arbitrariness of the choice of the distributions should not be cause of excessive concern (cf. Remark 10.4(1)). Indeed, suppose that a particular version of the model involves the four random variables $\mathbf{U}_{1,a}$, $\mathbf{U}_{2,x}$, $\mathbf{V}_{1,n}$, and $\mathbf{V}_{2,n'}$. Nothing changes in the predictions if these random variables are subjected to a real, strictly increasing, continuous transformation, provided that this transformation is the same for all four random variables. For example, let g be any strictly increasing, continuous, real-valued function on $\mathbb{R}$. We have, clearly,

$$\mathbb{P}\{\max\{\mathbf{U}_{1,a}, \mathbf{U}_{2,x}\} \geqslant \max\{\mathbf{V}_{1,n}, \mathbf{V}_{2,n'}\}\}$$
$$= \mathbb{P}\{g(\max\{\mathbf{U}_{1,a}, \mathbf{U}_{2,x}\} \geqslant g\{\max\{\mathbf{V}_{1,n}, \mathbf{V}_{2,n'}\}\}$$
$$= \mathbb{P}\{\max\{g(\mathbf{U}_{1,a}), g(\mathbf{U}_{2,x})\} \geqslant \max\{g(\mathbf{V}_{1,n}), g(\mathbf{V}_{2,n'})\}\}.$$

Thus, the prediction for the area under the ROC curve is invariant under the transformation g. (Actually, the exact form of the ROC curve is unaffected by the transformation; see Exercise 3.) Notice that this relative "robustness" of the predictions with regard to particular assumptions on the distributions cannot be extended to some other forms of the pooling function. Two examples of such pooling functions are briefly considered in the next section.

(2) As specified by Equations 8 to 11, probability summation assumes that the same criterion value λ_θ is used for both channels. According to (8) for example, a "yes" response occurs following the presentation of a stimulus (a,x) if

$$\text{either} \qquad \mathbf{U}_{1,a} \geqslant \lambda_\theta \qquad \text{or} \qquad \mathbf{U}_{2,x} \geqslant \lambda_\theta.$$

Occasionally (e.g., Nachmias, 1981), a model is used in which (8) and (10) are replaced by the forms

$$p_{ax}(\theta) = 1 - \mathbb{P}\{\lambda_{\theta,1} \geqslant \mathbf{U}_{1,a}\}\mathbb{P}\{\lambda_{\theta,2} \geqslant \mathbf{U}_{2,x}\}, \tag{12}$$

$$p_{nn'}(\theta) = 1 - \mathbb{P}\{\lambda_{\theta,1} \geqslant \mathbf{V}_{1,n}\}\mathbb{P}\{\lambda_{\theta,2} \geqslant \mathbf{V}_{2,n'}\}. \tag{13}$$

Thus, for a given payoff matrix θ, the criterion values $\lambda_{\theta,1}$ and $\lambda_{\theta,2}$ corresponding to the two channels may be different. The extra generality is only apparent, however. This may be understood as follows. Let Θ be the set of all payoff matrices. We assume thus that there are two functions $\theta \mapsto \lambda_{\theta,1}$ and $\theta \mapsto \lambda_{\theta,2}$, each of which maps Θ onto a real interval. It is reasonable to suppose that, even though these functions may be different, they generate the same order on the set Θ of all payoff matrices. That is, for any two θ and θ' in Θ, we have

$$\lambda_{\theta,1} < \lambda_{\theta',1} \qquad \text{iff} \qquad \lambda_{\theta,2} < \lambda_{\theta',2}$$

By a simple mathematical argument, this means that there exists a continuous, strictly increasing function g such that $g(\lambda_{\theta,2}) = \lambda_{\theta,1}$. But then (12) implies

$$\begin{aligned} p_{ax}(\theta) &= 1 - \mathbb{P}\{\mathbf{U}_{1,a} \leqslant \lambda_{\theta,1}\}\mathbb{P}\{g(\mathbf{U}_{2,x}) \leqslant g(\lambda_{\theta,2})\} \\ &= 1 - \mathbb{P}\{\mathbf{U}_{1,a} \leqslant \lambda_{\theta,1}\}\mathbb{P}\{g(\mathbf{U}_{2,x}) \leqslant \lambda_{\theta,1}\}. \end{aligned}$$

Similarly, (13) yields

$$p_{nn'}(\theta) = 1 - \mathbb{P}\{\mathbf{V}_{1,n} \leqslant \lambda_{\theta,1}\}\mathbb{P}\{g(\mathbf{V}_{2,n'}) \leqslant \lambda_{\theta,1}\}.$$

Thus, after transforming $\mathbf{U}_{2,x}$ into $g(\mathbf{U}_{2,x})$ and $\mathbf{V}_{2,n'}$ into $g(\mathbf{V}_{2,n'})$, the criteria are identical for both channels. We conclude that the two models are equivalent. Obviously, the distributional forms of $\mathbf{U}_{2,x}$ and $\mathbf{V}_{2,n'}$ may be modified by the transformation. For example, if both $\mathbf{U}_{2,x}$ and $\mathbf{V}_{2,n'}$ are normal, then $g(\mathbf{U}_{2,x})$ and $g(\mathbf{V}_{2,n'})$ are normal only if g is a linear function. This means that if particular forms of distributions are imposed by the model, the above equivalence does not necessarily hold.

(3) The notion of probability summation is often formalized differently (e.g. Nachmias, 1981), in terms of a two-state threshold model similar to that of Luce (1960, 1963a, 1963b), which we discussed in Chapter 10. This model is defined by the two equations

$$p_{ax}(\theta) = 1 - (1 - p_{1,a})(1 - p_{2,x})[1 - \gamma(\theta)] \tag{14}$$

$$p_{nn'}(\theta) = 1 - (1 - p_{1,n})(1 - p_{2,n'})[1 - \gamma(\theta)], \tag{15}$$

and is sometimes referred as the *high threshold* model. In (14), $p_{1,a}$ and $p_{2,x}$ are two parameters specifying the probabilities, when stimulus (a,x) is presented, that the threshold is exceeded in at least one of the two channels. A "yes" response may also result from a guess, in a case in which neither of the two thresholds is exceeded. The probability of this positive guess is $\gamma(\theta)$, the value of which may vary with the payoff matrix. A similar interpretation holds for (15), which corresponds to the noise trials and introduces two additional parameters $p_{1,n}$ and $p_{2,n'}$.

The popularity of this model is difficult to justify, since it makes the unescapable, but unlikely, prediction that the ROC curves in the binaural situation are straight lines (Exercise 4). For visual contrast detection data, this model was rejected convincingly by Nachmias (1981) in the framework of particular assumptions on the parameters $p_{1,a}$, $p_{2,x}$, $p_{1,n}$, and $p_{2,n'}$.

A discussion of probability summation can be found in Watson (1984).

TWO ADDITIVE POOLING RULES

For the same two-channel paradigm, we consider here two other possibilities for the form of the pooling function F in the general model defined in 11.3. In both cases, we assume that the distributions of all the random variables are Gaussian.

11.9. An additive, equal variance, Gaussian model. Suppose that $(U_{1,a}, U_{2,x}, V_{1,n}, V_{2,n'})$ is a joint random representation of the triple of ROC curves $(\rho_{12}, \rho_1, \rho_2)$ in the sense of Definition 11.3, and that the pooling function F is a binary addition, that is,

$$F(s,t) = s + t.$$

The area under the ROC curve ρ_{12} becomes

$$\mathbb{P}\{U_{1,a} + U_{2,x} > V_{1,n} + V_{2,n'}\}. \tag{16}$$

Let $\mu_{1,a}$, $\mu_{2,x}$, $\mu_{1,n}$, and $\mu_{2,n'}$ be the expectations of these random variables, and suppose that their common variance is equal to 1. Assume, moreover, that all four random variables are normally distributed. From (16), we obtain

$$\mathbb{P}\{U_{1,a} + U_{2,x} - V_{1,n} - V_{2,n'} > 0\} = \Phi[(\mu_{1,a} + \mu_{2,x} - \mu_{1,n} - \mu_{2,n'})/2]$$
$$= \Phi(d'_{12}/\sqrt{2}).$$

The last equation defines a detectability index for the two-channel situation consistent with that introduced in 10.10 for the one-channel situation. Let d'_1 and d'_2 be the detectability indices of ρ_1 and ρ_2, respectively. That is,

$$\mathbb{P}\{U_{1,a} > V_{1,n}\} = \Phi[(\mu_{1,a} - \mu_{1,n})/\sqrt{2}]$$
$$= \Phi(d'_1/\sqrt{2}),$$
$$\mathbb{P}\{U_{2,x} > V_{2,n'}\} = \Phi[(\mu_{2,x} - \mu_{2,n'})/\sqrt{2}]$$
$$= \Phi(d'_2/\sqrt{2}).$$

By simple algebra, it follows that

$$d'_{12} = (d'_1 + d'_2)/\sqrt{2}, \tag{17}$$

a prediction that can be tested by methods discussed in Chapter 10. Notice that Axiom 5 in Definition 11.3 (the three random representations of the ROC curves ρ_{12}, ρ_1, and ρ_2 have the same criterion), was not used to obtain (17).

It is worth remarking that Equation 17 does not imply Equation 4. In other words, the model described here does not necessarily formalize an improvement in performance. We leave to the reader to establish this fact (see Exercise 12.)

11.10. The integration model.   (See Green & Swets, 1974.) Let f_{ax} be the joint density of $U_{1,a}$ and $U_{2,x}$, and let $f_{nn'}$ be the joint density of $V_{1,n}$ and $V_{2,n'}$. Let $f_{1,a}, f_{2,x}, f_{1,n}$, and $f_{2,n'}$ be the densities of $U_{1,a}, U_{2,x}, V_{1,n'}$, and $V_{2,n'}$, respectively. As in 10.5, we suppose that the subject behaves as a statistician and bases his or her decision on the computation of a likelihood ratio. In other terms, we assume that the pooling function F has the form

$$F(s,t) = \frac{f_{ax}(s,t)}{f_{nn'}(s,t)} \tag{18}$$

$$= f_{1,a}(s)f_{2,x}(t)/f_{1,n}(s)f_{2,n'}(t),$$

by the independence of the random variables. This leads to

$$p_{ax}(\theta) = \mathbb{P}\{f_{1,a}(U_{1,a})f_{2,x}(U_{2,x})/f_{1,n}(U_{1,a})f_{2,n'}(U_{2,x}) > \lambda_\theta\}$$

and

$$p_{nn'}(\theta) = \mathbb{P}\{f_{1,a}(V_{1,n})f_{2,x}(V_{2,n'})/f_{1,n}(V_{1,n})f_{2,n'}(V_{2,n'}) > \lambda_\theta\}.$$

Green and Swets (1974, p. 271) show that if all four random variables are Gaussian and that

$$\text{Var}(U_{1,a}) = \text{Var}(V_{1,n}),$$

$$\text{Var}(U_{2,x}) = \text{Var}(V_{2,n'}),$$

then

$$d'_{12} = [(d'_1)^2 + (d'_2)^2]^{1/2}, \tag{19}$$

a special case of Equation 4.

Applications of this model to visual perception data are discussed in Kristofferson and Dember (1958) and Green and Swets (1974). Another combination rule,

$$d'_{12} = d'_1 + d'_2$$

is also considered there.

ADDITIVE CONJOINT MEASUREMENT—
THE ALGEBRAIC MODEL

A central notion in a number of models encountered in this book is that the sensory system of the subject, when confronted with a multidimensional stimulus, performs a simple operation akin to one of arithmetic, such as addition, multiplication, subtraction, etc. Often, this operation is at the kernel of a process modeling other aspects of the subject's performance (e.g., probabilistic, cognitive). The analysis of such operations, to the extent that they are used to model fundamental aspects of scientific data, is the concern of measurement theory, an introduction to which was given in Chapters 1 and 2. This section discusses an important special case, in which the effect on the organism of a two-dimensional stimulus (a,x) is captured by the addition of two numbers

$$f(a) + g(x).$$

11.11. The task and the representation.   Consider a 2AFC paradigm. On each trial, the subject is presented with two stimuli (a,x) and (b,y). For concreteness suppose that, as earlier in this chapter, these stimuli are pairs of intensities of a pure tone presented binaurally.

Thus, a and b denote the intensities of the tone in the left auditory channel, and x and y are the intensities in the right auditory channel. The subject is asked which of (a,x) and (b,y) seems loudest. If (b,y) is not chosen, the experimenter writes

$$by \lesssim ax$$

as the data for the trial. It is assumed that the effect of component a of stimulus (a,x) can be represented by some number, denoted by $f(a)$. Similarly, the effect of component x is represented by a number $g(x)$. If one wishes, these numbers can be interpreted as representing the intensities of the activations induced by the stimulus in some neural location. The model, however, is noncommital in that respect. The basic assumption is that

$$by \lesssim ax \qquad \text{iff} \qquad f(b) + g(y) \leqslant f(a) + g(x). \tag{20}$$

This model is in the spirit of those discussed in the last section, except that, somewhat unrealistically, it is deterministic: the presentation of (a,x) always results in evoking the same number $f(a) + g(x)$. (By comparison, in the model of 11.9, each presentation of (a,x) determines a sample of the random variable $U_{1,a} + U_{2,x}$.) This implies that each presentation of a pair of stimuli (a,x) and (b,y) results in the same choice by the subject, a prediction that may be reasonable for some carefully selected set of stimuli, but would certainly not be acceptable in general. It is not assumed that the numbers $f(a)$, $g(x)$, $f(b)$, etc. are accessible to direct investigation.

11.12. Some necessary conditions.   It is clear that $\lesssim$ must be a weak order (i.e. a transitive and connected relation; cf. 1.14). Beyond that, it may not be immediately obvious that this model imposes strong constraints on the data. But it does. Suppose indeed that the experimenter observes

$$bz \lesssim ay \quad \text{and} \quad cy \lesssim bx.$$

According to the model, this can arise only if

$$f(b) + g(z) \leqslant f(a) + g(y)$$

and

$$f(c) + g(y) \leqslant g(b) + g(x).$$

Adding these two inequalities and canceling appropriately yields

$$f(c) + g(z) \leqslant f(a) + g(x),$$

which in turn predicts that

$$cz \lesssim ax.$$

Summarizing this argument, we see that the model specified by (20) holds only if

whenever $bz \lesssim ay$ and $cy \lesssim bx$, then $cz \lesssim ax$.

In the measurement literature, this condition is known as the (*algebraic*) *double cancellation condition*. The term "double cancellation condition" was actually used in Chapter 6 to capture essentially the same property, but in the probabilistic framework of psychometric functions. This condition is illustrated in the following diagram.

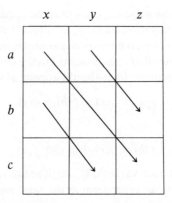

Additionally, a pair of *independence conditions* are easily shown to be necessary:

1. $ax \lesssim bx$ iff $ay \lesssim by$.
2. $ax \lesssim ay$ iff $bx \lesssim by$.

The double cancellation condition and the two independence conditions are the key axioms of a system that, measurement theory tells us, implies the existence of the two scales f and g satisfying (20). As indicated, the deterministic nature of this model limits its application to psychophysical data, and we will not enter into technical details (see e.g., Roberts, 1979; or Krantz et al., 1971). It suffices it to remember that if the data are to be explained by (20), then the double cancellation and the independence conditions must be satisfied.

An experimental test of these conditions in binaural perception can be found in a paper by Levelt, Riemersma, and Bunt (1972). However, Levelt et al.'s positive conclusions have recently (and rightly, in the opinion of this writer) been challenged by Gigerenzer and Strube (1983).

The appeal of measurement models of this kind is that they offer the possibility of getting at what many consider to be the essential determinants of the subject's performance: the scale(s) transforming the physical inputs into sensory intensities, and the basic operation(s) performed by the sensory system. A serious weakness of such models is that they are ill equipped to deal with the data variability that characteristically results from psychophysical experimentation. In the next two sections, we discuss some probabilistic versions of the conjoint measurement model considered here.

RANDOM ADDITIVE CONJOINT MEASUREMENT

11.13. The Matching Task. As in the 2AFC paradigm for binaural loudness, the subject is presented at each trial with a binaural stimulus (a,x) followed by another stimulus (b,y). The task is to modify the intensity of b (e.g., by turning a dial) until, by successive approximations, the two binaural stimuli appear equally loud. Typically, this value varies across trials (for fixed a,x, and y).

11.14. The Model. Let us write $U_{xy}(a)$, a random variable, for the final value of b yielding a match. This notation seems appropriate since this value depends on a,x, and y. (The reason for the asymmetry in the notation — x,y as indices and a in parentheses — will become clear in a moment.) In the deterministic framework of additive conjoint measurement, (a,x) should appear as loud as (b,y) iff

$$f(a) + g(x) = f(b) + g(y),$$

or equivalent, iff

$$f(b) = g(x) - g(y) + f(a).$$

If b is replaced by the random variable $U_{xy}(a)$, it seems reasonable to balance the above equation by adding an error term in the right member, which gives

$$f[U_{xy}(a)] = g(x) - g(y) + f(a) + \varepsilon_{xy}(a). \tag{21}$$

The error term $\varepsilon_{xy}(a)$ is assumed to be a random variable with a (uniquely defined) median equal to zero. This model is in the spirit of the additive conjoint measurement model just discussed, but may be applied to noisy data.

Since the scales f and g are unknown and no assumption is made regarding the distributions of the random variables $U_{xy}(a)$ and $\varepsilon_{xy}(a)$, one may ask how (21) is constraining the data. Or in other terms, under which (necessary/sufficient) conditions do scales f and g exist satisfying (21)? It turns out that (21) imposes strong, highly testable constraints on the medians of the random variables $\mathbf{U}_{xy}(a)$. A simple argument demonstrating this fact is given in 11.15.

11.15. Some key necessary conditions. If $\mathbf{T}$ is a random variable having a unique median v, we write $M(\mathbf{T}) = v$. The following fact will be useful: if h is a real, strictly increasing function, then $M[h(\mathbf{T})] = h[M(\mathbf{T})]$. (This follows immediately from the definition of the unique median of T; cf. Exercise 5.) We adopt the abbreviation

$$m_{xy}(a) = M[\mathbf{U}_{xy}(a)],$$

for the median of the matching random variable $\mathbf{U}_{xy}(a)$. Taking medians on both sides of (21) yields

$$M\{f[\mathbf{U}_{xy}(a)]\} = f\{M[\mathbf{U}_{xy}(a)]\} = g(x) - g(y) + f(a),$$

or equivalently

$$m_{xy}(a) = f^{-1}[g(x) - g(y) + f(a)], \tag{22}$$

in which f^{-1} is the inverse of the scale f. From this equation, a number of necessary conditions are easily derived. For example, take any x, y, $z \in X$, and $a \in A$. Successively,

$$\begin{aligned}
f\{m_{xy}[m_{yz}(a)]\} &= g(x) - g(y) + f[m_{yz}(a)] \\
&= g(x) - g(y) + f\{f^{-1}[g(y) - g(z) + f(a)]\} \\
&= g(x) - g(y) + g(y) - g(z) + f(a) \\
&= f[m_{xz}(a)].
\end{aligned}$$

Since f is a one-to-one function, we conclude that

$$m_{xz}(a) = m_{xy}[m_{yz}(a)],$$

whenever all three medians are defined, a condition illustrated in Figure 11.2. We

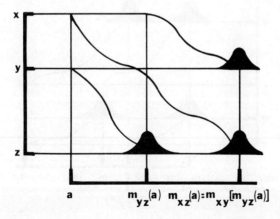

FIGURE 11.2. Cancellation rule. (The three distributions of the figure are those of $\mathbf{U}_{xz}(a)$, $\mathbf{U}_{xy}[m_{yz}(a)]$, and $\mathbf{U}_{yz}(a)$. The three curves are the "isoloudness curves" of (a, x), $[m_{yz}(a), x]$, and (a, y).)

will see that it is the counterpart, in this probabilistic setting, of the (algebraic) double cancellation condition encountered in the last section. It is worth noticing that it only concerns the "observable" medians of the matching random variables (the unknown scales f and g have been eliminated). A further understanding of this condition will be obtained from a discussion, which we give in a moment, of how it can be tested. Another condition of a similar nature is also introduced in Definition 11.16.

11.16. Definition.   Let A,X be   two   real   nondegenerate   intervals.   Let $\mathcal{U} = \{\mathbf{U}_{xy}(a) | x,y \in X, a \in A\}$ be a collection of random variables, with uniquely defined medians

$$m_{xy}(a) = M[\mathbf{U}_{xy}(a)],$$

for all $x,y \in X$ and $a \in A$. Then $\mathcal{U}$ satisfies the *cancellation rule* iff

$$(m_{xy} \circ m_{yz})(a) = m_{xz}(a)$$

whenever both members are defined. The collection $\mathcal{U}$ satisfies the *commutativity rule* iff

$$(m_{xy} \circ m_{zw})(a) = (m_{zw} \circ m_{xy})(a)$$

whenever both members are defined. Since m_{xy}, m_{yx}, and m_{zw} are functions, these two rules can be written more compactly as

$$m_{xy} \circ m_{yz} = m_{xz}$$

and

$$m_{xy} \circ m_{zw} = m_{zw} \circ m_{xy},$$

respectively. The commutatively rule is illustrated in Figure 11.3. The proof that

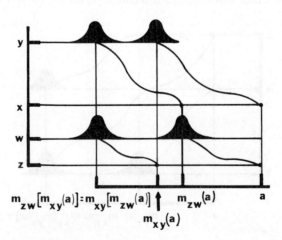

FIGURE 11.3.   Commutativity rule. (The conventions are similar to those of Figure 11.2. The four distributions are those of $\mathbf{U}_{xy}(a)$, $\mathbf{U}_{zw}(a)$, $\mathbf{U}_{xy}[m_{zw}(a)]$, and $\mathbf{U}_{zw}[m_{xy}(a)]$. The four curves are the "isoloudness curves" of (a,x), (a,z), $[m_{zw}(a), x]$, and $[m_{zy}(a), w]$.)

this condition follows from Equation 22 is left to the reader (Exercise 6). It turns out that, in the framework of appropriate side conditions, the cancellation rule implies the commutativity rule (Theorem 11.18) and, moreover, guarantees the existence of the functions f and g satisfying Equation 21. A list of such conditions is given in Definition 11.17.

11.17. Definition. Let A,X be two real nondegenerate intervals. Let $\mathcal{U} = \{U_{xy}(a) \mid x,y \in X, a \in A\}$ be a collection of random variables, with uniquely defined medians. Then $\mathcal{U}$ is a *random structure for additive conjoint measurement* iff for all $x,y \in X$ and $a \in A$ the medians $m_{xy}(a) = M[U_{xy}(a)]$:

1. Are continuous in all three variables.
2. Are strictly increasing in a,X and strictly decreasing in y.
3. Map A into A.
4. Satisfy the cancellation rule.

11.18. Theorem.   *A random structure for additive conjoint measurement satisfies the commutativity rule.*

The proof of this result is fairly long and will be postponed (see 11.29).

11.19. Theorem.   *Suppose that* $\mathcal{U} = \{U_{xy}(a) \mid x,y \in X, \ a \in A\}$ *is a random structure for additive conjoint measurement. Then, there exists two real-valued, continuous, strictly increasing functions* f, g, *respectively defined on* A,X *such that for any* $U_{xy}(a) \in \mathcal{U}$,

$$f[U_{xy}(a)] = g(x) + f(a) - g(y) + \varepsilon_{xy}(a) \tag{23}$$

where $\varepsilon_{xy}(a)$ *is a random variable with a unique median equal to zero. Moreover, if* f^*, g^* *are two other functions satisfying the above conditions, then necessarily*

$$f^* = \alpha f + \beta$$

and

$$g^* = \alpha g + \beta'$$

for some constants $\alpha > 0$, β, *and* β'.

Only a sketch of a proof will be given, the basic idea of which is contained in Theorem 11.20.

11.20. Theorem.   *Suppose that* $\mathcal{U} = \{U_{xy}(a) \mid x,y \in X, \ a \in A\}$ *satisfies all the conditions of a random structure for additive conjoint measurement. Define a relation* $\precsim$ *on* $A \times X$ *by*

$$ax \precsim by \qquad iff \qquad m_{xy}(a) \leqslant b. \tag{24}$$

Then $\precsim$ *is a weak order satisfying the Double Cancellation Condition and the Independence Conditions of 11.12.*

   Proof. The connectedness of $\precsim$ is clear. The cancellation rule implies that, for any $x,y \in X$ and $a \in A$, $(m_{yx} \circ m_{xx})(a) = m_{yx}(a)$. If we assume that $m_{xx}(a) \neq a$, strict monotonicity yields a contradiction. Thus we have $ax \lesssim ax$; that is, $\lesssim$ is reflexive. To show that $\lesssim$ also satisfies double cancellation, suppose that

$$ay \lesssim bz \quad \text{and} \quad bx \lesssim cy.$$

Thus, by definition

$$m_{yz}(a) \leqslant b \quad \text{and} \quad m_{xy}(a) \leqslant c.$$

Using the monotonicity of the function m_{xy}, this implies

$$m_{xy}[m_{yz}(a)] \leqslant m_{xy}(b) \leqslant c$$

and, by the cancellation rule,

$$m_{xz}(a) \leqslant c,$$

that is,

$$ax \lesssim cz.$$

We conclude that double cancellation holds. The rest of the proof ($\lesssim$ is transitive and satisfies the independence conditions of 11.12), is left to the reader. ∎

11.21. Sketch of Proof of Theorem 11.19.   Let $\lesssim$ be the relation defined on $A \times X$ by Formula 24. By Theorem 11.20, $\lesssim$ is a weak order on $A \times X$ satisfying double cancellation and the independence conditions of 11.12 (Exercise 7). It can be shown that the other conditions of an additive conjoint structure in the sense of Krantz et al. (1971, p. 256, Definition 7) also hold. Consequently, there exists real-valued functions f,g respectively defined on A,X such that

$$ax \lesssim by \quad \text{iff} \quad f(a) + g(x) \leqslant f(b) + g(y).$$

In particular, with $m_{xy}(a) = b$, we have

$$f[m_{xy}(a)] = g(x) + f(a) - g(y),$$

which implies that Equation 21 holds. The continuity and monotonicity of the functions f and g follow without difficulty from the axioms. The uniqueness properties of f and g are immediate consequences of Krantz et al.'s theorem. ∎

A complete proof can be found in Falmagne (1976).

11.22. An empirical test of the cancellation rule.   In the framework of the binaural loudness paradigm, such a test could proceed as follows.

Step 1.   Choose one intensity $a \in A$ in the left auditory channel, and three intensities $x,y,z \in X$ in the right auditory channel. Have the subject find an intensity b such that (b,z) matches (a,y) in loudness. Repeat $2p$ times. Order these $2p + 1$ values $b_1 \leqslant b_2 \leqslant \cdots \leqslant b_{2p+1}$. Then b_{p+1} is an estimate of $m_{yz}(a)$.

Step 2.   Have the subject find c such that (c,y) matches (b_{p+1},x). Repeat q times. The obtained empirical distribution is denoted by D.

Step 3. Have the subject find an intensity d, such that (d,z) matches (a,x). Repeat k times. The obtained empirical distribution is denoted by D'.

Step 4. Test whether $U_{xy}(b_{p+1})$ and $U_{xz}(a)$ have the same median by performing a median test comparing D and D'. (This test is known to be reasonably robust to a difference in the shape of the distributions; cf. J. W. Pratt, 1964.)

A similar test can be designed for the cancellation rule. A discussion regarding the soundness of this procedure can be found in Falmagne (1976).

11.23. Application. Gigerenzer and Strube (1983), have applied this model to binaural loudness data. The hypothesis that the two auditory channels are additive in the sense of Equation 21 is convincingly rejected. The data favors a model in which one channel dominates when its intensity sufficiently dominates that of the other.

PROBABILISTIC CONJOINT MEASUREMENT

In a number of papers, Falmagne and his co-workers have investigated another way of injecting statistical considerations into additive conjoint measurement (Falmagne, 1978; Falmagne & Iverson, 1979; Falmagne, Iverson, & Marcovici, 1979, Iverson & Falmagne, 1983).

11.24. A general model. Suppose that, in a 2AFC paradigm, the subject must select one of the two-component stimuli (a,x) and (b,y). As before, we assume that a, b, x, and y denote numbers representing physical intensities. Let $P_{ax,by}$ be the probability that (a,x) is chosen over (b,y). A general additive model is embodied in the equation

$$P_{ax,by} = H[f(a) + g(x), f(b) + g(y)], \tag{25}$$

in which the real-valued functions H, f, and g in the right member are unspecified, except for their monotonicity and continuity properties: all three functions are continuous, H is strictly increasing in the first variable and strictly decreasing in the second variable, and f and g are strictly increasing. We also assume that the function H in (25) satisfies the property

$$H(s,t) = .5 \quad \text{iff} \quad s = t.$$

The connections between this model and that discussed in 11.23 must be appreciated. Consider a situation in which the experimenter, an expert in adaptive methods (cf. Chapter 9), fixes the values of a,x, and y in (25), and induces the subject's performance—say, using stochastic approximation—to converge to a point β satisfying

$$P_{ax,\beta y} = H[f(a) + g(x), f(\beta) + g(y)] = .5 \tag{26}$$

The estimated value of β is actually a random variable, the distribution of which depends on a,x, and y. Using reasonable differentiability assumptions (cf. 9.4), the asymptotic distribution of this random variable is normal, with an expectation equal to β. Let us denote this asymptotic random variable by $\mathbf{U}_{xy}(a)$. Notice that, using (25) and (26),

$$f(a) + g(x) = f(\beta) + g(y)$$

and thus

$$\beta = E[\mathbf{U}_{xy}(a)] = f^{-1}[g(x) + f(a) - g(y)],$$

which is equivalent to the equation (22) constraining the medians, in our discussion of random conjoint measurement. (Indeed, for a normal random variable, the expectation and the median are equal.) The model specified by (25) can thus be tested by checking whether the cancellation and the commutativity rules are satisfied, to an acceptable approximation, by the estimates obtained experimentally for the expectations $E[\mathbf{U}_{xy}(a)]$.

11.25. Special cases. A number of cases of this model are of interest, the defining equations of which are listed below. Note that the function k in (27) is assumed to be continuous and strictly increasing.

$$P_{ax,by} = H\{k[f(a) + g(x)] - k[f(b) + g(y)]\} \tag{27}$$

$$P_{ax,by} = H[f(a) + g(x) - f(b) - g(y)] \tag{28}$$

$$P_{ax,by} = H\left[\frac{f(a) + g(x)}{f(b) + g(y)}\right] \tag{29}$$

$$P_{ax,by} = H[f(a)g(x) - f(b)g(y)] \tag{30}$$

Diagnostic properties distinguishing these models have been developed (Falmagne, 1979). The behavior of the function $a \mapsto P_{ax,bx}$ is particularly instructive in this respect. Assuming that (27) holds, it can be shown, for example (Falmagne et al., 1979), that for $a > b$, the function

$$k \text{ is} \begin{Bmatrix} \text{linear} \\ \text{strictly convex} \\ \text{strictly concave} \end{Bmatrix} \quad \text{iff} \quad P_{ax,bx} \text{ is} \begin{Bmatrix} \text{independent of } x; \\ \text{strictly increasing in } x; \\ \text{strictly decreasing in } x. \end{Bmatrix}$$

Important examples of strictly convex and strictly concave functions are the logarithmic and exponential functions. Observe in this connection that each of (28), (29), and (30) follows from (27) by assuming that k is a linear, logarithmic, or exponential function, respectively. (Obviously, a change of notation vis-à-vis the functions H, f, and g is taking place.)

Falmagne et al. (1979) applied these models to binaural loudness data collected in a series of experiments using the 2AFC paradigm. A special case of (29) was found to yield a good fit (see, however, the results of Gigerenzer & Strube, 1983, mentioned in the last section). More will be said about this study in Chapter 12.

BISECTION

This heading refers to a class of paradigms in which a subject is confronted with a pair (a,b) of stimuli and is required to produce (in a way depending on the particular situation) a stimulus appearing midway between a and b. As stated before in this chapter, a and b are numbers measuring physical intensities. The midway intensity $\mathbf{B}_{ab}$ produced by the subject is assumed to be a random variable taking its values in the same physical scale as a and b. In some situations, the subject may be asked to produce $\mathbf{B}_{ab}$ by manipulating a dial. The midway intensity $\mathbf{B}_{ab}$ may also be obtained by applying an adaptive procedure. This case seems to lead to a more natural treatment of the errors, and will be considered in some detail. We will discuss a model that will eventually lead to a representation of the medians $M(\mathbf{B}_{ab})$ of the random variables $\mathbf{B}_{ab}$ by the equation

$$u[M(\mathbf{B}_{ab})] = [u(a) + u(b)]/2 \tag{31}$$

in which the function u is strictly increasing and differentiable.

11.26. The task. At each trial of an experiment, the subject is presented with three stimuli $c \leqslant b \leqslant a$, and is required to decide which of a and c appears closest to b. It is reasonable to suppose that the subject's choice will not necessarily be the same over repeated presentations of a given triple (a,b,c).

11.27. A model. The basic theoretical notion is the probability P_{abc}, with $c \leqslant b \leqslant a$, that the subject will chose a as closest to b in the set $\{a,c\}$.

An interesting model for such a situation is formalized by the Fechnerian-type equation

$$P_{abc} = H[u(a) - u(b), u(b) - u(c)], \tag{32}$$

in which u is a real-valued, strictly increasing, differentiable function, and H is differentiable, strictly decreasing in the first variable, and strictly increasing in the second variable. Thus, for fixed a and c, the function $b \mapsto P_{abc}$ is differentiable and strictly increasing. As in 11.22, we assume that the function H satisfies

$$H(s,t) = .5 \quad \text{iff} \quad s = t. \tag{33}$$

Suppose that the experimenter is applying a stochastic approximation procedure. For fixed a and c, the procedure induces the value of b in (32) to converge to a point β such that

$$P_{a\beta c} = H[u(a) - u(\beta), u(\beta) - u(c)] = .5. \tag{34}$$

Using (33), this gives

$$u(a) - u(\beta) = u(\beta) - u(c). \tag{35}$$

Using familiar arguments based on the strict monotonicity and differentiability of the function $b \mapsto P_{abc}$ (cf. Chapter 9), we can assert that the estimated value of β is a normally distributed random variable $\mathbf{B}_{ab}$ with an expectation equal to β. Writing $m(a,b)$ for the expectation or the median of B_{ab}, we have $m(a,b) = \beta$, and, from (35),

$$m(a,b) = u^{-1}\{[u(a) + u(b)]/2\} \tag{36}$$

This equation, which occurred in our discussion of functional equations in Chapter 3, is considered here from an axiomatic viewpoint. We show that it puts severe constraint on the medians $m(a,b)$ of the random variables $\mathbf{B}_{ab}$. A simple example is the commutativity equation

$$m(a,b) = m(b,a), \tag{37}$$

which immediately results from (36) by observing that the terms $u(a)$ and $u(b)$ commute in the right member. Equation 36 also implies that m must be *idempotent*; that is, we must have

$$m(a,a) = a \tag{38}$$

for all stimuli a. This follows from the fact that

$$m(a,a) = u^{-1}\{[u(a) + u(a)]/2\} = u^{-1}[u(a)] = a.$$

A less obvious consequence of (36) is the condition

$$m[m(a,b), m(c,d)] = m[m(a,c), m(b,d)] \tag{39}$$

which is often referred to as *bisymmetry*. The easy proof that (36) implies bisymmetry is left to the reader. These implications can be reversed: under general continuity and monotonicity, properties on the median $m(a,b)$ of the random variable $\mathbf{B}_{ab}$ (this median being considered as a function of the two variables a and b), commutativity, idempotency, and bisymmetry together imply the existence of a continuous, strictly increasing function u satisfying (36) (see Krantz et al., 1971). No proof of these facts will be given here.

In some cases, commutativity may not hold. Consider a situation in which a and b are two intensities of a pure tone presented monaurally and successively. It is conceivable (in fact, likely), that the produced midway value will depend on which of a and b is presented first. (For example, the midway operation has to be performed between two stimuli, one of which has to be kept in memory for some time, and is thus subject to the effects of a possible decay.) The idempotency may also fail. In such cases, Equation 36 may be generalised as follows. If bisymmetry and idempotency hold, but not necessarily commutativity, then an appropriate model is

$$m(a,b) = u^{-1}[\alpha u(a) + (1 - \alpha)u(b)], \tag{40}$$

with $\alpha > 0$, a constant. If neither idempotency nor commutativity are assumed to hold, but bisymmetry is satisfied, we have the still more general model

$$m(a,b) = u^{-1}[\alpha u(a) + \gamma u(b) + \delta], \tag{41}$$

with $\alpha > 0, \gamma > 0$. Both of these representations are analyzed in Krantz et al. (1971).

11.28. Applications. An experimental test of bisymmetry in auditory perception is reported in Cross (1965; cited by Coombs, Dawes, & Tversky, 1970). Bypassing such a test, it is also possible to "search" directly for a function u satisfying (36). This is done by Weiss (1975) and Anderson (1976, p. 107; 1981, p. 37). A good fit is obtained for a power function $u(a) = \lambda a^\gamma$. We recall that, by Theorem 3.12, the power function $u(a) = \lambda a^\gamma + \beta$ is one of the two functional forms consistent with both (36) and the homogeneity equation

$$m(\alpha a, \alpha b) = m(a,b)$$

(cf. our discussion of Plateau's experiment in Chapter 3). A discussion of homogeneity laws in psychophysics is contained in the next chapter.

*PROOFS

11.29. Proof of Theorem 11.18. For $x, y \in X$ and $a \in A$, let $m_{xy}(a)$ be the median of $U_{xy}(a)$. Let $K = \{m_{x,y} | x, y \in X\}$.

   Lemma 1. m_{xx} *is the identity on A, for any* $x \in X$.

Indeed, $m_{xx} \circ m_{xx} = m_{xx}$ by the cancellation rule.

   Lemma 2. $(K, \circ)$ *is a group with identity element* m_{xx} *and inverses* $m_{xy}^{-1} = m_{yx}$.

It is straightforward to check that all the conditions are satisfied. The cancellation rule gives the inverses, since it implies, in particular, $m_{xy} \circ m_{yx} = m_{xx}$.
   Define a relation $\precsim$ on K by

$$m_{xy} \precsim m_{zw} \qquad \text{iff} \qquad m_{xy}(a) \leqslant m_{zw}(a)$$

for some $a \in A$.

   Lemma 3. $(K, \precsim)$ *is a simple order (transitive, connected, and antisymmetric; Definition 1.14).*

   Proof. We only have to show that $\precsim$ is well defined. We proceed by contradiction and assume that for some $b < a$,

$$m_{xy}(a) < m_{zw}(a) \qquad \text{and} \qquad m_{zw}(b) \leqslant m_{xy}(b).$$

(The argument is similar if $a \leqslant b$).) Applying m_{wz} on both sides of the above inequalities, we obtain, using Lemma 2,

$$b \leqslant (m_{wz} \circ m_{xy})(b) < (m_{wz} \circ m_{xy})(a) < a.$$

Writing $m = m_{wz} \circ m_{xy}$ leads to

$$b \leqslant m^n(b) \leqslant m^{n+1}(b) < a,$$

which yields

$$\lim_{n \to \infty} m^n(b) = a^* \leqslant a,$$

for some $a^* \in A$. It is easily shown that

$$b \leqslant m^{-1}(a^*) < a.$$

Take some positive integer k such that

$$m^{-1}(a^*) < m^k(b) \leqslant a^*.$$

This gives

$$a^* < m^{k+1}(b),$$

a contradiction.   ■

Lemma 4. $(K, \circ, \leqslant)$ *is an Archimedean, simply ordered group* (*see Exercise* 15 *in Chapter* 2 *for the definition*).

Proof.   All the conditions are immediate, except for the Archimedean, which is obtained by an argument similar to that used in the proof of Lemma 3. Proceeding by contradiction, suppose that

$$m_{xx} < m_{zw}^n < m_{st}$$

for some $x, z, w, s, t \in X$ and all positive integers n. Take $a \in A$ arbitrarily. Then,

$$a < m_{zw}^n(a) < m_{zw}^{n+1}(a) \leqslant m_{st}(a)$$

and thus

$$\lim_{n \to \infty} m_{zw}^n(a) = a^* \leqslant m_{st}(t),$$

for some $a^* \in A$. We have $a \leqslant m_{wz}(a^*) < a^*$, and for some positive integer k,

$$m_{wz}(a^*) < m_{zw}^k(a) \leqslant a^*.$$

which gives

$$a^* = (m_{zw} \circ m_{wz})(a^*) < m_{zw}^{k+1}(a),$$

a contradiction.   ■

By Hölder's theorem (see Exercise 15 in Chapter 2), any Archimedean ordered group is isomorphic to a subgroup of the additive real numbers and is thus commutative. In other terms, for all $x, y, z, w \in X$

$$m_{xy} \circ m_{zw} = m_{zw} \circ m_{xy'}$$

that is, the commutativity rule is satisfied.   ■

EXERCISES

1. Show by a counterexample that a probability summation model (in the sense of Definition 11.5) does not necessarily satisfy Equation 4.
2. Check the details of the derivations for the prediction of the ROC curve obtained in 11.7.

3. In the case where the pooling function F is the maximum function, show that the prediction for the ROC curve is not affected by a strictly increasing, continuous transformation of all four random variables involved (cf. 11.8(1)).

4. Compute the predictions for the ROC curve in the high threshold model (cf. 11.8(3)).

5. Show that if T is a random variable with a uniquely defined median $M(T)$, and h is any real, strictly increasing function, then $h[M(T)] = M[h(T)]$ (cf. 11.14).

6. Show that the commutativity rule follows from Equation 22 (cf. 11.15).

7. Prove that the conditions defining a random structure for additive conjoint measurement (Definition 11.17) imply that the relation $\precsim$ defined by (24) is transitive and satisfies the independence conditions of 11.12 (cf. 11.20, 11.21).

8. While only one model was formulated for algebraic conjoint measurement, embodied in Equation 20, several nonequivalent models were proposed for probabilistic conjoint measurement. Reflect on this discrepancy and propose an explanation.

*9. Find sufficient conditions on the probabilities P_{abc} analyzed in 11.25 for representation (32) to hold, under the stated continuity and monotonicity conditions of the functions u and H. Specify the uniqueness of the functions u and H. Provide proofs of these results. Generalize the results to the representation

$$P_{abc} = H[u(a) - g(b), g(b) - h(c)],$$

with H, u, g, and h, strictly increasing and continuous. (These are unsolved problems.)

10. Show by a counterexample that, in the framework of the other conditions defining a random structure for additive conjoint measurement (Definition 11.17), the commutativity rule does not imply the cancellation rule.

11. Prove that bisymmetry is a necessary condition for Equation 36.

12. Show by a counterexample that Equation 17 does not imply Equation 4. This means that the model defined in 11.9 does not formalize an improvement in performance.

12

Homogeneity Laws[†]

There is a class of empirical laws that deserves a serious consideration by the psychophysicist.[1] Examples of such laws are provided by the two forms of Weber's law encountered in Chapter 8. As specified in 8.9, this law constrains the psychometric functions and takes the form

$$p_{\lambda a}(\lambda x) = p_a(x),$$ (1)

with $\lambda, x > 0$, and a a real vector. In words: the value of a psychometric function is invariant under multiplication of the intensities of the stimulus and the standard by the same constant $\lambda > 0$. Equivalently (Theorem 8.12), Weber's law concerns the Weber functions, and states that

$$\Delta_\pi(\lambda a) = \lambda \Delta_\pi(a).$$ (2)

We recall that a real-valued function f defined on a subset T of a real vector space is called *homogeneous of degree β on T* iff for any real number $\lambda \neq 0$

$$f(\lambda a) = \lambda^\beta f(a)$$

whenever a, $\lambda a \in T$ (see Definition 8.8). In this terminology, (1) states that the function p is homogeneous of degree zero, and (2) states that the Weber function $a \mapsto \Delta_\pi(a)$ is homogeneous of degree one. Plateau's bisection experiment (discussed in Chapter 3) offers still another case of a homogeneous function. Plateau's results were formalized by the equation

$$M(\lambda a, \lambda b) = \lambda M(a,b),$$ (3)

in which λ, a, b are positive real numbers and M is a real-valued, continuous function, strictly increasing in both variables. Thus, M is homogeneous of degree one. The following "averaging" representation was assumed:

$$u[M(a,b)] = \frac{u(a) + u(b)}{2},$$ (4)

[†] Parts of this chapter are based on "Conjoint Weber Laws and Additivity" by Jean-Claude Falmagne and Geoffrey Iverson, *Journal of Mathematical Psychology*, Vol. 20, No. 2, October 1979, Academic Press, Copyright © 1979.

1. Let us avoid both a misunderstanding and a philosophical trap. By "law" I mean here an important equation, purporting to explain a body of data. This equation derives its importance, and thus the label "law," from that of the data to be explained, from the consequences of the equation regarding feasible theories, and possibly also from the simplicity of its form. Scientific usage indicates that complete accuracy of the prediction is not a major requirement (e.g., the failure of Boyle's law at low temperature).

in which u is some unknown continuous, strictly increasing function. It was then shown (Theorem 3.12) that if both (3) and (4) are assumed to hold, then u could only have one of two possible forms

$$u(a) = \alpha a^\gamma + \delta,$$

for some constants α, γ and δ, with $\alpha\gamma > 0$, or

$$u(a) = \alpha \log a + \gamma$$

for some constants $\alpha > 0$ and γ.

Equations 1, 2, and 3 provide examples of homogeneity laws. Other examples will be discussed in this chapter. The importance of such laws is due to a number of factors. Their predictions have a simple form and are easy to test. For reasons that we are beginning to understand (see Chapter 14), they tend to occur with a remarkable regularity not only in psychophysics, but in science in general. Finally, as demonstrated by the results in Plateau's experiment, homogeneity laws typically set very severe constraints on the possible models for a body of data. This chapter discusses a few additional examples in detail.

The results discussed in the next four sections were obtained by Falmagne and Iverson (1979) and Falmagne, Iverson, and Marcovici (1979).

THE CONJOINT WEBER'S LAWS—OUTLINE

Let us go back to the 2AFC paradigm used by Falmagne et al. (1979), and discussed in Chapter 11, in which the subject had to compare two binaural stimuli (a,x) and (b,y). (Thus, a and b are positive real numbers representing the physical intensities of a pure tone in the left auditory channel, and x, y are the intensities of the tone in the right channel.) The basic notion is a probability

$$P_{ax,by}$$

that the subject chooses (a,x) as the loudest stimulus. A test of the following generalization of Weber's law was performed

$$P_{(\lambda a)(\lambda x),(\lambda b)(\lambda y)} = P_{ax,by}. \tag{5}$$

Using the decibel scale, this result can be described by stating that the choice probability is invariant under addition of the same number of decibels to all four intensities. This prediction, which was christened the *conjoint Weber's law*, was found to be well supported by the data, at least for the relatively modest range of stimulus intensities considered in the experiment (see Figure 12.1). The importance of this result from a theoretical standpoint should not be underestimated. Researchers in this field are concerned with the hypothesis that the two auditory channels may be "additive." As indicated in 11.22, a possible formalization of this notion lies in the equation

$$P_{ax,by} = H[f(a) + r(x), f(b) + r(y)], \tag{6}$$

in which all three functions in the right member are unspecified, except for some

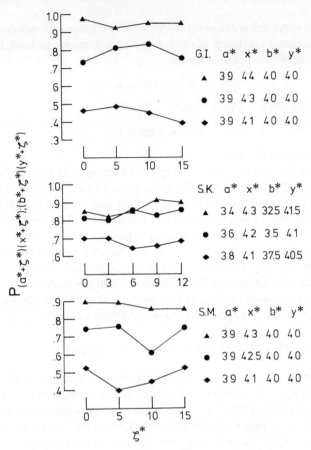

FIGURE 12.1. Summarized data of the three subjects in Experiment 2 of Falmagne, Iverson, and Marcovici (1979). The stimuli were gated 6000-Hz sinusoidal tones, presented binaurally with different intensities in the two auditory channels. The intensities are given in the dB scale. The data were collected and analyzed to test the conjoint Weber's law, which in the dB scale, reads

$$P_{a^*x^*,b^*,y^*} = P_{(a^*+\zeta^*)(x^*+\zeta^*),(b^*+\zeta^*)(y^*+\zeta^*)}.$$

The observed frequencies corresponding to these probabilities are in ordinate. For each subject four values of ζ^* were considered, which are given in abscissa. The prediction is well supported by the data. Note in passing that the first two lines of subject S.M.'s data were generated by two quadruple differing only by .5 dB in the value of x^*. From "Binaural 'Loudness' Summation: Probabilistic Theory and Data" by J.-C. Falmagne, G. Iverson, and S. Marcovici, 1979, *Psychological Review*, 86(1), pp. 25–43. Reprinted with permission of authors and publisher.

natural monotonicity and continuity properties. Falmagne and Iverson (1979) show that if both (6) and the conjoint Weber's law hold, then the choice probabilities must have one of the following three forms

$$P_{ax,by} = G\left(\frac{a^\beta + \delta x^\beta}{b^\beta + \delta y^\beta}\right) \tag{7}$$

$$P_{ax,by} = G\left(\frac{a^\beta x^\gamma}{b^\beta y^\gamma}\right) \tag{8}$$

$$P_{ax,by} = Q\left(\frac{a}{x}, \frac{b}{y}\right) \tag{9}$$

(see Theorem 12.6).

In these equations, β, γ, and $\delta > 0$ are constants, G is strictly increasing and continuous, and Q is continuous, strictly increasing in the first variable, and strictly decreasing in the second variable. These three equations are easy to discriminate experimentally. For examply, (9) can be eliminated immediately as a model for binaural loudness, since it predicts that $P_{ax,by}$ is decreasing in x and increasing in y. A different way of separating these equations leads us two introduce two other homogeneity laws, each of which is a strengthening of the conjoint Weber's law:

$$P_{ax,by} = P_{(\lambda a)(\lambda x),(\tau b)(\tau y)}; \tag{10}$$

$$P_{ax,by} = P_{(\lambda a)(\tau x),(\lambda b)(\tau y)}. \tag{11}$$

These equations are assumed to hold for all positive real numbers a, b, x, y, λ, and τ. These two laws, which we call the *strong conjoint Weber's laws*, provide a sharp method to distinguish between (7), (8), and (9) from an experimental standpoint. In particular, it is not difficult to prove that (9) is equivalent to (10) (Theorem 12.8). It can also be shown that the additive form (6) together with (11) is equivalent to (8) (Theorem 12.11). A useful conclusion follows: if the conjoint Weber's law holds, but both (10) and (11) fail, then (6) is necessarily of the form of equation (7). The details of these and related results, which are due to Iverson and Falmagne (1979), are given in the next three sections.

These examples illustrate how the experimental testing of homogeneity laws (with positive or negative outcomes) may result in a considerable strengthening of the hypotheses of a model.

*THE CONJOINT WEBER'S LAW—RESULTS

12.1. Definition. Let D be an open, convex subset of the real plane; let $(a, x, b, y) \mapsto P_{ax,by}$ be a continuous mapping of D^2 into the closed interval $[0,1]$, strictly monotonic in all four variables, increasing in the first variable, satisfying

$$P_{ax,by} = 1 - P_{by,ax} \tag{12}$$

for all $(a,x), (b,y) \in D$. Then, (D,P) is called a *probabilistic conjoint comparison system*, or more simply, a *system*. Two special cases will be considered.

(i) $D = I^2$ for some nonempty real, open interval I.

(ii) D is a nonempty, positive convex cone.

$V = \{(a,x) | t_- x < a < t_+ x, \text{ for some constants } t_-, t_+ \text{ with } 0 < t_- < 1 < t_+\}$.

In the sequel, these cases will be distinguished by the notation adopted for the system, that is, (I,P) or (V,P). Notice that, by (12), $P_{ax,by}$ is decreasing in b; and increasing in x iff it is decreasing in y. A system (D,P) is called *isotone* iff $P_{ax,by}$ is increasing in x. A system is called *antitone* iff it is not isotone. (Thus, the binaural loudness paradigm offers an example of an isotone system.) A system (D,P) satisfies the *conjoint Weber's law*, or equivalently, *is a conjoint Weber's system*, iff

$$P_{ax,by} = P_{(\lambda a)(\lambda x),(\lambda b)(\lambda y)}$$

holds whenever both members are defined.

We begin with a straightforward characterization of the conjoint Weber systems.

12.2. Theorem.   *Let* (I^2,P) *be a system, with* $I = (0,\alpha)$ *an open interval; then* (I^2,P) *is a conjoint Weber system iff there exists a real-valued function* Q *on* $\mathbb{R}^3_+$, *strictly increasing in the first variable, and strictly decreasing in the third variable, such that*

$$P_{ax,by} = Q(a/x, x/y, b/y) \tag{13}$$

for all a, x, b, $y \in I$. *Moreover,* (I^2,P) *is isotone iff* Q *is increasing in the second variable.*

The proof of this result is straightforward and will be left to the reader (Exercise 2).

All the representations of interest (e.g., Equations 6, 7, 8, and 9) postulate a basic mechanism combining the effects in the two channels, prior to comparing the binaural pairs (a,x) and (b,y). This suggests examining the impact of the conjoint Weber's law on the equation

$$P_{ax,by} = F[g(a,x), g(b,y)]. \tag{14}$$

Thus, the function g plays a role similar to that of the pooling function in Chapter 11.

12.3. Definition.   A system (D,P) is *simply scalable* iff there exists a pair (g,F) of functions satisfying (14) for all $(a,x), (b,y) \in D$, with F strictly increasing in the first argument, and strictly decreasing in the second argument (Krantz, 1964; Tversky & Russo, 1969). By Definition 12.1, the function g is strictly increasing in the first argument and strictly decreasing in the second argument. Note that the domain of F is of the form $I \times I$, where I is an open interval. A pair of functions (g,F) will be called a *simple scale representation* of (D,P).

We state a preparatory result.

12.4. Theorem.   *Let* (V,P) *be a system. Then, the following conditions are equivalent:*

(i) (V,P) *is a simply scalable, conjoint Weber system.*

(ii) *(V,P) has a simple scale representation (h,H) such that h is homogeneous of degree β for some constant β; moreover, if β ≠ 0, then H is homogeneous of degree 0; that is, we have*

$$P_{ax,by} = G[h(a,x)/h(b,y)]$$

for some continuous, strictly increasing function G.

Proof. Clearly, (ii) implies (i). Assume that

$$P_{ax,by} = F[g(a,x), g(b,y)]$$

for some continuous functions F,g. Since the cone V contains all pairs (a,a), $g(a,a)$ is defined and continuous for all $a > 0$. For the moment we suppose either that $g(a,a)$ is constant, or that it is strictly monotone in a. If $g(a,a)$ is constant, we obtain successively

$$
\begin{aligned}
P_{aa,by} &= F[g(a,a), g(b,y)] \\
&= F[g(\lambda a,\lambda a), g(\lambda b,\lambda y)] \qquad \text{(conjoint Weber's law)} \\
&= F[g(a,a), g(\lambda b,\lambda y)]
\end{aligned}
$$

and by monotonicity of F we thus derive

$$g(\lambda b,\lambda y) = g(b,y)$$

for all $(b,y) \in V, \lambda > 0$. In other words, g is homogeneous of degree zero on V, and (ii) follows, with $H = F$, $h = g$, and $\beta = 0$.

If, on the other hand, $g(a,a)$ is strictly monotone, we show that there exists a solution $\alpha \in \mathbb{R}_+$ of the equation

$$g(\alpha,\alpha) = g(a,x) \tag{15}$$

for each $(a,x) \in V$. To establish this fact we proceed by contradiction. Suppose, for instance, that $g(t,t)$ is strictly increasing in t, and further that for some $(a,x) \in V$

$$g(t,t) > g(a,x), \qquad \text{for all } t > 0.$$

Define

$$L = \inf\{g(t,t) | t > 0\} \geqslant g(a,x).$$

Since the range of g is an interval, the function F is defined at every point $[L, g(b,y)]$ for $(b,y) \in V$. In particular, using the conjoint Weber's law, and the continuity of F,

$$
\begin{aligned}
F[L, g(a,a)] &= \lim_{t \to 0} F[g(t,t), g(a,a)] \\
&= \lim_{t \to 0} F[g(\lambda t,\lambda t), g(\lambda a,\lambda a)] = F[L, g(\lambda a,\lambda a)],
\end{aligned}
$$

for all $a \in \mathbb{R}_+$. Again, by the monotonicity of F, we derive $g(\lambda a,\lambda a) = g(a,a)$, that is, $g(a,a)$ is constant, a contradiction. Thus, it cannot be the case that $g(t,t) > g(a,x)$ for all $t > 0$. If we assume that there is a point (a,x) for which

$$g(t,t) < g(a,x), \qquad \text{for all } t > 0,$$

a similar contradiction is reached by allowing $t \to \infty$. Finally, in case $g(t,t)$ is strictly decreasing, an argument symmetrical to the above is readily constructed. Thus we have shown that if $g(t,t)$ is strictly monotone, a solution $\alpha(a,x) \in \mathbb{R}_+$ of (15) exists. Moreover, the function $\alpha(a,x)$ is continuous on V; for $j(t) = g(t,t)$ is continuous and strictly monotone so that j^{-1} exists, is continuous and strictly monotone, and hence $\alpha(a,x) = (j^{-1} \circ g)(a,x)$ is continuous on V, and possesses monotonicity determined by that of g. Repeated application of the conjoint Weber's law now yields, with $\alpha = \alpha(a,x)$, $\beta = \alpha(b,y)$,

$$\begin{aligned} P_{ax,by} &= P_{\alpha\alpha,\beta\beta} \\ &= P_{(\lambda\alpha)(\lambda\alpha),(\lambda\beta)(\lambda\beta)} \\ &= P_{(\alpha/\beta)(\alpha/\beta),11} \qquad (\lambda = 1/\beta) \\ &= M(\alpha/\beta), \end{aligned}$$

where $M(s) = P_{ss,11}$ is strictly monotone (since $g(t,t)$ is strictly monotone). Thus,

$$\begin{aligned} P_{ax,by} &= M[\alpha(a,x)/\alpha(b,y)] \\ &= M[\alpha(\lambda a,\lambda x)/\alpha(\lambda b,\lambda y)]. \end{aligned}$$

With $A(\lambda) = \alpha(\lambda,\lambda)/\alpha(1,1)$, this implies

$$\alpha(\lambda a,\lambda x) = A(\lambda)\,\alpha(a,x).$$

Notice that A is continuous on $\mathbb{R}_+$. It is immediate that $A(\lambda\lambda') = A(\lambda) \cdot A(\lambda')$, $A(\lambda) = \lambda^\beta$ for some $\beta \neq 0$. Thus α is homogeneous of degree $\beta \neq 0$. If $g(t,t)$ is strictly increasing, then M is strictly increasing and α is strictly increasing in the first variable. Thus (ii) obtains with $h = \alpha$, $G = M$, and $\beta \neq 0$. In the other case, we define $h = \alpha^{-1}$ and $G(s) = M(1/s)$.

We now prove that if $g(t,t)$ is not constant, it must be strictly monotone. Let a_0, a_1, with $a_0 < a_1$, be two points such that, say

$$g(a_0,a_0) < g(a_1,a_1).$$

By the continuity of g, it follows that there exists an interval $(a_2,a_1]$, $a_2 \geqslant a_0$ such that if $a_2 < s \leqslant a_1$,

$$g(a_2,a_2) < g(s,s).$$

For any $t \in \mathbb{R}_+$ and $1 \leqslant \lambda \leqslant a_1/a_2$, we have by the conjoint Weber's law, successively

$$\begin{aligned} P_{a_2 a_2,tt} &= P_{(\lambda a_2)(\lambda a_2),(\lambda t)(\lambda t)} \\ &> P_{a_2 a_2,(\lambda t)(\lambda t)}, \end{aligned}$$

since (g,F) is a simple scale representation of (V,P), yielding

$$g(\lambda t,\lambda t) > g(t,t).$$

Observing that any real number $\lambda > 1$ can be written in the form $\lambda = \lambda_1^n \lambda_2$ for some integer $n \geqslant 0$ and some $\lambda_1,\lambda_2 \in (1,a_1/a_2]$, we conclude that $g(t,t)$ is strictly increasing. In the case $g(a_0,a_0) > g(a_1,a_1)$, $a_0 < a_1$, a similar argument gives $g(t,t)$ strictly decreasing. ∎

12.5. Theorem. *If (V,P) is a simply scalable conjoint Weber's system, then one of the following three possibilities must hold:*

(i) *There are some real-valued, continuous, strictly monotone functions $T > 0$ and M satisfying*

$$P_{ax,by} = M\left[\frac{T(a/x)x}{T(b/y)y}\right];$$ (16)

(ii) *There are some real-valued, continuous, strictly monotone function $\kappa > 0$ and G, with G increasing, and a constant $\beta \neq 0$, satisfying*

$$P_{ax,by} = G\left[\frac{\kappa(a/x)(a^\beta + x^\beta)}{\kappa(b/y)(b^\beta + y^\beta)}\right];$$ (17)

(iii) *There is a continuous function Q_0, strictly increasing in the first argument, strictly decreasing in the second argument, such that*

$$P_{ax,by} = Q_0(a/x,b/y).$$

Moreover, (i) and (ii) are equivalent.

Thus, Equation (16) particularizes Equation (13). This result suggests that, when a system (V,P) satisfies the hypotheses of the theorem, a simple scale representation (g,F) can be found in which the function g has some of the properties of the addition of the reals. This obviously holds for case (iii). In case (ii), defining a binary operation $*$ by

$$a * x = [\kappa(a/x)(a^\beta + x^\beta)]^{1/\beta},$$

we have for any (a,x), $(\xi a, \xi x) \in V$,

$$\xi(a * x) = \{\kappa(\xi a/\xi x)[(\xi a)^\beta + (\xi x)^\beta]\}^{1/\beta}$$
$$= \xi a * \xi x;$$

that is, real multiplication is distributive with respect to the operation $*$. As it is easy to see, essentially the same information is conveyed by case (i) and Equation 16. Notice two special cases of the function κ in (17) encountered implicitly in the outline:

$$\kappa(a/x) = \frac{(a^\beta x^\beta)^{\beta/(\beta + \delta)}}{a^\beta + x^\beta},$$ (18)

$$\kappa(a/x) = \frac{a^\beta + \delta x^\beta}{a^\beta + x^\beta}.$$ (19)

Equations 17 and 18 lead to Equation 8, while Equation 7 follows from Equations 17 and 19. It is easy to verify that in case Equation 18 or 19 holds (and moreover, it can be shown that only in these cases) the operation $*$ satisfies bisymmetry:

$$(a * x) * (b * y) = (a * b) * (x * y).$$

Proof. Clearly, case (iii) is compatible with the hypothesis of the theorem. Let (h,F) be the simple scale representation of (V,P) obtained in Theorem 12.4. Thus, h is homogeneous of degree β. Assume that case (iii) does not hold. It is easy to verify that we must have $\beta \neq 0$. Defining $r(a,x) = h(a,x)/(a^\beta + x^\beta)$, $r(a/x, 1) = \kappa(a/x)$, we have $r(\xi a, \xi x) = r(a,x) = r(a/x, 1) = \kappa(a/x)$, yielding $h(a,x) = \kappa(a/x)(a^\beta + x^\beta)$.

Thus, (ii) is implied by the hypotheses of the theorem if (iii) does not hold. Finally, the equivalence of (i) and (ii) follows immediately from the definitions

$$T(s) = [\kappa(s)(s^\beta + 1)]^{1/\beta}. \tag{20}$$

$$M(s) = G(s^\beta). \quad \blacksquare$$

We now turn to the first result announced in our introductory remarks—that under the conjoint Weber's law (and technical conditions such as continuity and monotonicity), Equations 7, 8, and 9 are the only possible cases of Equation 6.

12.6. Theorem.   *Let (V,P) be a conjoint Weber's system satisfying*

$$P_{ax,by} = H[f(a) + r(x), f(b) + r(y)] \tag{21}$$

for some real-valued, continuous, strictly monotone functions f and r, with f strictly increasing, and some continuous function H strictly increasing in its first argument and strictly decreasing in its second. Then, one of the three equations

$$P_{ax,by} = G\left(\frac{a^\beta + \delta x^\beta}{b^\beta + \delta y^\beta}\right), \tag{22}$$

$$P_{ax,by} = G\left(\frac{a^\beta x^\gamma}{b^\beta y^\gamma}\right), \tag{23}$$

$$P_{ax,by} = Q_0\left(\frac{a}{x}, \frac{b}{y}\right), \tag{24}$$

must hold for all (a,x), $(b,y) \in V$. In (22) and (23), G is continuous and strictly increasing; $\beta > 0$ and $\delta \neq 0$ are constants, with $\delta > 0$ iff (V,P) is isotone. In (24), Q_0 is continuous, strictly increasing in its first argument and strictly decreasing in its second argument (so that (V,P) is necessarily antitone).

Proof.   The hypotheses of the theorem imply that (V,P) is a simply scalable conjoint Weber's system. From Theorem 12.5, either (24) obtains, which with $f = -r = \ln$ and $H(s,t) = Q_0(e^s, e^t)$, is clearly of the additive form (21), or else

$$P_{ax,by} = M\left[\frac{T(a/x)x}{T(b/y)y}\right].$$

Setting $b = y = 1$ and defining $v(s) = H[s, f(1) + r(1)]$, $\tau(t) = T(t)/T(1)$, we obtain, by combining (21) with the equation above,

$$M[\tau(a/x)x] = v[f(a) + r(x)].$$

Notice that

$$\tau(a/x)\xi x = (M^{-1} \circ v)[f(a\xi) + r(\xi x)]$$
$$= \xi(M^{-1} \circ v)[f(a) + r(x)]. \tag{25}$$

Fixing $\xi \in \mathbb{R}_+$ and defining

$$f_\xi(a) = f(a\xi), \qquad r_\xi = r(x\xi), \qquad M^{-1} \circ v = K, \qquad K_\xi(s) = K(s)/\xi,$$

Equation 25 becomes, with $s = f(a)$ and $t = r(x)$,

$$(K_\xi^{-1} \circ K)(s + t) = (f_\xi \circ f^{-1})(s) + (r_\xi \circ r^{-1})(t).$$

It is easy to check that the three functions $K_\xi^{-1} \circ K$, $f_\xi \circ f^{-1}$, and $r_\xi \circ r^{-1}$ are continuous. Without loss of generality, we can assume that 0 is a possible value of the functions f and r. Standard functional equations methods apply, and we obtain, by Theorem 3.6,

$$(f_\xi \circ f^{-1})(s) = A(\xi)s + B(\xi),$$
$$(r_\xi \circ r^{-1})(t) = A(\xi)t + C(\xi),$$

where A, B, and C are continuous functions on $\mathbb{R}_+$; $A(1) = 1$; $B(1) = C(1) = 0$.
    In other terms,

$$f(\xi a) = A(\xi)f(a) + B(\xi),$$
$$r(\xi x) = A(\xi)r(x) + C(\xi).$$

Applying 3.10(iv) yields the two solutions

$$\text{(i)} \quad f(a) = A_1 a^\beta + B_1, \qquad r(x) = A_2 x^\beta + B_2, \tag{26}$$

where A_1, B_1, A_2, B_2 and β are constants, $A_1\beta > 0$, $A_2 \neq 0$;

$$\text{(ii)} \quad f(a) = A_1 \ln a + B_1, \qquad r(x) = A_2 \ln x + B_2, \tag{27}$$

where A_1, B_1, A_2, B_2 are constants, $A_1 > 0$, $A_2 \neq 0$.
The first of these systems immediately leads to Equation 22; the second likewise leads to (23). ■

    This theorem is closely related to a result of Luce (1977). A summary of the results of this section is given schematically in Figure 12.2.

*THE STRONG CONJOINT WEBER'S LAWS

12.7. Definition.   In a system (D, P) the equations

$$\text{(I)} \quad P_{ax,by} = P_{(\lambda a)(\lambda x),(\tau b)(\tau y)}, \tag{28}$$
$$\text{(II)} \quad P_{ax,by} = P_{(\lambda a)(\tau x),(\lambda b)(\tau y)}, \tag{29}$$

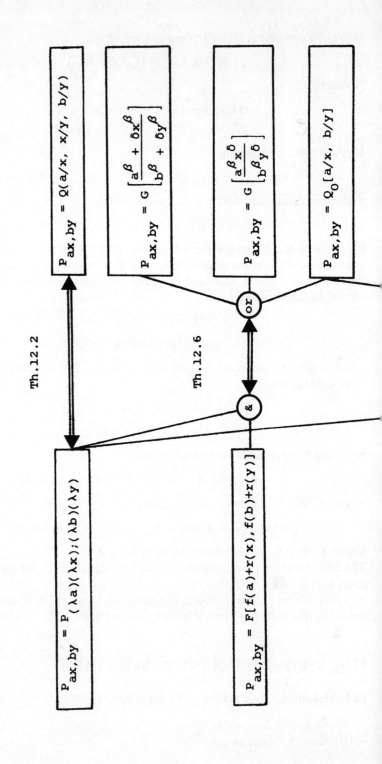

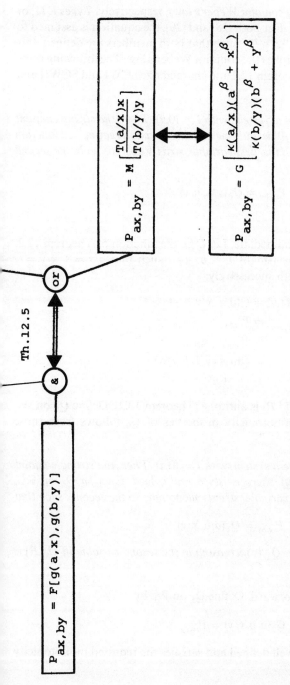

FIGURE 12.2. The conjoint Weber's law. Summary of the implications.

293

will be referred to as the *strong conjoint Weber's laws*, respectively, *Types I, II*; or more briefly as SCWI, SCWII. For both (28) and (29), the equation is assumed to hold for all (a,x), $(b,y) \in D$ and $\lambda,\gamma \in \mathbb{R}_+$ such that both members are defined. It is clear that each of these laws implies the conjoint Weber's law. The following three theorems are in the style of Theorem 12.2 and characterize SCWI and SCWII and their logical conjunction.

12.8. Theorem. *Let (I^2,P) be a System, with $I = (0,\alpha)$. Then, the strong conjoint Weber's law type I holds iff (I^2,P) is antitone and there exists a real-valued function Q_0 on $\mathbb{R}^2_+$, strictly increasing in the first variable, strictly decreasing in the second variable, such that*

$$P_{ax,by} = Q_0(a/x, b/y)$$

for all a, x, b, $y \in I$.

   Proof. The sufficiency is immediate. Let Q be the function of Theorem 12.2. For any s, t, $u \in \mathbb{R}_+$, there are (small) a, x, b, $y \in I$ such that $a/x = s$, $x/y = t$, $b/y = u$, and ay, xy, $bx \in I$, with successively

$$
\begin{aligned}
Q(s,t,u) &= Q(a/x, x/y, b/y) \\
&= P_{ax,by} \\
&= P_{(ay)(xy),(bx)(yx)} \\
&= Q(ay/xy, 1, bx/yx) \\
&= Q(s,1,u),
\end{aligned}
$$

implying, in particular, that (I^2,P) is antitone (Theorem 12.2). Define Q_0 on $\mathbb{R}_+$ by $Q_0(s,u) = Q(s,1,u)$. The monotonicity properties of Q_0 follows from those of Q.

12.9. Theorem. *Let (I^2,P) be a system, with $I = (0,\alpha)$. Then, the strong conjoint Weber's law Type II holds iff there exists a real-valued function Q_1 on $\mathbb{R}^2_+$, strictly increasing in the first variable, strictly monotonic in the second, such that*

$$P_{ax,by} = Q_1(a/b, x/y)$$

for all a, x, b, $y \in I$. Moreover, Q_1 is increasing in the second variable iff (I^2,P) is isotone.

   The sufficiency is straightforward. Define Q_1 on $\mathbb{R}^2_+$ by

$$Q_1(a/b,x/y) = P_{ax,by}.$$

It is easy to check that Q_1 is well defined and satisfies the required monotonicity properties (Exercise 5).

12.10. Theorem. *Let (I^2,P) be a system with $I = (0,\alpha)$. Then both strong conjoint Weber's laws hold iff (I^2,P) is antitone, and there exists a real-valued, strictly* *increasing function Q_2 on $\mathbb{R}_+$, such that*

$$P_{ax,by} = Q_2(ay/bx)$$

for all $a, x, b, y \in I$.

Proof. For any $s \in \mathbb{R}_+$, there are $a, x, b, y \in I$ such that $s = ax/by$. Define

$$Q_2(s) = P_{ax,by},$$

and show that Q_2 is well defined (Exercise 6). The sufficiency is clear. ∎

Next, we consider the impact of the strong conjoint Weber's laws on Equations 6 and 14. In the style of Theorems 12.6 and 12.5, we have the following two results.

12.11. Theorem. *Let (V,P) be a system, satisfying*

$$P_{ax,by} = F[f(a) + r(x), f(b) + r(y)] \tag{30}$$

for some real-valued, continuous, strictly monotonic functions f,r and some continuous functions F of two variables, strictly increasing in its first argument, strictly decreasing in its second. Then, the strong conjoint Weber's law, Type II, holds iff

$$P_{ax,by} = G_0(a^\beta x^\delta / b^\beta y^\delta) \tag{31}$$

for some continuous, strictly increasing, function G_0, and some constants $\beta > 0$, and $\delta \neq 0$.

Notice that a similar theorem involving SCWI would be of no interest, since by Theorem 12.8 SCWI implies (24).

Proof. The sufficiency is obvious. By Theorem 12.6, one of (22), (23), (24) must hold, since SCWII implies the conjoint Weber's law. It is easy to show that (22) contradicts SCWII. Equation 20 is already of form (31). Suppose, therefore, that

$$P_{ax,by} = Q_0(a/x, b/y).$$

With $a/x = s, b/y = t$, we obtain

$$\begin{aligned} P_{ax,by} &= Q_0(s,t) \\ &= P_{(\lambda a)x,(\lambda b)y} \\ &= Q_0(\lambda s, \lambda t), \end{aligned}$$

yielding $P_{ax,by} = G_0(ay/bx)$ with $\lambda = y/b$ and $G_0(z) = Q_0(z,1)$; this is particular case of (31), with $\beta = -\delta = 1$. ∎

Our next theorem is a specialization of Theorem 12.5. The fact that isotonicity is required eliminates SCWI from consideration.

12.12. Theorem. *Let (V,P) be an isotone simply scalable system. Then, the following two conditions are equivalent.*

(i) *The strong conjoint Weber's law, Type II, hold.*

(ii) *There exists a real-valued, strictly increasing function M, and a constant*
$\beta, 0 < \beta < 1$, *such that*

$$P_{ax,by} = M(a^\beta x^{1-\beta}/b^\beta y^{1-\beta}).$$

Proof.   Clearly, (ii) implies (i). By Theorem 12.5 we have

$$P_{ax,by} = M\left[\frac{T(a/x)x}{T(b/y)y}\right] \tag{32}$$

for some real-valued, continuous function $T > 0$, $T(1) = 1$, and some function M.
By SCWII, we obtain

$$\frac{T(a/x)}{T(b/y)} = \frac{T(\lambda a/\tau x)}{T(\lambda b/\tau y)}; \qquad \lambda > 0, \tau > 0.$$

Setting $b/y = 1$, $a/x = s$, $\lambda/\theta = t$, we obtain

$$T(s)\,T(t) = T(st).$$

We note that this equation is satisfied on an open interval containing 1. Applying
Theorem 3.4 yields

$$T(s) = s^\beta$$

for some constant $\beta > 0$. Replacing T in (32) by its expression above, the result
follows.   ■

The results of this section and the next one are summarized in Figure 12.3.

*THE CONJOINT WEBER'S INEQUALITY

In some situations, it may not be realistic to suppose that the conjoint Weber's
law holds for all values of the stimulus variables. A natural generalization of this
law (cf. the "near-miss-to-Weber's-law," see 8.16; Jesteadt et al., 1977; McGill &
Goldberg, 1968; Rabinowitz et al., 1976 is proposed below.

12.13. Definition.   In a system (D,P), we refer to the *conjoint Weber's inequality*
as the formula

$$P_{ax,by} \leqslant P_{(\lambda a)(\lambda x),(\lambda b)(\lambda y)}.$$

assumed to hold for all (a,x), $(b,y) \in D$ and $\lambda \in \mathbb{R}_+$ such that $a \geqslant b$, $x \geqslant y$, and
$(\lambda a, \lambda x)$, $(\lambda b, \lambda y) \in D$. In view of the weakness of such a constraint, one may ask
whether it puts any interesting restriction on the unknown functions in Equations
6 and 14. An example of what can be expected is given in Theorem 12.14.

Suppose that, in the conditions of Theorem 12.5, we replace the conjoint
Weber's law by the conjoint Weber's inequality. Since P is a bounded function, it

may perhaps be conjectured that the conjoint Weber's inequality implies

$$\lim_{\lambda \to \infty} P_{(\lambda a)(\lambda x),(\lambda b)(\lambda y)} = G\left[\frac{\kappa(a/x)(a^\beta + x^\beta)}{\kappa(b/y)(b^\beta + y^\beta)}\right], \tag{33}$$

with G, κ, and β as in Theorem 12.5. This conjecture is false. Suppose, indeed, that

$$P_{ax,by} = G\left(\frac{e^{a+x}}{e^{b+y}}\right).$$

The conjoint Weber's inequality holds, but with $a + x > b + y$, we have

$$\lim_{\lambda \to \infty} \frac{e^{\lambda(a+x)}}{e^{\lambda(b+y)}} = \infty,$$

contradicting (33). If, however, the function $h(a,a)$ of Condition (ii) in Theorem 12.4 is dominated by *some* power function, then (33) can be derived. More precisely:

12.14. Theorem. *Let (V,P) be an isotone simply scalable system satisfying*

$$P_{ax,by} = G\left[\frac{g(a,x)}{g(b,y)}\right]$$

for some continuous, strictly increasing function G, and some continuous function $g > 0$, mapping V onto $\mathbb{R}_+$, strictly increasing in both variables. Suppose also that for sufficiently large a, $g(a,a) \leqslant \gamma a^\mu$ for some constants γ, $\mu > 0$ and that the conjoint Weber's inequality is satisfied. Then

$$\lim_{\lambda \to \infty} P_{(\lambda a)(\lambda x),(\lambda b)(\lambda y)} = G\left[\frac{\kappa(a/x)(a^\beta + x^\beta)}{\kappa(b/y)(b^\beta + y^\beta)}\right],$$

for some function $\kappa > 0$, and some constant $\beta > 0$.

We omit the proof (see Falmagne & Iverson, 1979), which is similar to that of Theorem 12.5, but uses a result of Falmagne (1977) to deal with the conjoint Weber's inequality.

SHIFT INVARIANCE IN LOUDNESS RECRUITMENT

A tone embedded in noise does not appear as loud as the same noise in quiet. As the intensity of the tone increases, however, the subjective difference tends to disappear. In psychoacoustics, this phenomenon is known as *loudness recruitment*. Let $\psi(x,n)$ denote the intensity of a tone in quiet matching an intensity x of the same tone embedded in a noise of intensity n. These matching functions were investigated by Pavel (1980) and Iverson and Pavel (1980, 1981; see also Pavel & Iverson, 1981), who demonstrated that, to an excellent approximation, the following property was satisfied by the data: for some $\gamma > 0$ and all $\lambda > 0$

$$\psi(\lambda s, \lambda^\gamma n) = \lambda \psi(x,n). \tag{34}$$

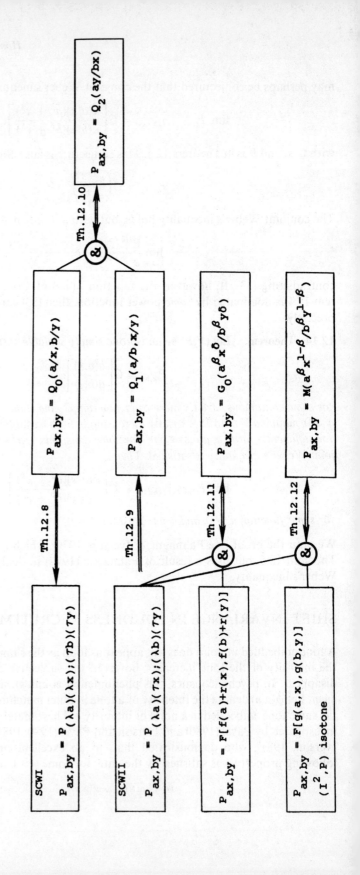

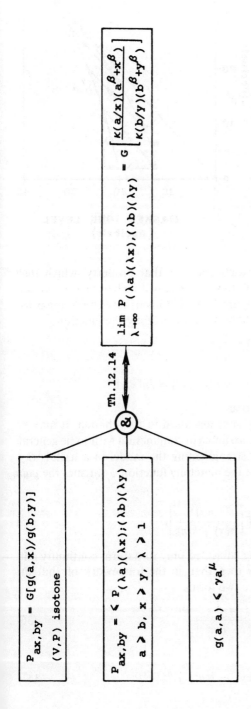

FIGURE 12.3. The strong conjoint Weber's law and the conjoint Weber's inequality. A summary of the implications.

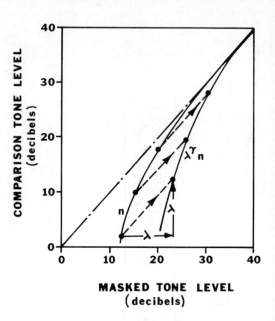

FIGURE 12.4. The property of shift invariance illustrated by two hypothetical loudness matching curves. The right curve representing loudness matching with noise $\lambda^\gamma n$ can be obtained by a rigid shift of the left curve (generated by loudness matching with noise n) along the first bisector. From *Homogeneity in Complete and Partial Masking* by M. Pavel, 1980, unpublished doctoral dissertation, New York University. Reprinted with permission of author.

They investigated the theoretical consequences of that property, which they called *shift invariance*. The choice of this name is justified by a geometrical interpretation of (34), illustrated in Figure 12.4. Shift invariance can be regarded as a homogeneity property under a slight disguise: defining the function

$$\eta(x,y) = \psi(x,y^\gamma),$$

it follows that

$$\eta(\lambda x, \lambda y) = \psi(\lambda x, \lambda^\gamma y^\gamma) = \lambda \psi(x, y^\gamma) = \lambda \eta(x, y).$$

That is, η is homogeneous of degree one.

As in other cases of homogeneity laws discussed in this chapter, it may be asked whether shift invariance may be assumed in conjunction with some general, reasonable model with the effect of strengthening the model in a useful way. Iverson and Pavel (1981) assume that the matching function ψ satisfies the *gain control* equation

$$\psi(x,n) = F\left[\frac{g(x)}{h(x) + k(n)}\right], \tag{35}$$

with the functions g, h, k, and F being subjected only to natural continuity and monotonicity properties. They show then that, in the framework of shift invariance, (35) can only take one of the two forms

$$\psi(x, y) = \left[\frac{Ax^\alpha}{x^{\alpha'} + Kn^{\alpha/\gamma}}\right]^{1/(\alpha-\alpha')} \tag{36}$$

or

$$\psi(x,n) = A[x^\alpha(x^{\alpha'} - Kn^{\alpha'/\gamma}]^{1/(\alpha+\alpha')}, \tag{37}$$

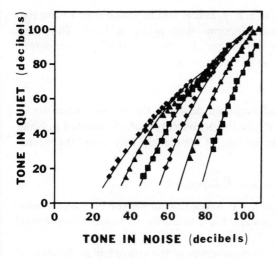

FIGURE 12.5. Least square fit of Equation 36, with $A = 1$, to Stevens and Guirao's (1967) data. The stimuli are 1000-Hz tones embedded in a wide-band Gaussian noise. The subject was matching the level of the tone in noise to that of the tone in quiet. The experimental points are obtained by averaging over subjects. From "On the Functional Form of Partial Masking Functions in Psychoacoustic" by G. J. Iverson and M. Pavel, 1981, *Journal of Mathematical Psychology*, 24, pp. 1–20. Reprinted with permission of authors and publisher.

where A, K, α, α' and γ are appropriately chosen constants. We will not enter here into the technical details of Iverson and Pavel's results, which can be found in their paper.

It is remarkable that both (36) and (37) are capable of providing excellent fits to the available data, such as that of Stevens and Guirao (1967) and Iverson and Pavel (1980), who note that distinguishing between these two classes of functions from an empirical standpoint would require a careful investigation of near-threshold data.

A special case of (37) was proposed by Lochner and Burger (1961) as an extension of the power law (see Chapter 13), incorporating the effects of a masking noise. Objections to (37) as a possible model for loudness recruitment can be found in Scharf (1978). A plot of a least square fit of (36) to the Stevens and Guirao's (1967) data is presented in Figure 12.5, reproduced from Iverson and Pavel (1981).

EXERCISES

1. Consider the law $M(a,b,c) = G(a^\alpha b^\beta c^\gamma)$, in which M is a real-valued, continuous function of three positive real variables, G is strictly increasing and continuous, and α, β, and γ are three constants $\neq 0$. In what sense can we say that an homogeneity law is involved here?

2. Prove Theorem 12.2.

3. Check that if we define a binary operation $*$ by

$$a * x = [\kappa(a/x)(a^\beta + x^\beta)]^{1/\beta},$$

then (19) implies that $*$ satisfies bisymmetry.

*4. Suppose that a system (D,P) satisfies the condition

$$P_{ax,by} = P_{[\mu(\lambda)a][\nu(\lambda)x],[\mu(\lambda)b][\nu(\lambda)y]}$$

for all positive real numbers a, x, b, y, and λ, and in which μ and v are two strictly increasing, continuous functions with $\mu(1) = v(1) = 1$. Thus, this condition generalizes the conjoint Weber's law. Investigate the consequences of this condition in the context of Equation 21.

5. Prove Theorem 12.9.
6. Prove Theorem 12.10.
7. Let $c \leqslant b \leqslant a$ be positive real numbers, denoting the physical intensity of three stimuli. As in 11.27, let P_{abc} be the probability that a is selected as being subjectively closest to b, in the set $\{a,c\}$. Consider the following "Weberian" law

$$P_{abc} = P_{(\lambda a)(\lambda b)(\lambda c)},$$

which we assume to hold for all $\lambda > 0$. Argue that, in view of Plateau's results, this equation formalizes a reasonable conjecture in some experimental situations.

8. (*Continuation.*) Investigate the consequences of the above law in the style of Theorem 12.2.
*9. (*Continuation.*) Assuming that this law holds, together with representation (32) in Chapter 11, what are the possible forms of function u? (The reader is thus asked to state and prove a result in the style of Theorem 12.6.)
*10. (*Continuation.*) Along the same lines, investigate the impact of the above "Weberian" law on the more general representation

$$P_{abc} = H[u(a) - g(b), g(b) - v(c)],$$

with u, g, and v, three real-valued, strictly increasing, continuous functions and H continuous, strictly decreasing in the first variable, and strictly increasing in the second variable. (As far as I know, the results in the last three exercises are unpublished.)

11. (Iverson & Pavel, 1981.) Show that shift invariance and the existence of a gain control representation are independent conditions.

13

Scaling and the Measurement of Sensation

This chapter covers a collection of models, procedures, and empirical analyses purporting to provide a representation of some data in terms of one or more numerical scales. Such is also the aim of measurement theory, a field in which (as we have seen in Chapters 1 and 2) axioms systems are given justifying specific methods of scale construction. In the work usually classified under "scaling," however, acquiring the scales is typically considered as an end in itself, and the theoretical underpinnings are of secondary importance.[1]

After an introduction to scale types, the most common unidimensional scaling methods and data will be reviewed. Two theoretical approaches will then be considered: the Krantz-Shepard *relation theory*, and the *functional measurement* procedures introduced by Norman Anderson. The chapter ends with a discussion of the celebrated, but controversial, issue of the measurement of sensation.

As the reader will surely notice, this chapter is written in a different, more discursive style. There will be few formal definitions, theorems, and proofs. Our aim is to outline an important aspect of psychophysics in which intensive empirical research is taking place, but which is still, from the viewpoint of this book, in the early stages of its theoretical development.

TYPES OF SCALES

13.1. Common types of scales. In most cases, numerical scales constructed from (and explaining) some empirical data are not defined uniquely. It is usually agreed, for example, that the numerical scale used for the measurement of length is a *ratio scale*, which means that the numerical values assigned to the objects are defined up to a multiplication by a positive constant (e.g., a change of units from centimeters to meters is admissible). In this exemplary case, the exact degree of arbitrariness is a consequence derivable from a completely axiomatized theory. One assumes that the data satisfy the axioms of the theory, which in turns provides a procedure for the construction of the scale and specifies the degree of

---

1. Objections have deservedly been made to that state of affairs. The use of scales without a firm theoretical foundation are limited. For example, if the *type* of a scale is unknown, it may be difficult to decide whether a given model or mathematical expression using this scale makes sense from a certain logicophilosophical standpoint. This question is usually referred to as *meaningfulness*, and we discuss it in detail in Chapter 14.

TABLE 13.1. *The most commonly used types of scales. Each type is defined by the class of admissible transformations of the scale; for example, the ratio scale type is that defined by all the transformations of the form:* $x \mapsto \alpha x$, *with* $\alpha > 0$. *The case for density and other fundamental physical quantities to be log-interval scales is made by Krantz et al. (1971).*

Scale type	Admissible Transformations	Examples
Absolute	Identity: $x \mapsto \phi(x) = x$	Counting
Ordinal (increasing)	Monotone increasing $x < y \Rightarrow \phi(x) < \phi(y)$	Moh's hardness scale
Ratio	Similarity: $x \mapsto \phi(x) = \alpha x$ With $\alpha > 0$	Length Mass
Interval	Positive affine: $x \mapsto \phi(x) = \alpha x + \beta$ With $\alpha > 0$	Temperature
Log interval	$x \mapsto \phi(x) = \alpha x^{\beta}$ With $\alpha > 0$ and $\beta > 0$	Density

arbitrariness of such construction. How this applies in the case of length was discussed in detail in Chapter 2. The degree of arbitrariness of the scale is referred to as its *type*. Despite the variety of forms of data, only a few types of scales are actually used in scientific practice. The reasons for this scarcity are not very well understood (see however, Narens, 1981). The most commonly used types of scales are listed in Table 13.1.

UNIDIMENSIONAL SCALING METHODS

13.2. Overview. The psychophysical procedures encountered in earlier chapters of this book (such as that used in the yes-no paradigm), are rather painstaking. In a typical experiment, several hundred observations per data point are collected for each subject. By contrast, the methods considered here may use only a few observations per point (sometimes, as few as one or two observations per subject). However, the subject's responses tend to be much more elaborate. For example, he or she may be asked to identify the stimulus presented using a label previously attached to that stimulus (as in the *absolute identification* method); or he or she may be required to evaluate the stimulus numerically, according to some rule (as in *magnitude estimation*). There are a number of such scaling methods, and more than one way to classify them. In the following paragraphs, we classify the methods by the type of response required from the subject. Each subsection contains a brief description of the procedures and of the typical empirical results.

Under the impetus of S. S. Stevens, an impressive array of experimental results were collected that generally gave credence to the contention that, through subjective judgments, the sensory continua are related to each other and to the number continuum by power laws (at least to a first approximation). Stevens offered the "power law" as a substitute for Fechner's logarithmic relation (cf. 8.13(2)). The merit of this proposal is discussed in 13.5 and 13.6. In this connection, the reader should bear in mind that the psychophysical methods considered in this section were often introduced in a spirit of criticism of the "classical" methods, such as the yes-no paradigm and its close relatives. These were thought to lack realism, to the extent that the data were focusing on "local" effects (e.g., the discrimination of neighboring stimuli) while the natural environment involved the simultaneous apprehension of a large collection of widely distributed stimuli. The terms *local* and *global* are sometimes used to denote the two classes of procedures.

13.3. Absolute identification.   In a preliminary period, the subject is trained to associate one of n labels (say the numbers from 1 to $n = 10$) to each of n stimuli. During the main phase of the experiment, the subject is presented a stimulus on each trial and is required to produce the appropriate label. The subject's response is recorded. The succession of the stimuli is random. Occasionally, immediate repetitions are avoided.

A straightforward analysis of the data is in terms of the proportion of correct responses. Another measure of performance, not often used now, is the *average information transmitted by the responses* (cf. Coombs et al. 1970; Garner, 1962; Miller, 1953). More recently, a measure based on the index d' of signal detection theory (cf. Chapter 10) has been proposed (Luce, Green, & Weber, 1976).

For stimuli varying along one sensory continuum, the main finding is that the maximum number of stimuli that can be identified perfectly by an untrained subject is between 5 and 9, depending on the continuum (Pollack, 1952; Garner, 1953). (See Miller, 1956, for a review of the facts. Obviously, specialists, such as professional musicians identifying pitch, may score much better than that.) This result is regarded as puzzling since it appears to be at variance with the data of "local" studies. For instance, only stimuli that are very close on the physical scale (say less that a couple of decibels apart in loudness discrimination) are ever confused in a two-alternatives-forced-choice paradigm (2AFC). An extrapolation would lead to predict a perfect identification of several dozen, suitably located stimuli, in an absolute identification experiment. The discrepancy may be due, at least in part, to the fact that efficient guessing strategies can be used in a 2AFC situation, which are no longer available in absolute identification.

At first, the absolute identification paradigm may seem straightforward. Actually, the data are plagued with a variety of sequential effects and "anchoring" effects that render the analysis extremely difficult. Regarding "anchoring" or "edge" effects, see, for example, Berliner and Durlach (1973), Berliner, Durlach, and Braida (1977), Braida and Durlach (1972), Durlach and Braida (1969), Gravetter and Lockhead (1973), Lippman, Braida, and Durlach (1976), and Weber, Green, and Luce (1977). Sequential effects in absolute identification have been explored, for example, by Holland and Lockhead (1968), Ward and Lockhead (1970, 1971), and Purks, Callaghan, Braida, and Durlach (1980).

13.4. Category rating.   As is absolute identification, one stimulus from a sensory continuum is presented at each trial. The subject is instructed to assign each stimulus to one of m ordered categories, for example, the numbers 1 to m. These categories are assumed to be subjectively "equally spaced," that is, the subjective distance between category 3 and 4 is identical to that between 10 and 11. The number m of categories is often smaller than the number of stimuli and may vary from a few (5 to 7) to several dozens.

In variations of this methods, pairs of stimuli are presented at each trial, and the subject is required to rate (i.e., to assign a category to) subjective "differences" or "ratios" of these stimuli. In a rather extreme version, four stimuli are presented simultaneously, and the subjects are asked to make very sophisticated judgments, such as rating the "ratio of differences" or the "difference of ratios" (Birnbaum, 1982).

The most startling result is, perhaps, that the subjects not only are capable of performing such tasks without major difficulties, but they provide surprisingly regular data: the average rating values often appear to vary smoothly with stimulus intensity. The data may be analyzed in various ways. In an exemplary case, the subjects rate subjective "differences" between stimuli, and it is assumed that the average rating $D_{x,y}$ corresponding to physical intensities x,y satisfies a Fechnerian-type relation

$$D_{x,y} = F[u(x) - u(y)], \tag{1}$$

in which u and F are strictly increasing functions. In some cases, F is shown to be well approximated by a linear function. Unfortunately, the subject's performance in these tasks varies markedly with the context. For example, the value of $D_{x,y}$ in (1) strongly depends on the distribution of all the stimuli used in the experiment: specifically the range, the spacing, and the frequencies of these stimuli. Such facts, which are well documented, may create problems for psychophysical theorizing, depending on the locus of the effects. To pursue our example, a major concern is which of the two functions u,F in the right member of (1) is affected by the context. The available evidence suggests that only F is affected (Parducci, 1963, 1965, 1974; Parducci & Perrett, 1971; see Birnbaum, 1982, for a general discussion and further references). Since the function u is a candidate for the psychophysical scale (i.e., the key invariant), this would leave open the possibility of a general theory.

13.5. Magnitude estimation.   In this widely used method, the main advocate of which was S. S. Stevens, the subject is required to provide "direct" numerical estimates of the magnitude of the sensation evoked by the stimulation. Two variants of the method have been employed.

In one variant, the subject is initially presented with a stimulus (the *standard*) and told that the sensory magnitude of that stimulus is assigned a certain value (*modulus*), say 100. Other stimuli are then presented in random order, and the subject is instructed to estimate their sensory magnitude to preserve ratios. For instance, if the second stimulus presented seems to have a sensory magnitude that is half of that of the standard, its sensory magnitude should be estimated to be 50.

Typically, only a couple of observations are taken from each subject, and the data of all subjects are combined by computing the median or the geometrical mean.

The second variant has the favor of many investigators. No standard and modulus are provided. The subject is simply told to assign to any stimulus presented any number that seem suitable as an estimate of the sensation magnitude.

Interestingly, the results are very similar for the two methods. For intensive continua, the mean or median response $\phi(x)$ is approximately a power function of the physical intensity x:

$$\phi(x) = \alpha x^\beta. \tag{2}$$

In log-log coordinates, (2) becomes the equation of a linear function with slope β, which can be fitted to the data by linear regression. As exemplified in Figure 13.1, this prediction holds reasonably well for many data, at least for moderate to large intensities (see Marks, 1974 or S. S. Stevens, 1975, for a presentation of the evidence). A better overall fit may be obtained, at the cost of one extra parameter, by forms such as

$$\phi(x) = \alpha x^\beta + \gamma$$

or

$$\phi(x) = \alpha(x - \gamma)^\beta,$$

both of which are capable of handling the data at low intensities (cf. Ekman, 1956, 1961; Fagot, 1963; Galanter & Messick, 1961; Luce, 1959; S. S. Stevens, 1959).

The magnitude estimation procedure is also used in other paradigms. For example, in *ratio estimation*, the observer is asked to evaluate the subjective

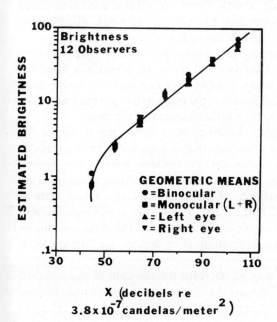

FIGURE 13.1. Magnitude estimates of brightness. In abscissa, the luminance of the stimuli in decibels *re* 3.8×10^{-7} candelas/meter². From "Brightness Function: Binocular versus Monocular Stimulation" by J. C. Stevens, 1967, *Perception & Psychophysics, 2*, pp. 189–192. Adapted and reprinted with permission of author and publisher.

"ratio" of two stimuli. At least to a first approximation, the experimental results are consistent with those reported for the magnitude estimation of single stimuli.

S. S. Stevens, (1957, 1959, 1961a, 1961b, 1961c) strongly argued that Equation 2 should be taken as the fundamental psychophysical law, rather than the logarithmic "Fechnerian" form derived from Weber's law together with the difference representation for choice probabilities. Accordingly, serious consideration is given to the estimated value of the exponent β in Equation 2, which some believe could measure some basic feature of the subject's sensory system. Several dozen sensory continua, were investigated by Stevens and others, and the values of the exponent β were tabulated (see, for example, Table 1 in Stevens, 1975). The claim that the exponent in (2) is fundamentally important for psychophysical theory encounters difficulties with various data, however, which indicate that its estimated value strongly depends on the experimental conditions, or even on the instructions given to the subject. Among other studies, we mention: Teghtsoonian (1971), for example, who showed that the estimated values of β are correlated with the range of the set of stimuli used in the experiment; and Robinson (1976), who demonstrated how the instructions can systematically affect this exponent. Poulton (1968) reviewed some of these effects. In the light of available evidence, it is clear that no single, basic sensory factor is responsible for the variations of the exponent. In particular, as Green and Luce (1974) argued, its value may reflect some aspects of the subject's decision-making process.

13.6. Production and matching methods.   In this class of experiment, the subject is requested to react to the stimulation by "producing" a value of a sensory variable, for example, by turning a dial. There are several commonly used procedures, some of which were encountered earlier in this book. The *bisection* method described in Chapter 11 also belongs to that category.

The *magnitude production* reverses the procedure used in magnitude estimation. The subject is given a number and asked to produce a matching intensity. As in magnitude estimation, a power law can be fitted to the data. However, as observed by many investigators, the estimated exponent tends to be larger (see Stevens & Greenbaum, 1966, for a summary of the data).

In the *ratio production* method, the observer is instructed to adjust the intensity of the stimulus in such a manner that it appears to be a particular multiple or fraction of a standard. (In this last case, the term *fractionation* method is also used.) For example, the subject may be required to produce a tone intensity appearing half as loud as standard tone of the same frequency. These methods have a long but scattered history, and were regarded with some suspicion until Steven's major contribution to the field. By and large, the data are similar to that obtained with magnitude estimation. (For details, see Marks, 1974; S. S. Stevens, 1975.)

A rather startling prediction may be obtained for the data of the so-called *cross-modality matching* method. Suppose that for two sensory continua, denoted below as 1 and 2, the magnitude estimation data are adequately summarized by the two power laws

$$\phi_1(x) = \alpha_1 x^{\beta_1}, \qquad \phi_2(y) = \alpha_2 y^{\beta_2}. \tag{3}$$

For concreteness, suppose that the two sensory continua are loudness and brightness. Imagine now that in a third experiment the subject, rather than matching physical quantities to numbers as in a magnitude estimation experiment, is requested to directly match the values from one sensory continuum to the other, say from loudness to brightness. At first, this instruction may seem rather bizarre. Actually, not only are the subjects capable of performing such a task without undue hardship but, once again, they provide reasonably regular data. Assuming that the matching of brightness to loudness is achieved by equating the values of the two psychophysical scales, that is, the two right members in (3), we obtain

$$\alpha_1 x^{\beta_1} = \alpha_2 y^{\beta_2}. \tag{4}$$

Writing ϕ_{12} for the cross-modality matching function (thus $\phi_{12}(x) = y$) and rearranging, yields

$$\phi_{12}(x) = \alpha_{12} x^{\beta_{12}}, \tag{5}$$

a power law with

$$\beta_{12} = \beta_1/\beta_2. \tag{6}$$

The prediction that the cross-modality matching function is a power law has been verified by several authors for many continua, and it holds rather well (cf. Fig. 13.2). For a number of reasons, verifying the specific relation linking the exponents in cross-modality matching and magnitude estimation is not as straightforward as it may seem. While S. S. Stevens (1975) and Marks (1974) concluded that (6) is well supported by the facts, Baird, Green, and Luce, (1980) and Mashour and Hosman (1968) have expressed doubt, based on their analysis of their own data.

THE KRANTZ-SHEPARD THEORY

Despite their limitations, the array of results collected by S. S. Stevens and his followers, and summarized in the last two paragraphs, contain enough regularities to require a systematic explanation.

The *relation theory* outlined in this section represents the most satisfactory effort made to account for a substantial part of the data. Some seminal ideas were first proposed by Shepard,[2] in an unpublished manuscript, and were then elaborated and axiomatized by Krantz (1972; see also Shepard, 1981). In presenting this theory, we make a number of idealizations. For example, we omit

---

2. Actually, as pointed out by Krantz (1984), Shepard's idea's had been anticipated by others, notably Junge (1966, 1967) and Stevens (1957), and can be traced back to Hering.

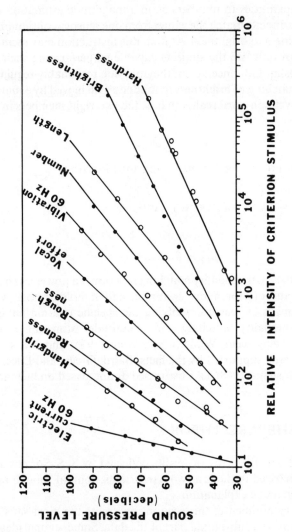

FIGURE 13.2. Cross-modality matching data between loudness and 10 other sensory continua. From "Matching Functions between Loudness and Ten Other Continua" by S. S. Stevens, 1966, *Perception & Psychophysics, 1*, pp. 5–8. Reprinted with permission of author and publisher.

that the data are noisy, are the locus of important contextual and sequential effects, and so forth. To simplify and shorten the exposition, we also specify the theory by properties actually derivable from the more abstract axioms in Krantz's paper. (To some extent, our presentation "trivializes" the theory, but hopefully renders key notions easier to understand.)

13.7. Notation.   The data concern n sensory continua, numbered $1, 2, \ldots, n$. The letters $x, y, \ldots$ (or sometimes $x_i, y_i, \ldots, 1 \leqslant i \leqslant n$, to avoid ambiguities) will stand for positive real numbers representing the physical intensities of the stimuli (energy level). We use the following symbols:

$N_i(y|x,p)$ — Magnitude estimation of stimulus y, with standard x and modulus p, in the sensory continuum i, $1 \leqslant i \leqslant n$;

$P_i(x,y)$ — Ratio estimate of the pair (x,y) in the sensory continuum i; thus, the subject is presented with a pair (x,y) of stimuli in the sensory continuum i, and is required to provide a numerical estimate of their subjective ratio; this number is denoted by $P_i(x,y)$;

$C_{ji}(y_j|x_j,x_i)$ — Cross-modality matching value of stimulus y_j, from sensory continuum j into sensory continuum i, with modulus (x_j,x_i).

Note that in Krantz's system, the cross-modality matching modulus may be taken to be the stimulus response pair of the preceding trial.

13.8. Axioms.   Six axioms specify the theory, labeled RT1 to RT6.

RT1.   For every sensory continuum i, $1 \leqslant i \leqslant n$, there is a function

$$(x,y) \mapsto \ell_i(x,y)$$

mapping the pairs of stimuli onto an interval of positive real numbers, independent of i. These functions are continuous, strictly increasing in the first variable, and strictly decreasing in the second variable. Moreover, the functions ℓ_i are assumed to satisfy the following two conditions.

(i) $\ell_i(x,y) \geqslant \ell_j(z,w)$ implies $\ell_j(w,z) \geqslant \ell_i(y,x)$.
(ii) If $\ell_i(x,y) \geqslant \ell_j(x',y')$ and $\ell_i(y,z) \geqslant \ell_j(y',z')$, then $\ell_i(x,z) \geqslant \ell_j(x',z')$.

This is the basic notion. Every pair (x,y) in a sensory continuum i is mapped into a *sensation continuum* by the function ℓ_i. We will see that the two conditions (i) and (ii) ensure that the quantities $\ell_i(x,y), \ell_j(z,w) \ldots$ etc., behave in a certain sense like arithmetical ratios (cf. Equation 7). In the sequel, we refer to the quantity $\ell_i(x,y)$ as the *sensation 'ratio'* of (x,y). Any estimation or production task is then carried out through the mediation of the sensation 'ratios' of the pairs of stimuli involved. Examples are given in the next two axioms.

RT2.   There is a positive-valued, strictly increasing function H such that for every sensory continuum i,

$$P_i(x,y) = H[\ell_i(x,y)].$$

That is, the ratio estimates are strictly increasing with the sensation 'ratios'.

RT3. For every pair (j,i) of sensory continua, $C_{ji}(y_j|x_j,x_i) = y_i$ implies $\ell_j(y_j,x_j) = \ell_i(y_i,x_i)$.

That is, with cross-modality matching modulus (x_j,x_i), y_j is matched to y_i only if the sensation 'ratios' of (y_j,x_j) and (y_j,x_i) coincide.

The next two axioms emphasize the special role played by one sensory continuum, arbitrarily numbered 1.

RT4. For the sensory continuum 1,

$$P_1(x,y) \cdot P_1(y,z) = P_1(x,z).$$

RT5. If $\ell_i(y,x) = \ell_1(z,w)$, then

$$N_i(y|x,p) = p\,P_1(z,w).$$

The special continuum is assumed to be length. Axiom *RT4* essentially states that mental estimation of length ratios behave like physical measurements, an assumption which, Krantz argues, is supported by the fact that the estimated exponents of the power law for judgments of distance are often close to 1. (Some would question that fact. We postpone criticisms at this point.) Axiom *RT5* is consistent with a mechanism in which magnitude estimation in any sensory continuum i is obtained through computation in the length continuum.

RT6. For any sensory continuum i, and any positive real numbers x,y, and λ,

$$\ell_i(\lambda x,\lambda y) = \ell_i(x,y).$$

Note that this last axiom, which will procure the power law, has the form of Weber's law but applies also to discriminable stimuli.

13.9. Some consequences.   A number of predictions can be derived from these six axioms, examples of which follow. To an attentive reader of this book, the type of arguments leading to these results should be familiar. Only a broad sketch of the proofs will be given. (The details will be left for the exercises.)

If we set $i = j$ in Condition (ii) in RT1, this condition has the form of the bicancellation axiom of Definition 4.10. Notice, moreover, that, except for minor details, the sensation 'ratio' ℓ_i for a continuum i satisfies the conditions of a discrimination system in the sense of Definition 4.7. In fact, Theorem 4.13 can be applied, to yield

$$\ell_i(x,y) = G[f_i(x)/f_i(y)], \tag{7}$$

for some strictly increasing functions G and f_i. Combining this result and RT2, we obtain

$$P_i(x,y) = H\{G[f_i(x)/f_i(y)]\}. \tag{8}$$

Using both (8) and RT4 and applying a standard functional equation argument, results in the function $H \circ G$ having the form

$$H[G(s)] = s^\gamma, \tag{9}$$

for some positive constant γ. From Equation 7 and RT6, we deduce

$$f_i(\lambda x)/f_i(\lambda y) = f_i(x)/f_i(y),$$

a functional equation that (in the conditions of monotonicity and continuity of f_i) has only the solutions

$$f_i(x) = \alpha_i x^{\beta_i},$$

for some constant $\alpha,\beta > 0$. From (7), we thus obtain

$$\ell_i(x,y) = G[(x/y)^{\beta_i}]. \tag{10}$$

Replacing the sensation magnitudes in RT2, RT5, and RT3 by their expressions as given by (10), and using also (9), gives the expected predictions

$$P_i(x,y) = (x/y)^{\beta_i\gamma};$$

$$N_i(y\,|\,x,p) = p(x/y)^{\beta_i\gamma};$$

$$C_{ji}(y_j\,|\,x_j,x_i) = x_i(y_j/x_j)^{\beta_j/\beta_i}.$$

Notice that the cross-modality matching exponents β_j/β_i can be predicted by the ratio of the magnitude estimation exponents of the preceding equation.

Various criticisms can be made against this theory. In particular: (i) it is deterministic, while the data are highly variable, within or across observers; (ii) it omits important sequential and contextual effects, which some believe to be important enough to seriously bias the picture; (iii) the special role of the length continuum can be questioned, specifically the contention that the estimated exponent of the power law is approximately equal to one (Baird, 1970).

Even though the predictions of relation theory may not be fully supported by the data, they certainly represent useful approximations. If nothing more, relation theory may be taken as a good summary of the way a sizable part of the psychophysical community idealizes important data, still a highly serviceable device.

FUNCTIONAL MEASUREMENT

For some psychophysicists, the data of magnitude estimation and production are hopelessly biased by uncontrollable nuisance effects and such methods should be abandoned. Such is Anderson's position when he advocates an alternative collection of procedures and models, which he calls *functional measurement* (see Anderson 1974, 1976, 1981 for numerous references).

In a typical application of functional measurement, the subject is presented with stimuli varying along several dimensions or aspects, in a factorial design, and is required to produce a rating value, say on a 20-category rating scale. In one experiment, for example, designed to assess the so-called *size-weight* illusion, subjects were asked to rate the subjective heaviness of cubical blocks varying in weight and size (Anderson, 1970b). One or more algebraic models are then

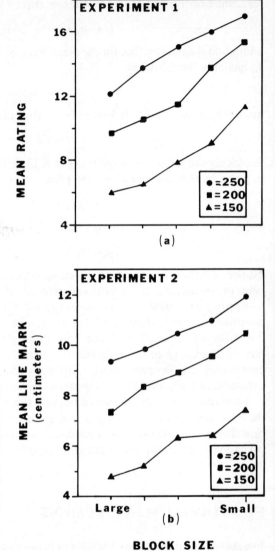

FIGURE 13.3. Anderson's data for the size-weight illusion. Subjects lift and judge heaviness of cubical blocks in a 3 × 5, gram weight × block size design. Verbal rating response is plotted in the upper graph; graphic rating response in the lower graph. From "Averaging Model Applied to the Size-Weight Illusion" by N. H. Anderson, 1970, *Perception & Psychophysics, 8,* pp. 153–170. Reprinted with permission of author and publisher.

applied, symbolizing different combination rules for the factors. Let r_{ij} stand for the (average) rating in cell (i,j) of a two-factor design. The most frequently used models are:

The adding model $\qquad r_{ij} = \alpha_i + \beta_j;$

The averaging model $\qquad r_{ij} = \dfrac{w_i \alpha_i + w_j \beta_j}{w_i + w_j};$

The multiplying model $\qquad r_{ij} = \alpha_i \cdot \beta_j.$

Assuming appropriate distributions for the variances of the errors, these models can be tested through standard analysis of variance techniques. A graphic plot of the data is also used to validate a model. In the case of the adding model for instance, since $r_{ik} - r_{jk} = \alpha_i - \beta_j$, independent on k, a check of "parallelism" can be made. This is illustrated in Figure 13.3, for the size-weight illusion experiment mentioned above (Anderson, 1970b, 1981). This analysis favors a model in which subjective heaviness (as evaluated by the ratings) is represented as the sum of subjective weight and appearance.

Occasionally, the standard models cannot be fitted to the rating data. A monotonic rescaling of the ratings is then carried out by numerical techniques. When the fit of a model is taken to be acceptable, the estimated values of the parameters α_i, β_j can be plotted against the corresponding physical measure. The resulting relation is called the *psychophysical law* for that sensory continuum. It is assumed, or hoped, that this relation will hold across situations varying the experimental design, the instructions, and the model, but involving the same sensory continuum.

Over the years, Anderson and his followers have applied functional measurement methods to a large body of data in psychophysics and elsewhere, and have often succeeded in parsing out the effects of the factors on the ratings, through one or the other of the standard models.

A number of criticisms of Anderson's approach have been made, however. The major point of contention concerns the rating response used, and in particular the status of that response measure with respect to scale type. The mathematical form of the adding and averaging models is invariant under affine transformations (i.e., transformations $x \mapsto \gamma x + \delta$). This property led Anderson to argue that, when one such model is found to fit some data, it can be concluded that the rating response, as well as the estimated parameters, are interval scales. Birnbaum (1982) reviewed the objections to this controversial claim.

THE MEASUREMENT OF SENSATION—SOURCES OF THE CONTROVERSY

To the outsider, the diversity of positions advocated by respected scientists regarding the measurement of sensation and the form of the "psychophysical scale" is bewildering. These positions range from a rejection of the issue (sensation cannot be measured) by James (1890), and more recently Savage (1966, 1970), Zuriff (1972), and Tumarkin (1981) among others, to a strongly held opinion that, given careful experimental control, some particular method yields the desired "psychophysical scale" (see, for example, Anderson, 1981 or S. S. Stevens, 1975). A representative sample of these positions can be found in the commentaries following the paper by Warren (1981), where no less than 29 active researchers give their current thoughts on the matter. A consensus is not in sight. There are four main sources of conflict, which are examined in the next four paragraphs.

13.10. The label "sensation." This unfortunate choice of term is probably at the origin of much disagreement. For reasons that we need not go into here, Fechner's particular combination of scientific skills and philosophical inclination led him to search for ways of measuring sensation by rigorous methods. Sensation, he claimed, cannot be measured directly. His Jnd-counting procedure was intended to measure sensation indirectly: one jnd is interpreted as the difference between two sensations. But the focal meaning of "sensation" is *conscious experience*, and it is far from clear that Fechner's methods, based on discrimination data, depend in any way on the awareness of the stimulation. (For example, these methods are routinely applied in animal psychophysics. Whether or not animals are conscious of their sensory experiences is not a dispute likely to be productive.)

The use of the term "sensation" is probably responsible for the rejection of Fechner's approach by James (1890). Stevens's choice of psychophysical methods, designed to appeal to the subject's conscious experience of the stimulation, was a critical reaction to Fechner's indirect methods of measuring sensation. If Fechner had stated as his goal the measurement of sensory intensities, it may very well be that tone of the debate would have been much less passionate.

The interpretation of "sensation" as meaning "conscious experience" is by no means universal in sensory psychology, which is, of course, a major cause of dissension regarding which data is most relevant to the measurement of sensation. For example, Piéron writes: "There is sensation when the effect of a stimulation is revealed—or is proved to be revealable through conditioning—by a global reaction of the organism, a particular modality of activity, a form of conduct, or a modification resulting from some behaviors, when the effect of this stimulation may thus be integrated in the psychological system governing the adaptation of the animal to the external conditions of the environment" (Piéron, 1967, p. 14). [Translation by the author.]

13.11. The data. There is a divergence of opinions regarding which is to be considered as the primary data of psychophysics. While some favor the discrimination or detection data of classical psychophysics, others advocate the introspective data provided by the "direct" methods of S. S. Stevens and his followers, or that obtained with Anderson's functional measurement procedures. Still others regard physiological recordings as providing the ultimate information.

It is true that some psychophyscists are willing to take all the available data, or at least a large part of it, as the experimental basis of the psychophysical enterprise (e.g., Baird, 1981). There is, however, an unfortunate tendency to consider that the data collected by the methods of an adversary school of psychophysics are either biased, or irrelevant to "the" important problems to be solved. Tumarkin, for example, writes, in reaction to a text of S. S. Stevens (1962): "It will suffice to state explicitly that in the decade that has followed Stevens's pronouncement no light whatsoever has been thrown on the workings of the central nervous system or on the ultimate mystery of the mind by the sone or any other psychometric function, and there are no grounds for hoping that any further work along those lines will be any more fruitful" (Tumarkin, 1972).

13.12. The problem(s) to be solved by the psychophysical scale.   The fact that this is not always addressed with precision produces another occasion of discord. For example, Fechner did not state, perhaps even did not realize clearly, that his method was essentially a partial construction of a function u solving, for some function F, the functional equation

$$P_{a,b} = F[u(a) - u(b)]. \tag{11}$$

Since the function P is constrained by the experimental data, it could not be a priori certain that the construction was feasible. It was shown in Chapter 4 that (11) had a solution—u can be constructed—only if P satisfies some conditions. One such condition is the quadruple condition

$$P_{a,b} \leqslant P_{a',b'} \qquad \text{iff} \qquad P_{a,a'} \leqslant P_{b,b'}.$$

A study of the available data indicates that the quadruple condition would be hard to reject, which gives credence to Equation 11 as a model for discrimination. In turn, this suggests that the scale u merits serious consideration.

A quite different problem is the following. *Construct a scale ψ providing a medium of communication with the general public on practical questions regarding subjective impressions of sensory intensities.* This is a legitimate concern, which leads to introspective methods such as those developed by S. S. Stevens.

My interpretation of the problem tackled by Anderson's functional measurement methods is as follows. Anderson's goal is similar to S. S. Stevens's, but he realizes that the data generated by magnitude estimation and related methods is the locus of important experimental biases. The problem is then: *Construct a scale Ψ using introspective methods in which the artefacts are minimized or controlled experimentally.*

A fourth problem might be this: *Find a scale η that simplifies the notation of psychophysical facts, laws, and models.*

Assuming that the first three scales u, ψ, and Ψ are available, they may or may not coincide. If they do not, which appears to be the case, one or the other, or all three, may be chosen by the scientific community for some useful purpose. For semantic reasons, the scales ψ and Ψ have a more valid claim to the label "sensation" than does the scale u of Equation 11. By itself, this fact does not warrant the adoption of the power function say, for scientific uses. We note, however, that the scales u, ψ, and Ψ are, typically, pairwise related by some simple, monotonically increasing transformation, such as a logarithmic, exponential, or power function, and that either the logarithmic function or the power function would be an adequate solution to the fourth problem—to provide a simple scientific notation.

13.13. The model used to generate the scale.   Granting, for a moment, the legitimacy of selecting some data to be of primary importance in the construction of a particular scale, analyzing such data often depends on an implicit, but testable, model, which may or not be satisfied at an acceptable level. More important, such a model typically has equivalent versions, and the form of the scale may vary critically from one version to another. These facts are not always well understood. In Warren (1981), for example, we read the following.

> Plateau (1872) was the first to try to measure sensation directly. When he instructed eight artists to mix white and black pigments and paint what they considered to be a midgray, it was found that there was close agreement in the shades they selected. He also noted that the same percentage reflectance corresponded to a mid-gray regardless of the level of illumination. This invariance corresponded to the simple relation: *Equal stimulus ratios produce equal sensory ratios.* This relation was used by Plateau to derive his psychophysical power rule [...] which was proposed as an alternative to Fechner's logarithmic rule. Plateau suggested that the power function applied not only to vision, but to all sensory modalities. [...]
>
> Fechner's objection to direct measurement of sensory intensity was not that responses could not be obtained, but that a valid measure of sensory intensity could not be obtained in this manner. Since he claimed that direct measurement of sensation was invalid, it was not possible either to verify or to refute his contention that JNDs were subjectively equal and additive.

Plateau's interpretation of his results, which is adopted by Warren in the quoted text (and by many others before him), was incorrect or at least misleading. The critical statement that

"equal stimulus ratios produce equal sensory ratios"

can be formalized by the functional equation

$$a/b = F[u(a)/u(b)] \qquad (12)$$

in which a and b denote stimulus values, u is the sensory scale, and F is a one-to-one function. Under reasonable side conditions, Equation (12) leads indeed, using standard functional equation techniques, to a power function as the unique form for the sensory scale u. But Equation 12 does not follow from Plateau's data.[3] It is in fact independent from it. Assuming (12) is thus begging the question. Let us establish this.

As in Chapter 3, we denote by $M(a,b)$ the midway gray produced by a typical subject. Thus, $M(a,b)$ is a positive real number in the same scale as a and b. A close reading of Plateau's text strongly suggests that he had in mind the following model of the subject mode of operation.[4]

---

3. It is possible that Plateau was aware of this fact. In a footnote of his paper, we read: "Fechner's formula leads to this consequence that, when the overall illumination increases, the differences in sensation remain constant; it seemed to me more rational, in order to explain the invariance of the general effect of the picture, to postulate *a priori* the constancy of the ratios, and not of the differences, of the sensations." (Plateau, 1872, pp. 382–383.) [Translation by the author; the emphasis is ours.]

4. Plateau writes: "Thus, even though we do not have the capability of directly estimating the ratio of the intensities of two sensations of light, we possess another faculty, which enable us to obtain the value of this ratio indirectly: this faculty consists in that we can sharply appreciate the equality between two contrasts". (Plateau, 1872, p. 380.) [Translated by the author.]

$$M(a,b) = c \qquad \text{iff} \qquad u(a)/u(c) = u(c)/u(b)$$

or equivalently,

$$M(a,b) = c \qquad \text{iff} \qquad u(c) = [u(a)u(b)]^{1/2}$$

or still equivalently,

$$u[M(a,b)] = [u(a)u(b)]^{1/2}. \tag{13}$$

In this model, it is assumed that a subject's response results from a two-step process: first, the physical intensities a and b corresponding to the white and black pigments are transformed into sensory intensities valued in the scale u; next, the subject searches for a midgray stimulus with intensity c such that the ratio $u(a)/u(c)$ is judged to be identical to the ratio $u(c)/u(b)$. This model was encountered earlier, and is testable. We know, for instance (cf. 11.27, 11.28), that for Equation 13 to hold, the function M must satisfy the bisymmetry condition

$$M[M(a,b), M(c,d)] = M[M(a,c), M(b,d)]. \tag{14}$$

In Chapter 3, Plateau's results were formalized by the statement that the midway gray function M is homogeneous of degree one, that is

$$M(\lambda a, \lambda b) = \lambda M(a,b). \tag{15}$$

This homogeneity law is independent of (13) (cf. Exercise 7). However, if both (13) and (15) are assumed to hold, there are two possible forms of the function u:

$$u(a) = \alpha a^{\beta}, \qquad \text{with } \alpha, \beta > 0, \tag{16}$$

$$u(a) = \alpha \exp(\gamma a^{\beta}), \qquad \text{with } \alpha > 0 \text{ and } \gamma\beta > 0 \tag{17}$$

(Theorem 3.13). Notice that, with $F(s) = s^{\beta}$, (16) implies (12), but (17) and (12) are not consistent.

Let us summarize. Plateau's data, taken alone or in the framework of the model specified by Equation 13, does not imply the power law. If this model is assumed, then the scale u appearing in (13) must have one of the two forms (16) and (17), only one of which is a power function.

Since Equation 13 is a reasonable model, this discussion seems to rule out Fechner's logarithmic function. Actually, the form of the sensory scale is even less constrained than the above argument suggests. On the basis of Plateau's data, the logarithmic function is still a viable candidate for the sensory scale. Suppose indeed that the subject's responses are based on checking the equality of differences of sensations, rather than that of ratios. In other terms, assume that

$$M(a,b) = c \qquad \text{iff} \qquad u(a) - u(c) = u(c) - u(b).$$

It is easy to show that this is equivalent to

$$u[M(a,b)] = \frac{u(a) + u(b)}{2} \tag{18}$$

This model is equivalent to (13): there is no way of distinguishing between (13) and (18) experimentally. However, depending on which of (13) or (18) is chosen, the possible forms of the sensory scale may differ. In particular, if both the homogeneity law (15) and (18) are holding, then the function u must have one of the two following forms.

$$u(a) = \alpha \log a + \beta, \qquad \text{with } \alpha > 0,$$

$$u(a) = \alpha a^{\beta} + \gamma, \qquad \text{with } \alpha\beta > 0$$

(Theorem 3.12). We end up with four possible forms for the sensory scale, only one of which satisfies (12).

Our conclusion must be that Plateau's data offer no support whatsoever for the choice of a power function over a logarithmic function. The logarithmic function is eliminated only if (13) is adopted as a model rather than the equivalent (18). The choice depends on whether a geometric or arithmetic mean is preferred, which is arbitrary.

Another part of the quoted text of Warren also deserves some reaction: "Since he [Fechner] claimed that direct measurement of sensation was invalid, it was impossible either to verify or to refute his contention that the JNDs were subjectively equal and additive" (Warren, 1981). But we have seen that Fechner's construction implicitly relies on representation (11). This model is testable since (in the presence of side conditions), it is equivalent to the quadruple condition, which only involves the choice probabilities.

The point to be stressed is that a sensory scale is typically obtained through the analysis of some data in terms of a model that, unfortunately, is sometimes left implicit, as in the important cases of Fechner and Plateau.[5] Moreover, the relative arbitrariness of the selection of one model among equivalent ones is often overlooked. These loose ends certainly contribute to our uncertainty regarding the foundation of sensory scaling.

TWO POSITIONS CONCERNING THE SCALING OF SENSORY MAGNITUDES

It is useful to distinguish two classes of adversary positions.

13.14. Uncovering the psychophysical law.   The psychophysicists in this class consider some particular data to be of primal value in *uncovering* the psychophysical law. The basic idea is that stimulus intensities have a *numerical* representation in the subject's organism, which can be accessed directly if the right response is elicited from the subject in the right paradigm. In the same vein, the logarithmic scale is rejected by observing, for example, that pairs of stimuli that are equidistant on the logarithmic scale do not appear to be equidistant subjectively, or by showing that this scale differs from that obtained by the selected "direct" methods. Many proponents of this position may be found

---

5. One might argue that no model need be postulated in some important methods of scale construction, such as magnitude estimation. Actually, even this apparently straightforward case may require nontrivial modeling, as illustrated by the Krantz-Shepard relation theory.

among S. S. Stevens's followers. When biases or experimental artifacts are observed, it is natural to search for more refined techniques, such as those developed by N. H. Anderson.

The belief in the existence, within the organism, of a numerical representation of sensory intensities may perhaps strike the philosopher as a severe case of reification. It may also annoy the mathematician, who will be puzzled by the multiplicity of different, but equivalent, numerical representations available for any set of sensory data. However, the surprising consistency of the results reported by different laboratories using the same "direct" method prevents a casual dismissal of the notion. As if some analog device were available to them, the subjects are indeed able to make sense of descriptions of stimuli such as "half as loud" or "twice as bright," or to provide regular magnitude estimation or rating data.

A major difficulty for the advocates of a particular "direct" method is that there is no agreement in the psychophysical community regarding the choice of such method. This is both understandable and justified, since the regularity and consistency of the data generated by any "direct" method (however remarkable they may be) are not such that these data could provide the foundation of a scientific scale.

13.15. Adopting a psychophysical scale. The psychophysicists in this second class take the position that the *adoption* of a psychophysical scale for a given sensory continuum is primarily a matter of scientific strategy. Given a large collection of data, considered important by the psychophysical community, a psychophysical scale should be *chosen* that renders simple or convenient the numerical expression of these data and of the models explaining them. In line with such a position, it is recognized that there is typically a degree of arbitrariness in the choice of a scientific scale, and that models and data can be recoded if a monotonic rescaling is taking place. Luce and Galanter (1963) and Ellis (1966) took this position, which is also that of the author.

In this connection, we note that there is a general tendency to plot psychophysical data in logarithmic coordinates, and that many models currently in use have their variables in decibel units, or could easily be recast in such terms. From this viewpoint, the Fechnerian logarithmic scale would yet appear—notwithstanding all the attacks—as a reasonable choice for the psychophysical scale.

One objection to this admittedly utilitarian position is, again, that there is no forseeable agreement regarding what constitutes the bulk of important psychophysical data.

WHY A PSYCHOPHYSICAL SCALE?

In view of the long-lasting debate, this question should be given some consideration. In physics, the adoption of a coherent set of scales was a fundamental step toward the construction of a quantitative representation of the world. The situation is very different in psychophysics, and an analogy—however tempting in view of the success of physics—would be misleading. There is no critical need in psychophysics for adopting a particular set of sensory scales for scientific purposes. The physical scales are available and are used routinely by psychophysicists to report their results and to code quantitative models. Moreover, these scales provide a reasonably simple picture of many important psychophysical data. To my knowledge, nobody ever argued convincingly that major progress would result in sensory research from using a standard set of psychophysical scales.

In my opinion, the only argument favoring the adoption of such a set lies on the practical side. In the last couple of decades, a consensus has emerged that subjects can, with a surprising degree of reliability, use numbers to quantify their experience of sensory intensities. A set of scales based on such "direct" assessment of sensory experience—thus constructed along the lines of S. S. Stevens's or N. H. Anderson's work—may have important practical uses. As mentioned earlier, such scales would provide a convenient medium of communication between experts and a lay public regarding matters of common concern, such as noise pollution or illumination in the working place.

If such a route is taken, a particulary sensory scale should then be regarded as a statistical entity, estimating a central tendency in a population with a nonnegligible variability resulting from many factors difficult to control, rather than as a scientific device evaluating sensory impressions with a specified physiological substratum. Obviously, one could also arbitrarily adopt such a scale for scientific purposes. The reasons for doing so are not compelling, however.

EXERCISES

1. Make the best possible case in favor of the statement: "Sensation grows as the logarithm of excitation."
2. Criticize the above statement.
3. Show that Equation 7 follows from an application of the axioms of the Krantz-Shepard theory, by an application of Theorem 4.13.
4. Using the equivalence of the quadruple condition and of the Bi-cancellation condition in Theorem 4.13, explore the possibility of modifying Axiom RT1(ii) in 13.8.
5. Derive Equation 9 from Equation 8 and RT4.
6. Derive Equation 10.
7. Prove by two counterexamples that (13) and (15) are independent.
8. Do you believe that the position advocated in 13.14 can be shown to be mistaken (logically or experimentally)? Elaborate your answer.

14

Meaningful Psychophysical Laws[†]

There is a view of quantitative science which goes roughly as follows. First, data are collected. Next, these data are summarized and organized along the lines of a mathematical theory, which provides a temporary explanation. Such an explanation never fits the data perfectly. The discrepancy between theory and data suggests alternative theories, and further experiments. Science pursues its course toward an increasingly reliable explanation of the world.

This outline of the quantitative approach to science is certainly correct, but important details are lacking. For example, a mathematical expression summarizing some data may be considered unacceptable, even though it provides a good fit.[1] An examination of scientific developments leads to the conclusion that the selection of a mathematical expression to describe a phenomenon follows implicit rules, which appear to favor a class of expressions called "meaningful." The study of "meaningfulness' is relatively recent.[2] There are several candidates for a definition of this concept, but as yet no general agreement on a choice. Nevertheless, a discussion of this topic deserves to be included here for two reasons.

1. Current definitions of "meaningfulness," even though they may capture formally independent concepts, tend to agree in practice on what "good" and "bad" expressions are.
2. More important, a consideration of this concept may lead the researcher to concentrate on aspects of the data that may otherwise have been neglected. The researcher may then be in position to draw more durable conclusions.

The viewpoint on "meaningfulness" presented here will be that of Falmagne and Narens (1983). Other discussions can be found in Suppes and Zinnes (1963), Roberts (1979) and Krantz et al. (in preparation).

We begin by observing that, in quoting quantitative empirical laws, scientists

---

† Parts of this chapter are based on "Scales and Meaningfulness of Quantitative Laws" by Jean-Claude Falmagne and Louis Narens, *Synthese*, Vol. 55, No. 3, June 1983, D. Reidel Publishing. Copyright © 1983.

1. Since a mathematical model can be regarded as a set of mathematical expressions, this remark also applies to models.

2. As far as I know, the first paper dealing specifically with this topic is that of Suppes (1959). On the other hand, some interpretation of "meaningfulness" render this concept essentially equivalent to a generalization of "dimensional invariance" in classical physics (Krantz et al., 1971). This is not the viewpoint taken in this chapter.

frequently omit to specify the various scales entering in the equations. Illustrations of this widespread habit abound in most scientific fields. Two examples are given as follows.

14.1. Examples. (a) *Visual Perception.* "A flash of light of short duration, presented to the eye in any condition of adaptation, provides a given effect (e.g., a brightness match against a standard) that can be achieved by the reciprocal manipulation of luminance and duration of the flash. This statement means that the given effect can be produced by a dim light that acts for a relatively long time, or by an intense flash that acts for a short time. Stated mathematically, $L \times t = C$, where L is the light intensity, t is the duration of the flash, and C is a constant. This relationship is sometimes known, for human vision, as Bloch's law (1885), or, because of its applicability to many other photochemical systems, as the Bunsen-Roscoe law" (Graham et al., 1965, p. 77).

(b) *Electromagnetism.* "The force in a homogeneous isotropic medium of infinite extent between two point charges is proportional to the product of their magnitude, divided by the square of the distance between them" (Coulomb's law, quoted from the *American Institute of Physics Handbook*, 1957.)

In addition to considerably simplifying the life of the student in quantitative sciences, such a practice fortunately makes good sense, in these and many other similar examples. Indeed, the mathematical forms of the quoted laws are unaffected by transformations of the scales entering in the equations formalizing the laws, provided that such transformations are "admissible." (We will be more specific in a moment.) Let us illustrate this remark in the case of (b). Each numerical assignment for the three variables involved in Coulomb's law—force, magnitude of charge, and distance—is a ratio scale, that is, these assignments are only defined up to multiplications by positive constants (Table 13.1). Such multiplications play the role of the "admissible" transformations. Let us formalize Coulomb's law by the expression

$$F = C\frac{q_1 q_2}{d_{12}^2}, \tag{1}$$

in which: F is the force acting on two point charges p_1, p_2; q_1, q_2 are the respective magnitudes of the charges; d_{12} is the distance between the point charges; and C is the constant of proportionality. Let α, β and γ be three positive constants. Then, obviously, Equation 1 holds if and only if

$$\alpha F = \frac{\gamma^2 \alpha C}{\beta^2} \times \frac{(\beta q_1)(\beta q_2)}{(\gamma d_{12})^2}. \tag{2}$$

Actually, Equation 2 is simply a restatement of Coulomb's law with the new assignments and a different constant of proportionality. Clearly, specific properties of the mathematical form of Coulomb's law were essential in reaching our conclusions. Similar arguments could be used in the case of (a). Notice in passing an important difference between these two examples. In Coulomb's law, the numbers assigned to two of the variables—the charges—are manipulated by the same admissible transformations. This situation does not arise in Bloch's law. We will see later that whether or not quantities entering into a law are manipulated by the same or by different admissible transformations will have a critical impact on the form of the law. To sum up, our discussion indicates that the following three concepts are intimately interrelated.

(i) The admissible transformations (scales) entering into an equation describing some empirical law.
(ii) The mathematical expression of this equation.
(iii) The invariance of this equation under the admissible transformations of the variables.

The label "meaningfulness" is attached to the last concept. A formal definition will be given in a moment. We argue that "meaningfulness" is a reasonable requirement for models or laws describing some empirical data. The strength of this requirement is deceptive, especially when the scales entering in the equations are ratio or interval scales, as is typically the case in psychophysics. The possible forms of the laws are then severely constrained. Several illustrations of this fact are given in this chapter.

We build up our definition of meaningfulness from the analysis of the following examples in psychopysics.

EXAMPLES

14.2. Example. (a) *Discrimination.* With a slight change of our usual notations, let $P(s,t)$ be the probability that stimulus s is judged as exceeding stimulus t, in a standard discrimination paradigm. The letters s and t denote positive real numbers representing physical intensities, measured in a ratio scale. Consider the following representation of these probabilities:

$$P(s,t) = F\left(\frac{s+1}{t+1}\right),\qquad(3)$$

where F is a strictly increasing function. As a model for the choice probabilities, Equation 3 is ambiguous, even if the function F is completely specified. The difficulty is that the constraints imposed on the probabilities by this equation depend on the scale used. This may be obvious. A detailed analysis of this case will nevertheless be informative. Let

$$a = 3 \qquad b = 2$$
$$c = 500 \qquad d = 400$$

be four stimulus values. From (3), we derive

$$P(a,b) = F\left(\frac{4}{3}\right) > F\left(\frac{501}{401}\right) = P(c,d).\qquad(4)$$

Suppose that a change of scale is taking place. Since we have a ratio scale, this involves multiplying all the stimulus values by a constant $\lambda > 0$. We take $\lambda = 100$. We have thus the transformation $s \mapsto \lambda s = s'$ for any $s > 0$. Notice that s and s' denote the same physical stimulus. The probability of judging that s exceeds t is thus identical to that of judging that s' exceeds t'. However, *we cannot write* $P(s,t) = P(s',t')$ since P, considered as a function of two real variables, does not denote the same function in the two members of that equation. Let P' denote the function representing the choice probabilities after the change of scale. We have thus, in general,

$$P(s,t) = P'(100s, 100t). \tag{5}$$

This leads to

$$P'(a,b) = P'(3,2) = P(.03, .02) = F\left(\frac{1.03}{1.02}\right) < F\left(\frac{6}{5}\right)$$

$$= P(5,4) = P'(500,400) = P'(c,d).$$

We conclude that

$$P'(a,b) < P'(c,d) \tag{6}$$

contrasting with (4). Obviously, there is no logical contradiction between (4) and (6). If the scale used in (3) is not known, however, the information contained in this equation is much less than what is intended. In particular, it cannot be decided which of the two inequalities (4) or (6) is predicted by the model for the particular values considered. We could, of course, remove all ambiguities by mentioning the scale in an appendix to Equation 3. This possibility would not be acceptable to the scientific community. As illustrated by Examples 14.1(a) and (b), important scientific laws, typically, do not specify the scale(s). Some reasons for this almost universal rule are examined later on in this chapter.

(b) *Continuation.* A better notation for the model symbolized by (3) is

$$P(s,t) = F\left(\frac{s + K}{t + K}\right), \tag{7}$$

in which $K > 0$ is a scale dependent constant, and all other notions are as in (3). This would be considered as the standard notation for this model. With the change of scale

$$s \mapsto \lambda s = s'$$

and the same convention as above regarding the function P', this leads to

$$P'(\lambda s, \lambda t) = F\left(\frac{\lambda s + \lambda K}{\lambda t + \lambda K}\right) = P(s,t).$$

In simple cases, this notational style is adequate, but ambiguities remain. The existence, and the form, of the dependence of the constant K on the scale is left implicit. Similarly, the function P also depends on the scale, but not the function F. The notation of (7) leaves to the educated common sense of the scientist to figure out these facts.

(c) *Continuation.* Any admissible change of scale in this model is completely specified by a positive constant λ. Using this fact, a more explicit notation for this model is

$$P_\lambda(s,t) = F\left[\frac{s + \kappa(\lambda)}{t + \kappa(\lambda)}\right], \tag{8}$$

with the function $\kappa(\lambda) = \lambda K$. The case $\lambda = 1$ in (8) may be interpreted as the *current scale* or the *initial scale*. Any $\lambda > 0$ corresponds to an admissible rescaling of the quantities. The difference between (7) and (8) may seem slight, but it is potent. We recommend that this style be adopted for the notation of a model, when questions regarding the effect of scales are discussed. One might perhaps object that such notation is needlessly heavy, and that the effect of a change of the scales entering in the mathematical expression of a model will be reasonably obvious to any sophisticated scientist. This is true in this simple case, but certainly not in general. Even a situation only slightly more complicated than that of the above example may raise nontrivial questions concerning the possible forms of a model, as determined by the admissible changes of the scales.

14.3. Example.   *Detection.* In a psychoacoustic paradigm, a subject is presented on each trial with a masking noise of intensity n. The stimulus to be detected is a click of intensity x, presented at a time τ measured from the end of the noise. Thus, the delay τ between the end of the noise and the presentation of the stimulus may be negative (the stimulus may be embedded in the noise). Let $P(x,n,\tau)$ be the probability of a correct detection. Consider the following model for this situation:

$$P(n,x,\tau) = F[x/n^{\delta(\tau)}], \tag{9}$$

in which F is a strictly increasing function, and δ is a function of the delay. This situation was investigated by Pavel (1980), who demonstrated that important predictions of the model specified by (9) were well supported by his data. Nevertheless, considerations of changes of scales lead to the conclusion that (9) is "meaningful" only if δ does not vary with τ, which is rejected by Pavel's data. Thus (9) is not a "good" form to summarize Pavel's data, a fact that may escape even sophisticated scientists. We return to this example later on in this chapter, and detailed proofs of these assertions will be provided (see 14.20 and 14.21).

14.4. Example.   *Discrimination.* In a standard loudness discrimination paradigm, two intensities of a 1000-Hz tone are presented successively to a subject. Let s,t be the intensities of the first and second stimulus, respectively. We assume that these numbers are measured on a ratio scale. Let $P(s,t)$ be the probability that the first stimulus is judged louder. Consider the following model for these probabilities:

$$P(s,t) = F(s^\beta - t^{\beta'}),\tag{10}$$

in which F is a strictly increasing function, and β, β' are positive constants, with possibly $\beta \neq \beta'$ accounting for a possible asymmetry (time-order error) in this paradigm. A change of scale $s \mapsto \lambda s$ can affect the function F, and the parameters β and β'. In the style of (8), we rewrite (10) as

$$P_\lambda(s,t) = F_\lambda[s^{\beta(\lambda)} - t^{\beta'(\lambda)}].\tag{11}$$

Let us assume that β and β' are distinct (whether or not they vary effectively as functions of the scale λ). It can be shown that (10) or the more explicit (11) does not satisfy the criterion of "meaningfulness" as we will define it (Definition 14.8): the form of (10) or (11) is not invariant with admissible transformations $s \mapsto \lambda s$. On the other hand, the slightly different

$$P(s,t) = F(s^\beta - \delta t^{\beta'}),\tag{12}$$

with the additional parameter δ, will be shown to be "meaningful."

14.5. Example.   *Bisection.* With the same stimuli as in Example 14.4, let $M_\lambda(s,t)$ be the stimulus sounding halfway between s and t. As before, λ denotes the scale. Consider the model

$$[M_\lambda(s,t)]^\beta = \frac{s^\beta + \delta(\lambda)t^\beta}{2},\tag{13}$$

in which $\delta(\lambda) = \lambda D > 0$, and $D, \beta > 0$ are parameters. This representation is closely related to that investigated in Chapters 3 and 11 for the bisection paradigm. The function δ is introduced to account for a possible asymmetry between the first and the second stimuli. Again, it can be established that (13) is not "meaningful" in the sense of Definition 14.8.

These examples provide some intuition for the concept that we are attempting to capture. In the next two sections, we introduce a precise terminology and notation, which will systematize and generalize the style used in writing (8), in which the dependence of the concepts on the scale is specified. "Meaningfulness" will then be defined as a type of invariance under changes of scales.

SCALE FAMILIES

The notions of *scale*, *ratio scale*, and *interval scale* were introduced in the preceding chapter. A tighter treatment is provided here.

14.6. Definition.   Let I be any nonempty, real, open interval. A strictly increasing, continuous function mapping I onto I will be called a *scale on I*. The identity scale $x \mapsto x$ will be denoted by ι_I. A set $\mathcal{K}$ of scales on I containing the identity scale ι_I will be called a *scale family with domain I*, or more briefly a *scale family on I*. Any subset of a scale family $\mathcal{K}$ containing the identity scale is a *scale* *subfamily of* $\mathcal{H}$. A scale family $\mathcal{H}$ is called a

$$\left.\begin{cases} \text{Ratio scale family} \\ \text{Interval scale family} \\ \text{Log interval scale family} \end{cases}\right\} \quad \text{iff, respectively,}$$

$$\begin{cases} \mathcal{H} = \{k\,|\,k(x) = \lambda_k x, \text{ for some } \lambda_k \in \mathbb{R}_+, \text{ and all } x \in \mathbb{R}_+\}, \\ \mathcal{H} = \{k\,|\,k(x) = \lambda_k x + \gamma_k, \text{ for some } \lambda_k \in \mathbb{R}_+, \gamma_k \in \mathbb{R}, \text{ and all } x \in \mathbb{R}\}, \\ \mathcal{H} = \{k\,|\,k(x) = \gamma_k x^{\lambda_k}, \text{ for some } \gamma_k, \lambda_k \in \mathbb{R}_+, \text{ and all } x \in \mathbb{R}_+\}. \end{cases}$$

Thus, a ratio scale family $\mathcal{H}$ is uncountable: to every positive real number λ_k, there exists a scale $k \in \mathcal{H}$ such that $k(x) = \lambda_k x$. A similar remark applies to interval and log interval scale families. Notice a fundamental resemblance between an interval scale family and a log interval scale family, which is expressed by the equation

$$\log(\gamma_k e^{\lambda_k x}) = \log \gamma_k + \lambda_k x.$$

This type of correspondence is explored in the Complements section of this chapter.

MEANINGFUL FAMILIES OF NUMERICAL CODES

We consider a situation in which the data collected have been coded numerically in terms of two input quantities

$$(a,x),$$

which are, respectively, evaluated in terms of two input scales

$$f \in \mathcal{F}, \qquad g \in \mathcal{G},$$

yielding an output quantity P, a function of (a,x). However, in the course of determining P, the input scales f and g are used. To express this dependence, we use the explicit notation

$$M_{f,g}(a,x),$$

to specify the output P. Thus, $M_{f,g}$ is a real-valued function of two real variables. This notation generalizes that of Equation 8. Clearly, the empirical situation is compatible with many numerical codes. To the extent that these numerical codes bear a "strong resemblance" to one another, in the sense that they formalize the same "essential information" in the data, one is tempted to describe the situation as "lawful." But what is the meaning of "strong resemblance" and "essential information"? The next and following definitions try to capture some important aspects of this concept.

14.7. Definition. Let $\mathcal{F}, \mathcal{G}$ be two scale families on A, X, respectively. Let R be a subset of $\mathcal{F} \times \mathcal{G}$, such that $(\iota_A, \iota_X) \in R$. Let $M_{f,g}$ be a real-valued, continuous function defined on $A \times X$, strictly increasing in the first argument, and strictly monotonic in the second argument. Then

$$\mathcal{M} = \{M_{f,g} | (f,g) \in R\}$$

is a *family of numerical codes*. (Some remarks on the role of R will be made shortly.) Each $M_{f,g} \in \mathcal{M}$ will be referred to as a *numerical code*. Since R is a binary relation, we often abbreviate $(f,g) \in R$ by fRg. Notice that, by definition, $\iota_A R \iota_X$. For simplicity, we adopt the abbreviation

$$M = M_{\iota_A, \iota_X}.$$

We will occasionally refer to M as the *initial code*. We are now in a position to formulate a very general invariance property for families of numerical codes.

14.8. Definition. A family $\mathcal{M} = \{M_{f,g} | fRg\}$ of numerical codes is *order-meaningful* iff whenever fRg, f^*Rg^*, then

$$M_{f,g}[f(a), g(x)] \leqslant M_{f,g}[f(b), g(y)]$$

iff

$$M_{f^*,g^*}[f^*(a), g^*(x)] \leqslant M_{f^*,g^*}[f^*(b), g^*(y)],$$

for all points a,b in the domain of f, f^* and all points x,y in the domain of g, g^*. By abuse of language, we sometimes say that a particular numerical code, or a particular numerical law is *order-meaningful* to signify that the corresponding family $\mathcal{M}$ of numerical codes, with a domain made clear by the context, is (order) meaningful. A similar convention will be used freely throughout this chapter for other properties of a family $\mathcal{M}$ of numerical codes. Moreover, the specification "order" in "order-meaningful" will be dropped for simplicity.

14.9. Remarks. (1) The relation R allows for a suitable generality in our definition. In Bloch's law, we have $R = \mathcal{F} \times \mathcal{G}$: this law can be formulated for any choice of two scales, measuring light intensity and duration. In the case of Coulomb's law, if the distance is kept constant, we have $\mathcal{F} = \mathcal{G}$ and R is the identity function on $\mathcal{F}$: the magnitudes of the two charges are measured using the same scale.

(2) We stress that, in one important respect, the definition of "meaningfulness" adopted here, which is that of Falmagne and Narens (1983), differs from that most frequently encountered in the measurement literature. A key feature of this definition is that it applies to a family of relations (the family of numerical codes), rather than to a single relation.

(3) Some reflection will probably convince the reader that the concept of meaningfulness, as defined here, represents a rather minimal (yet essential) requirement for a family of numerical codes to be worthy of consideration for scientific purposes. This may not be obvious. The following remarks may help the reader's examination of this notion.

Any numerical code $M_{f,g}$ is a translation, depending on the chosen scales f,g, of a collection of empirical facts. To be specific, to the Cartesian product

$A \times X$ corresponds a set $A^\circ \times X^\circ$ of empirical situations (inputs). Thus, $(\alpha, \xi) \in (A^\circ \times X^\circ)$ is an empirical situation characterized by two aspects that are in general nonnumerical. There is also an empirical set E° (of outputs), and a mapping

$$(\alpha, \xi) \mapsto \rho(\alpha, \xi)$$

of $A^\circ \times X^\circ$ onto E°. The notation $\rho(\alpha, \xi)$ symbolizes the output in E° generated by the input (α, ξ). We assume that some initial scaling has taken place, involving two real-valued mappings

$$\alpha \mapsto \alpha', \quad \xi \mapsto \xi'$$

respectively of A° onto A and X° onto X.

From an empirical viewpoint, the critical information is contained in the function ρ. This information should be preserved by any numerical translation. In particular, the fact that two inputs $(\alpha, \xi), (\beta, \zeta)$ generate the same output should be preserved no matter which numerical code $M_{f,g}$ is chosen. Symbolically,

$$\rho(\alpha, \xi) = \rho(\beta, \zeta) \tag{14}$$

iff

$$M_{f,g}[f(\alpha'), g(\xi')] = M_{f,g}[f(\beta'), g(\zeta')]. \tag{15}$$

Since (14) does not depend on the scales, this immediately yields

$$M_{f,g}[f(a), g(x)] = M_{f,g}[f(b), g(y)]$$

iff

$$M_{f*,g*}[f*(a), g*(x)] = M_{f*,g*}[f*(b), g*(y)].$$

This is a weaker form of the meaningfulness condition defined in 14.8, and is certainly a natural requirement for a family of numerical codes. We consider here a case in which we have an ordering $\precsim$ on the set E° of outputs, containing important empirical informations. It is reasonable to require then that this ordering be preserved under any numerical coding. Symbolically.

$$\rho(\alpha, \xi) \precsim \rho(\beta, \zeta)$$

iff

$$M_{f,g}[f(\alpha'), g(\xi')] \leqslant M_{f,g}[f(\beta'), g(\zeta')],$$

leading to Definition 14.8.

We apply Definition 14.8 to some of the examples discussed earlier.

14.10. Examples. Equation 3 in Example 14.2(a) is not meaningful. Indeed, the only possible dependence on the scale in the right member of

$$P(s,t) = F\left(\frac{s+1}{t+1}\right) \tag{16}$$

is in the function F. We rewrite (16) as

$$P_\lambda(s,t) = F_\lambda\left(\frac{s+1}{t+1}\right), \tag{17}$$

with $\lambda > 0$, a constant symbolizing the scale. Let $\mathcal{M} = \{P_\lambda\}$ be the corresponding family of numerical codes. The two scale families used to measure the two variables s and t in (16) are identical. We are thus in a case of Definition 14.8 in which the relation R is the identity on the scale family $\mathcal{F} = \mathcal{G}$. We write P_λ rather than $P_{\lambda,\lambda}$ for simplicity. The family $\mathcal{M}$ of numerical codes is meaningful iff

$$P_\lambda(\lambda a, \lambda b) \leqslant P_\lambda(\lambda c, \lambda d)$$

$$\text{iff} \tag{18}$$

$$P_\gamma(\gamma a, \gamma b) \leqslant P_\gamma(\gamma c, \gamma d),$$

for all $a, b, c, d, \lambda, \gamma > 0$. Applying (17), and using the assumption that the function F_λ is strictly increasing, (18) is equivalent to

$$\frac{\lambda a + 1}{\lambda b + 1} \leqslant \frac{\lambda c + 1}{\lambda d + 1}$$

$$\text{iff} \tag{19}$$

$$\frac{\gamma a + 1}{\gamma b + 1} \leqslant \frac{\gamma c + 1}{\gamma d + 1},$$

and it is clear that (19) cannot hold for all $a, b, c, d, \lambda, \gamma > 0$ (Exercise 1). On the other hand, it is easy to check that Example 14.2(b), or the more explicit 14.2(c), is meaningful.

14.11. Example.   We consider Example 14.4. The family $\mathcal{M}$ of numerical codes defined by

$$P_\lambda(s,t) = F_\lambda[s^{\beta(\lambda)} - t^{\beta'(\lambda)}],$$

with F_λ strictly increasing, is not meaningful if β and β' are distinct functions. By definition, $\mathcal{M}$ is meaningful if and only if we have

$$(\lambda a)^{\beta(\lambda)} - (\lambda b)^{\beta'(\lambda)} \leqslant (\lambda c)^{\beta(\lambda)} - (\lambda d)^{\beta'(\lambda)}$$

$$\text{iff} \tag{20}$$

$$(\gamma a)^{\beta(\gamma)} - (\gamma b)^{\beta'(\gamma)} \leqslant (\gamma c)^{\beta(\gamma)} - (\gamma d)^{\beta'(\gamma)}$$

for all $a, b, c, d, \lambda, \gamma > 0$. We suppose first that β and β' are constant, with $\beta \neq \beta'$. Fix $\gamma = 1$. Then (20) implies the existence of a strictly increasing function H_λ satisfying

$$H_\lambda(a^\beta - b^{\beta'}) = (\lambda a)^\beta - (\lambda b)^{\beta'}. \tag{21}$$

Varying a and b, while keeping $a^\beta - b^{\beta'} = 1$, we can rewrite this equation in the form

$$H_\lambda(1) = [\lambda(1 + b^{\beta'})^{1/\beta}]^\beta - (\lambda b)^{\beta'}$$
$$= \lambda^\beta + b^{\beta'}(\lambda^\beta - \lambda^{\beta'})$$

and the right member is independent of b only if $\beta = \beta'$, contradicting the hypothesis. The general case in which β and β' vary effectively with λ uses a similar line of argument and is left to the reader.

On the other hand,

$$P_\lambda(s,t) = F_\lambda[s^\beta - \delta(\lambda)t^{\beta'}]$$

is meaningful with $\delta(\lambda) = \lambda^{\beta-\beta'}$, since

$$P_\lambda(\lambda a, \lambda b) \leqslant P_\lambda(\lambda c, \lambda d)$$

iff

$$(\lambda a)^\beta - \lambda^{\beta-\beta'}(\lambda b)^{\beta'} \leqslant (\lambda c)^\beta - \lambda^{\beta-\beta'}(\lambda d)^{\beta'}$$

iff

$$a^\beta - b^{\beta'} \leqslant c^\beta - d^{\beta'},$$

independent of λ.

14.12. Example. The bisection model

$$[M_\lambda(s,t)]^\beta = \frac{s^\beta + \lambda D t^\beta}{2}$$

of Example 14.5 is not meaningful. Indeed, successively

$$[M_\lambda(\lambda a, \lambda b) \leqslant M_\lambda(\lambda c, \lambda d)$$

iff

$$\left[\frac{(\lambda a)^\beta + \lambda D(\lambda b)^\beta}{2}\right]^{1/\beta} \leqslant \left[\frac{(\lambda c)^\beta + \lambda D(\lambda d)^\beta}{2}\right]^{1/\beta}$$

iff

$$a^\beta + \lambda D b^\beta \leqslant c^\beta + \lambda D d^\beta,$$

and the dependence on the scale cannot be factored out.

The argument used to obtain the function H_λ in (21) can be generalized. The following simple consequence of Definition 14.8 will be useful in the sequel.

14.13. Theorem. *A family* $\mathcal{M} = \{M_{f,g} | fRg\}$ *of numerical codes is meaningful iff for all* $(f,g) \in R$, *there exists a strictly increasing, continuous function* $H_{f,g}$ *mapping the range of the initial code* M *onto the range of* $M_{f,g}$ *such that*

$$H_{f,g}[M(a,x)] = M_{f,g}[f(a),g(x)] \tag{22}$$

whenever both members are defined.

Indeed, if $\mathcal{M}$ is meaningful, it suffices to define $H_{f,g}$ by (22): with f^* and g^* as the two identity scales, the defining equivalence in 14.8 ensures that the function $H_{f,g}$ is well defined, strictly increasing, and continuous. However obvious, the following consequence of this theorem deserves explicit mention.

14.14. Theorem.   *If a family $\mathcal{M} = \{M_{f,g} \mid fRg\}$ of numerical codes is meaningful, and the range of each element of $\mathcal{M}$ is the same non empty open interval, then there exists a scale family $\mathcal{H}$ and a function $(f,g) \mapsto H_{f,g}$ from R onto $\mathcal{H}$, such that Equation (22) holds.*

Definition 14.8 provides a practically useful criterion for selecting acceptable mathematical expressions of laws or models. It must be clear that, taken by itself, the condition of meaningfulness has no empirical content. As a background axiom, however, this condition is powerful and can strengthen other, empirically relevant conditions.

We now introduce two conditions which formally resemble meaningfulness, but are nevertheless independent from it. These conditions may appear to be rather weak. In the context of meaningfulness, however, they considerably reduce the possible forms of empirical laws. Absorbing this material may require a serious effort. In case of difficulty, the reader is advised to go directly to the next section, where an application of these concepts in psychoacoustics is described. A glance at Table 14.1 may also be suggestive.

*ISOTONE AND DIMENSIONALLY INVARIANT FAMILIES OF NUMERICAL CODES

14.15. Definition.   Let $\mathcal{F}, \mathcal{G}$ be two scale family on A, X, respectively; let $\mathcal{M} = \{M_{f,g} \mid fRg\}$ be a family of numerical codes, with $R \subset \mathcal{F} \times \mathcal{G}$. A numerical code $M_{f,g} \in \mathcal{M}$ is called *dimensionally invariant* iff whenever f^*Rg^*, then

$$M_{f,g}[f^*(a), g^*(x)] \leqslant M_{f,g}[f^*(b), g^*(y)]$$

iff

$$M_{f,g}(a,x) \leqslant M_{f,g}(b,y)$$

for all $a, b \in A$ and $x, y \in X$. The family $\mathcal{M}$ is called *dimensionally invariant* iff all its numerical codes are dimensionally invariant. This definition generalizes the classical notion used in dimensional analysis (cf. Causey, 1969). Notice that a numerical code $M_{f,g} \in \mathcal{M}$ is dimensionally invariant iff for all f^*Rg^*, there exists a strictly increasing, continuous function $Q_{f,g;f^*,g^*}$ such that

$$M_{f,g}[f^*(a), g^*(x)] = Q_{f,g;f^*,g^*}[M_{f,g}(a,x)]$$

whenever both members of this equation are defined.

We shall say that $\mathcal{M}$ is *isotonically generated*, or more simply, *isotone*, iff there exists a real-valued function M^*, defined on $A \times X$ such that whenever fRg, then

$$M_{f,g} = m_{f,g} \circ M^* \tag{23}$$

for some strictly increasing, continuous function $m_{f,g}$ mapping the range of M^* onto the range of $M_{f,g}$. Notice that there is no loss of generality in assuming that $M^* = M$. Indeed, we have by definition of isotonicity

$$M = m_{\iota_{A},\iota_{X}} \circ M^*$$

which yields for any $(f,g) \in R$,

$$M_{f,g} = m_{f,g} \circ m_{\iota_{A},\iota_{X}}^{-1} \circ M,$$

and the function $m_{f,g} \circ m_{\iota_{A},\iota_{X}}^{-1}$ is strictly increasing, continuous, and maps the range of M onto the range of $M_{f,g}$. In other terms, if $\mathcal{M}$ is isotone, then any numerical code $M_{f,g}$ can be obtained by some strictly increasing, continuous transformation of M.

The reader should check the following facts.

(i) Example 14.5 is dimensionally invariant, but neither isotone nor meaningful.
(ii) Equation 17 is isotone, but neither dimensionally invariant nor meaningful.
(iii) Example 14.2(c) is meaningful, but neither isotone nor dimensionally invariant.

The interrelationship of these concepts is expressed in the following theorem, which also summarizes the above independence results.

14.16. Theorem. *The property of meaningfulness, isotonicity, and dimensional invariance are pairwise independent. However, any two of these conditions implies the third.*

Proof. Let $\mathcal{M} = \{M_{f,g} | fRg\}$ be a family of numerical codes.

(i) *Dimensional invariance and isotonicity imply meaningfulness.* For any $M_{f,g} \in \mathcal{M}$, using successively dimensional invariance and isotonicity,

$$\begin{aligned} M_{f,g}[f(a), g(x)] &= Q_{f,g;f,g}[M_{f,g}(a,x)] \\ &= (Q_{f,g;f,g} \circ m_{f,g})[M(a,x)] \\ &= H_{f,g}[M(a,x)], \end{aligned}$$

with $H_{f,g} = Q_{f,g;f,g} \circ m_{f,g}$ strictly increasing and continuous. By Theorem 14.13 we conclude that $\mathcal{M}$ is meaningful.

(ii) *Meaningfulness and isotonicity imply dimensional invariance.* Let $\mathcal{M}$ be a meaningful family of numerical codes. If $M_{f,g} \in \mathcal{M}$, we have by Theorem 14.13,

$$M_{f,g}[f(a), g(x)] = H_{f,g}[M(a,x)] \tag{24}$$

where $H_{f,g}$ is a strictly increasing, continuous function. Assuming that $\mathcal{M}$ is also isotone, we obtain

$$M_{f,g}[f(a), g(x)] = m_{f,g}\{M[f(a), g(x)]\}, \tag{25}$$

with $m_{f,g}$ again a strictly increasing, continuous function. Using successively (25) and (24), we have

$$M[f(a), g(x)] = m_{f,g}^{-1} \{M_{f,g}[f(a), g(x)]\}$$
$$= (m_{f,g}^{-1} \circ H_{f,g})[M(a,x)]$$

which implies that M is dimensionally invariant, since $m_{f,g}^{-1} \circ H_{f,g}$ is strictly increasing and continuous.

It follows that any numerical code $M_{f,g} \in \mathcal{M}$ is dimensionally invariant. Indeed, whenever $f*Rg*$,

$$M_{f,g}[f*(a), g*(x)] = m_{f,g}\{M[f*(a), g*(x)]\} \text{ (isotonicity)}$$
$$= Q_{f,g;f*,g*}[M_{f,g}(a,x)],$$

with strictly increasing and continuous

$$Q_{f,g;f*,g*} = m_{f,g} \circ Q_{\iota,\iota;f*,g*} \circ m_{f,g}^{-1},$$

where of course, by using the already established dimensional invariance of M, $Q_{\iota,\iota,f*,g*}$ is defined by

$$M(f*(a), g*(x)) = Q_{\iota,\iota,f*,g*}[M(a,x)].$$

(iii) *Dimensional invariance and meaningfulness imply isotonicity.* It is sufficient to assume that M is dimensionally invariant. With $J_{f,g} = Q_{\iota,\iota,f,g}$, we have

$$J_{f,g}[M[f(a), g(x)] = M(a,x). \tag{26}$$

Combining (24) and (26), we obtain

$$M_{f,g}[f(a), g(x)] = (H_{f,g} \circ J_{f,g})\{M[f(a), g(x)]\}$$

where $m_{f,g} = H_{f,g} \circ J_{f,g}$ is strictly increasing and continuous. Since any point (b,y) in the common domain $A \times X$ of $M_{f,g}$ and M can be written $f(a) = b, g(x) = y$ for some $a \in A, x \in X$, isotonicity follows. ∎

Remark. Notice that, in part (iii) of this proof, the isotonicity of $\mathcal{M}$ followed from the assumption of meaningfulness and the dimensional invariance of the initial code M.

In contrast to meaningfulness, dimensional invariance and isotonicity are testable properties. As an illustration, we consider a test of dimensional invariance in a detection paradigm. Let $P(x,n)$ be the probability of detecting a stimulus of intensity x embedded in a masking background of intensity n. We assume that the two intensities x and n are measured in distinct ratio scales. Verifying whether these detection probabilities satisfy dimensional invariance would involve checking whether the equivalence

$$P(x,n) \leqslant P(y,m)$$

$$\text{iff} \tag{27}$$

$$P(\lambda x, \gamma n) \leqslant P(\lambda y, \gamma m)$$

is satisfied empirically, for a reasonable sample of values $\lambda, \gamma, x, y, n, m > 0$. A model satisfying this condition is represented by the equation

$$P(x,n) = F(x^\theta/n^\delta), \tag{28}$$

in which θ and δ are positive constants and F is a strictly increasing function. Suppose that only meaningful models are considered. In that case, rather surprisingly, (28) is the only model satisfying dimensional invariance in this situation. This remarkable result stems from the combined strength of meaningfulness, dimensional invariance, and the fact that two distinct ratio scales are involved.

More generally, we have the following result.

14.17. Theorem. *Let $\mathscr{F}, \mathscr{G}$ be two ratio scale families, and suppose that $\mathscr{M} = \{M_{f,g} | f \in \mathscr{F}, g \in \mathscr{G}\}$ is a dimensionally invariant meaningful family of numerical codes. Then, there exist constants $\theta > 0$ and $\delta \neq 0$ such that for all $a \in A$ and $x \in X$,*

$$M(a,x) = G(a^\theta x^\delta),$$

where G is a strictly increasing, continuous function.

We postpone the proof of this theorem, which will be obtained by specializing a more abstract result in the Complements section.

The situation is considerably less constrained if only one scale family is involved, rather than two. To state this with precision, some preliminary material is needed.

Suppose that the numerical codes $M_{f,g}$ in a family $\mathscr{M}$ have multiplicative representations

$$M_{f,g}(a,x) = F^*[u(a)h(x)] \tag{29}$$

where the functions u, h and F^* are real valued, with $u, h > 0$, and have appropriate continuity and monotonicity properties. In general, the functions u, h and F^* may depend on the choice of the scales f, g. For isotone families of numerical codes however, it may be assumed that u, h do not depend on f, g. Indeed, with $m_{f,g}$ as in Definition 14.15, we have

$$M_{f,g}(a,x) = m_{f,g}[M(a,x)]$$
$$= (m_{f,g} \circ F)[u(a)h(x)],$$

where

$$M(a,x) = F[u(a)h(x)]$$

yielding

$$F^* = m_{f,g} \circ F.$$

This remark justifies the following definition.

14.18. Definition. Let $\mathscr{F}, \mathscr{G}$ be two scale families on A, X respectively; let $\mathscr{M} = \{M_{f,g} | f R g\}$, $R \subset \mathscr{F} \times \mathscr{G}$, be an isotone family of numerical codes. Then

(u,h) is a *multiplicative representation* of $\mathcal{M}$ iff u,h are continuous functions taking values in the positive reals and defined on A,X, respectively, such that for all $a \in A, x \in X$,

$$M(a,x) = F[u(a)h(x)]$$

where F is a strictly increasing, continuous function. Thus, u is strictly increasing, and h is strictly monotonic. Occasionally, when an isotone family $\mathcal{M}$ of numerical codes has a multiplicative representation, we simply say that $\mathcal{M}$ is *multiplicative*.

14.19. Theorem.   *Let $\mathcal{F}$ be a scale family, and let $\mathcal{M} = \{\mathcal{M}_{f,f} | f \in \mathcal{F}\}$ be a dimensionally invariant, meaningful, multiplicative family of numerical codes. Then,*

(i) *If $\mathcal{F}$ is a ratio scale family, then one of the two forms*

$$M(a,b) = F(a^{\theta}b^{\delta}), \qquad \theta > 0, \delta \neq 0 \qquad (30)$$

$$M(a,b) = F(\tau a^{\theta} + \xi b^{\theta}), \qquad \tau,\theta > 0, \xi \neq 0 \qquad (31)$$

must hold, with F, a strictly increasing, continuous function.

(ii) *If $\mathcal{F}$ is a log interval scale family, then (30) is the only possible form.*

(iii) *If $\mathcal{F}$ is an interval scale family, then we must have*

$$M(a,b) = F(\tau a + \xi b), \qquad \tau > 0, \xi \neq 0. \qquad (32)$$

The proof will be given in the Complements section. Let us apply this result to the standard discrimination paradigm. Suppose that the discrimination probabilities satisfy dimensional invariance. In other words, the equivalence

$$P(\lambda a, \lambda b) \leqslant P(\lambda c, \lambda d)$$

$$\text{iff} \qquad\qquad\qquad (33)$$

$$P(\gamma a, \gamma b) \leqslant P(\gamma c, \gamma d)$$

has been verified experimentally, on a number of values $a, b, c, d, \lambda, \gamma > 0$. We consider the general model

$$P(s,t) = F[u(s)/h(t)], \qquad (34)$$

which we assume to be meaningful, with the functions F, u, and h being strictly increasing and continuous. Finally, suppose that the stimulus intensities are measured in a ratio scale. All the conditions in Theorem 14.19(i) are satisfied. We conclude that (34) can only take one of the two forms:

$$P(s,t) = F(s^{\theta}/t^{\delta}), \qquad \theta,\delta > 0, \qquad (35)$$

$$P(s,t) = F(\tau s^{\theta} - \xi t^{\theta}), \qquad \theta,\xi,\tau > 0. \qquad (36)$$

If the balance condition

$$P(s,t) + P(t,s) = 1$$

is satisfied, we have in particular $P(s,s) = .5$ for all values of s, which further

TABLE 14.1. *Possible representations for meaningful, dimensionally invariant families of numerical codes. (Summary of Theorems 14.17 and 14.19)*

Case 1 Two distinct input scales:

$$\mathcal{M} = \{M_{f,g} \mid f \in \mathcal{F}, g \in \mathcal{G}\}$$

(Theorem 14.17)

$\mathcal{F}, \mathcal{G}$, two ratio scale families:

$$M(a,x) = G(a^\theta x^\delta) \qquad \theta > 0, \delta \neq 0$$

Case 2 Two identical input scales:

$$\mathcal{M} = \{M_{f,f} \mid f \in \mathcal{F}\}$$

(Theorem 14.19)

$\mathcal{F}$, a scale family

Log interval $\longrightarrow$	$M(a,b) = F(a^\theta b^\delta)$	$\theta > 0,$	$\delta \neq 0$
Ratio $\longrightarrow$	$M(a,b) = F(\tau a^\theta + \xi b^\theta)$	$\tau, \theta > 0,$	$\xi \neq 0$
Interval $\longrightarrow$	$M(a,b) = F(\tau a + \xi b)$	$\tau > 0,$	$\xi \neq 0.$

---

specializes these equations. In Equation (35), we have necessarily $\theta = \delta$, while $\tau = \xi$ must hold in Equation 36. In such a case, (35) and (36) can be rewritten respectively as

$$P(s,t) = F(s/t), \tag{37}$$

$$P(s,t) = F(s^\theta - t^\theta), \tag{38}$$

(the constants θ in (35) and τ in (36) being absorbed in the function F). Equation 37 is, of course, equivalent to Weber's law.

This argument offers a good example of how considerations of meaningfulness and of scale type may narrow down considerably the class of feasible models for a set of data. Another example is discussed in the next section.

The results of Theorems 14.17 and 14.19 are summarized in Table 14.1.

AN APPLICATION IN PSYCHOACOUSTICS

14.20. Dimensional invariance in a detection paradigm. We go back to a detection situation briefly discussed in 14.3. Each trial begins with the presentation of a masking noise of intensity n. The stimulus is a click of intensity x, which is presented at time τ, measured from the end of the noise. The click may be embedded in the noise in some conditions (i.e., τ may be negative). We denote by

$$P(x,n,\tau)$$

the probability that the subject detects the stimulus. This experiment was performed by Pavel (1980; see also Iverson & Pavel, 1981). As Iverson and Pavel (1981) described, the empirical results are consistent with the condition

$$P(x,n,\tau) \leqslant P(x',n',\tau)$$

$$\text{iff} \tag{39}$$

$$P(\lambda x, \mu n, \tau) \leqslant P(\lambda x', \mu n', \tau).$$

14.21. Discussion.   To frame this situation in the language developed in this chapter, we fix τ (temporarily), and assume that $P(x,n,\tau)$—an abbreviation of $P(x,n,\tau)$ are unrelated. Applying Theorem 14.17 (or consulting Table 14.1), we x,n are ratio scale measurements of physical intensities. Equation 39 states that the initial code is dimensionally invariant. We assume that $\mathcal{P}_\tau$ is meaningful. In view of the ratio scale character of the physical intensities, our knowledge of the possible forms of $P(x,n,\tau)$ is now considerable. We have, however, two cases to consider.

Case 1.   The intensities of the click and the noise are measured on distinct ratio scales. This means that the admissible transformations of the numbers x,n in $P(x,n,\tau)$ are unrelated. Applying Theorem 14.17 (or consulting Table 14.1), we obtain, as the only possible form,

$$P(x,n,\tau) = F_\tau[x/n^{\delta(\tau)}], \tag{40}$$

in which F_τ is a continuous, strictly increasing function. Notice that we cannot assume that F_τ does not depend on τ. Indeed, the equation

$$P(x,n,\tau) = F[x/n^{\delta(\tau)}] \tag{41}$$

together with the assumption that P varies effectively with τ, contradicts meaningfulness. To see this, we fix x and consider two admissible transformations $n \mapsto \lambda n$ and $\tau \mapsto \theta\tau$. Equation 40 becomes

$$P_{\lambda,\theta}(x,n,\tau) = F_{\lambda,\theta}[x/n^{\delta_{\lambda,\theta}(\tau)}],$$

where λ,θ denote the scales used to measure n,τ. Using meaningfulness, we obtain, via Theorem 14.13,

$$P_{\lambda,\theta}(x,\lambda n,\theta\tau) = (H_{\lambda,\theta} \circ F)[x/n^{\delta(\tau)}]$$
$$= F_{\lambda,\theta}[x/(\lambda n)^{\delta(\theta\tau)}]$$

for some strictly increasing, continuous function $H_{\lambda,\theta}$, which yields, with $x = 1$ and

$$G_{\lambda,\theta}(s) = [(F_{\lambda,\theta}^{-1} \circ H_{\lambda,\theta} \circ F)(1/s)]^{-1},$$

$$(\lambda n)^{\delta(\theta\tau)} = G_{\lambda,\theta}[n^{\delta(\tau)}]. \tag{42}$$

Setting $n = 1$ in (42) gives

$$\lambda^{\delta(\theta\tau)} = G_{\lambda,\theta}(1). \tag{43}$$

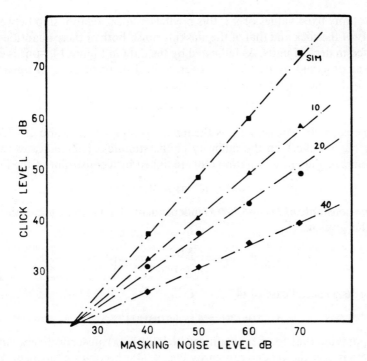

FIGURE 14.1. Pavel's data. The straight lines are a least square fit of Equation 40, plotted in decibels. From *Homogeneity in Complete and Partial Masking* by M. Pavel, 1980, unpublished doctoral dissertation, New York University. Reprinted with permission of author.

Since the right member of (43) does not depend on τ, it follows that δ is a constant function. This conclusion is not supported by the data (cf. Fig. 14.1).

We conclude that if a meaningful expression is to be chosen to describe Pavel's empirical results, it must be of the form (40), with the function F_τ effectively depending on τ. In fact, (40) is consistent with the data, some of which is displayed in Figure 14.1. Let us demonstrate this. Applying F_τ^{-1} on both sides of (40), we get

$$F_\tau^{-1}[P(x,n,\tau)] = x/n^{\delta(\tau)}. \tag{44}$$

setting

$$P(x,n,\tau) = \pi, \qquad \gamma(\tau,\pi) = F_\tau^{-1}(\pi)$$

and solving for x in (44), we obtain the form

$$x(n,\tau,\pi) = \gamma(\tau,\pi)n^{\delta(\tau)}, \tag{45}$$

or in decibel units, taking logs on both sides of (45), with obvious notation,

$$x^*(n,\tau,\pi) = \gamma^*(\tau,\pi) + \delta(\tau)n^*. \tag{46}$$

Thus, for any fixed values of π,τ, this predicts a linear relationship between the intensity of the click and that of the masking noise, both of these quantities being evaluated in decibel units. As indicated by the data in Figure 14.1 this is exactly what was observed by Pavel. Moreover, a fixed point property is apparent in Figure 14.1, which is expressed by the equation

$$x[n_0(\pi),\tau,\pi] = x[n_0(\pi),\tau',\pi] \qquad (47)$$

for some $n_0(\pi)$. In words: $n_0(\pi)$ is the intensity value of the noise at which the delay τ has no effect on the intensity of the stimulus. This indicates that the parameters of the linear equation (46) are linked by a constraint of the form

$$\gamma^*(\tau,\pi) = K^*(\pi) - \delta(\tau)n_0^*(\pi),$$

for some constants $n_0^*(\pi)$ and $K^*(\pi)$ independent of τ. Going back to the initial units, this gives us

$$F_\tau^{-1}(\pi) = \frac{K(\pi)}{n_0(\pi)^{\delta(\tau)}} = \gamma(\tau,\pi),$$

yielding, as a special case of (45),

$$x(n,\tau,\pi) = K(\pi)[n/n_0(\pi)]^{\delta(\pi)}. \qquad (48)$$

We point out that, for meaningfulness to hold, $n_0(\pi)$ must effectively vary with π. Otherwise, as the reader can easily check, (48) becomes equivalent to (41), which is not meaningful.

Case 2. The quantities x and n are physical quantities measured by the same ratio scale. That is, the admissible transformations $x \mapsto \gamma x, n \mapsto \theta n$ are linked: we must have $\gamma = \theta$. Meaningfulness arguments similar to those used for Case 1 (we omit the details), gives us two possible forms.

$$P(x,n,\tau) = F_\tau[x/n^{\delta(\tau)}], \qquad (49)$$

$$P(x,n,\tau) = F_\tau[x^{\delta(\tau)} + \xi(\tau)n^{\delta(\tau)}]. \qquad (50)$$

Equation 49 was analyzed in Case 1. With, as before, $\gamma(\tau,\pi) = F_\tau^{-1}(\pi)$, (50) gives

$$x(n,\tau,\pi) = [\gamma(\tau,\pi) - \xi(\tau)n^{\delta(\tau)}]^{1/\delta(\tau)}. \qquad (51)$$

A result for which the linearity in the data of Figure 14.1 will create difficulties.

Much more could be said about Pavel's empirical results, which are quite extensive and analyzed in great depth in his dissertation. Our purpose here was only to illustrate, by discussing this example, the impact of considerations of meaningfulness on the search for a suitable model for a body of data.

One may ask at this point why (or whether) forms of meaningfulness should be taken as required features for a family of numerical codes. After all, a family of numerical codes purports to be a description of some empirical phenomenon. Science is concerned with what is, not with what should be. We turn to this issue in the next section.

WHY MEANINGFUL LAWS?

The strong bias of the scientific community toward meaningful laws and models cannot be denied. The rationale for this bias, however, has never been fully analyzed. As far as can be seen, the importance of meaningful laws and models appears to be due to a mixture of practical and theoretical reasons.

On the practical side, it is clear that the adoption of a substantial number of nonmeaningful models would create serious difficulties of communication between scientists, except if a unique standard system of units for all important scientific scales is universally adopted, a prospect not easily realized.

On the theoretical side, meaningfulness appears to favor "coherent" systems of quantitative notations of scientific facts, over "incoherent" ones. An example of such "coherence" is provided by Theorem 14.14, in which meaningfulness results in linking input and output scales in a numerical code.

Finally (and this is perhaps the most important consideration), for some scientists, a model is a convincing explanation only if it is physically realizable. However, any physical realization is a scale-free construction. It seems that a nonmeaningful mathematical model—the form of which depends on the scales—cannot very well provide the blueprint for a physical, scale-free realization.[3]

In the next section, we generalize Theorems 14.17 and 14.19, and we provide proofs of these results.

COMPLEMENTS

Quite often the data, at an early stage of experimental research, are not coded in terms of ratio scale families or interval scale families. Effort is then exerted to recode the data in terms of such scales. The critical condition for a successful recoding is that the initial scaling shares certain basic structural properties with the intended final scaling. The next definition gives the general form of such recodings.

14.22. Definition. Two scale families $\mathscr{K}, \mathscr{H}$ are called *conjugate* iff there exists a strictly increasing, continuous function u mapping the domain of $\mathscr{K}$ onto the domain of $\mathscr{H}$ such that

$$\mathscr{H} = \{h \mid h = u \circ k \circ u^{-1}, \text{for some } k \in \mathscr{K}\}.$$

In such a case, we say that $\mathscr{H}$ is the *u-conjugate* of $\mathscr{K}$, and we write

$$\mathscr{H} = u\mathscr{K}u^{-1}.$$

---

3. An example was provided by Pavel (personal communication). For the detection situation discussed in the preceding section, Pavel tried to conceive a physical realization of the model defined by the equation $P(x, n, \tau) = F[x/n^{\delta(\tau)}]$. He did not succeed in imagining a physical system in which the function F did not depend on the variable τ, which made him uneasy about the model represented by that equation.

Clearly, $\mathcal{K}$ is then the u^{-1}-conjugate of $\mathcal{H}$. Conjugation is thus a symmetric relation. It is obviously reflexive and it is also transitive since if $\mathcal{F}$ is the v-conjugate of $\mathcal{H}$, then

$$
\begin{aligned}
\mathcal{F} &= v\mathcal{H}v^{-1} \\
&= v(u\mathcal{K}u^{-1})v^{-1} \\
&= (v \circ u)\mathcal{K}(u^{-1} \circ v^{-1}) \\
&= (v \circ u)\mathcal{K}(v \circ u)^{-1};
\end{aligned}
$$

that is, $\mathcal{F}$ is the $(v \circ u)$-conjugate of $\mathcal{K}$. We conclude that conjugation is an equivalence relation. A scale family is a *quasi ratio* (respectively, *quasi interval*) *scale family* iff it is conjugate to a ratio (respectively, interval) scale family. Notice in passing that if a scale family $\mathcal{F}$ is u-conjugate to some ratio scale family $\mathcal{H}$, then for any constants λ, θ such that $\lambda\theta > 0$, $\mathcal{F}$ is (λu^{θ})-conjugate to $\mathcal{H}$.

A scale family $\mathcal{F}$ on I is called *homogeneous* iff for every $x, y \in I$, there exists $f \in \mathcal{F}$ such that $f(x) = y$. It is clear that a ratio scale family is homogeneous. A scale family is called *commutative* iff it is commutative for the operation of composition of functions.

14.23. Examples.   (a) Any log interval scale family $\mathcal{K}$ is conjugate to some interval scale family $\mathcal{H}$. Actually, $\mathcal{H}$ is the log-conjugate of $\mathcal{K}$ since

$$
\log(\gamma_k e^{\lambda_k s}) = \log \gamma_k + \lambda_k s,
$$

for $\gamma_k, \lambda_k \in \mathbb{R}_+$ and $s \in \mathbb{R}$. More generally, a scale family $\mathcal{F}$ is u-conjugate to an interval scale family iff it is e^u-conjugate to a log interval scale family.

(b) Define

$$
\mathcal{K} = \{k \,|\, k(x) = [(x-1)^3 + \beta_k]^{1/3} + 1, \qquad \text{for some } \beta_k \text{ and all } x \text{ in } \mathbb{R}\}.
$$

Then $\mathcal{K}$ is a quasi ratio scale family. Indeed, with

$$
u(x) = e^{(x-1)^3}, \qquad \lambda_k = e^{\beta_k},
$$

we have

$$
u\mathcal{K}u^{-1} = \{f \,|\, f : x \mapsto \lambda_f x, \text{ for some } \lambda_f \text{ and all } x \text{ in } \mathbb{R}_+\}.
$$

(c) Notice that a quasi ratio scale family is commutative. More generally, many important properties of scale families are preserved under conjugation (cf. Falmagne & Narens, 1983). The following result generalizes Theorem 14.17.

14.24. Theorem.   *Let $\mathcal{F}, \mathcal{G}$ be two homogeneous scale families on A, X, respectively, and suppose that $\mathcal{M} = \{M_{f,g} \,|\, f \in \mathcal{F}, g \in \mathcal{G}\}$ is a dimensionally invariant family of numerical codes. Then, any two of the following three conditions implies the third.*

(i) *$\mathcal{M}$ is meaningful.*
(ii) *$\mathcal{M}$ has a multiplicative representative (u^{θ}, h^{δ}) where $\theta > 0$ and $\delta \neq 0$ are constants, and both u and h are strictly increasing.*
(iii) *$\mathcal{F}, \mathcal{G}$ are respectively u-conjugate and h-conjugate to ratio scale families.*

Proof. (i), (ii) *imply* (iii). Since $\mathscr{M}$ is dimensionally invariant, we can assert the existence, for any $f \in \mathscr{F}$ and $g \in \mathscr{G}$, of a strictly increasing continuous function $K_{f,g}$ such that

$$M(a,x) = K_{f,g}\{M[f(a), g(x)]\},$$

for all $a \in A$ and $x \in X$. By hypothesis, (u^θ, h^δ) is a multiplicative representation of $\mathscr{M}$; we have thus a continuous, strictly increasing function F such that

$$F[u^\theta(a)h^\delta(x)] = (K_{f,g} \circ F)\{u^\theta[f(a)]h^\delta[g(x)]\}, \tag{52}$$

for all $a \in A$, $x \in X$, $f \in \mathscr{F}$ and $g \in \mathscr{G}$. Let us assume (temporarily) that M is strictly increasing in the second váriable. Then, $\delta > 0$. In fact, since, as mentioned earlier, $\mathscr{F}, \mathscr{G}$ are respectively u-conjugate and h-conjugate to ratio scale families iff they are respectively u^θ-conjugate and h^δ-conjugate to ratio scale families, we may as well assume $\theta = \delta = 1$. Fixing f, g in (52) and writing

$$L_{f,g} = F^{-1} \circ K_{f,g}^{-1} \circ F$$

$$u_f = u \circ f \circ u^{-1}, \qquad h_g = h \circ g \circ h^{-1}$$

and

$$u(a) = s, \qquad h(x) = t,$$

(52) is transformed into

$$L_{f,g}(st) = u_f(s)h_g(t). \tag{53}$$

Without loss of generality, we may assume

$$1 \in \mathscr{R}(u) \cap \mathscr{R}(h),$$

where, as indicated earlier, $\mathscr{R}$ denotes the range of the functions. Notice that all three functions $L_{f,g}$, u_f and h_g in (53) are continuous. Using standard functional equation results (cf. chapter 3) we obtain for all $s \in \mathscr{R}(u) \cap \mathscr{R}(h)$,

$$L_{f,g}(s) = \beta_f \gamma_g s^{\alpha_{f,g}}, \tag{54}$$

$$u_f(s) = \beta_f s^{\alpha_{f,g}}, \tag{55}$$

$$h_g(s) = \gamma_g s^{\alpha_{f,g}}, \tag{56}$$

for some constants β_f, γ_g, $\alpha_{f,g} > 0$ which however may depend on the choice of scales $f \in \mathscr{F}$ and $g \in \mathscr{G}$ as suggested by our notation. The results in (54), (55) and (56) are readily extended to the whole domain of the function. (We leave it to the reader to check this.) Since the left members of (55), (56) do not depend on g, f, respectively, the same property applies to the right members, which yields

$$\alpha_{f,g} = \alpha,$$

a constant, for all $f \in \mathscr{F}$ and $g \in \mathscr{G}$. We obtain for (55)

$$(u \circ f \circ u^{-1})(s) = \beta_f s^\alpha,$$

with in particular, since $\iota_A \in \mathscr{F}$,

$$s = \beta_{\iota_A} s^\alpha,$$

which gives $\beta_{\iota_A} = \alpha = 1$. This establishes the fact that $u\mathscr{F}u^{-1}$ is a ratio scale family. A similar argument, using Equation 56 shows that $h\mathscr{G}h^{-1}$ is also a ratio scale family. In the case where M is strictly decreasing in the second variable, we have $\delta < 0$ and a ratio representation

$$M(a,x) = F[u^\theta(a)/h^{-\delta}(x)].$$

We assume $\theta = -\delta = 1$, which leads to

$$L_{f,g}(s/t) = u_f(s)/h_g(t),$$

replacing (53), with a practically identical development. We leave the details to the reader.

(ii), (iii) *imply* (i). Using successively isotonicity ($M_{f,g} = m_{f,g} \circ M$, $m_{f,g}$ strictly increasing and continuous), (ii) and (iii), we have for all $f \in \mathscr{F}$, $g \in \mathscr{G}$, $a, b \in A$ and $x, y \in X$,

$$M_{f,g}[f(a),g(x)] \leqslant M_{f,g}[f(b),g(y)]$$

iff

$$m_{f,g}\{M[f(a),g(x)]\} \leqslant m_{f,g}\{M[f(b),g(y)]\}$$

iff

$$(m_{f,g} \circ F)\{u^\theta[f(a)]h^\delta[g(x)]\} \leqslant (m_{f,g} \circ F)\{u^\theta[f(b)]h^\delta[g(y)]\} \tag{57}$$

iff

$$u^\theta(a)\beta_f^\theta h^\delta(x)\gamma_g^\delta \leqslant u^\theta(b)\beta_f^\theta h^\delta(y)\gamma_g^\delta \tag{58}$$

iff

$$u^\theta(a)h^\delta(x) \leqslant u^\theta(b)h^\delta(y),$$

which is independent of f,g. In (57), (58) we use the fact that, in view of (iii), any $f \in \mathscr{F}$ and $g \in \mathscr{G}$ are of the form

$$(u \circ f \circ u^{-1})(s) = \beta_f s, \qquad \beta_f > 0$$

$$(h \circ g \circ h^{-1})(s) = \gamma_g s, \qquad \gamma_g > 0.$$

This establishes the meaningfulness of $\mathscr{M}$.

(i), (iii) *imply* (ii). As a first step, we show that M satisfies double cancellation (cf. 11.12); that is,

$$M(a,x) \leqslant M(b,y) \tag{59}$$

$$M(b,z) \leqslant M(c,x) \tag{60}$$

imply

$$M(a,z) \leqslant M(c,y) \tag{61}$$

for all $a, b, c \in A$ and $x, y, z \in X$. Because $\mathcal{G}$ is conjugate to a ratio scale family, it is homogeneous. There are thus $g, g^* \in \mathcal{G}$ satisfying $g(x) = z$, $g^*(z) = g(y)$.

The fact that M is dimensionally invariant implies the existence of strictly increasing continuous functions Ψ_g, Ψ_{g^*} such that successively, using (59), (60),

$$
\begin{aligned}
M(a,z) = M[a,g(x)] &= \Psi_g[M(a,x)] \leqslant \Psi_g[M(b,y)] \\
&= M[b,g^*(z)] = \Psi_{g^*}[M(b,z)] \leqslant \Psi_{g^*}[M(c,x)] \\
&= M[c,g^*(x)] = M(c,y).
\end{aligned}
$$

Indeed, from the commutativity of $\mathcal{G}$ (which follows from the fact that $\mathcal{M}$ is conjugate to a ratio family) we have

$$
g^*(x) = (g^* \circ g^{-1})(z) = (g^* \circ g^{-1} \circ g^{*-1} \circ g)(y) = y.
$$

We conclude that (59), (60) imply (61); that is, double cancellation holds. In view of the isotonicity and continuity properties of M, we can assert, using standard measurement results (Krantz et al., 1971), the existence of a multiplicative representation (v, p) satisfying

$$
M(a,x) = F[v(a)p(x)] \tag{62}
$$

for some strictly increasing, continuous function F and all $a \in A, x \in X$. Using the result that (i) and (ii) imply (iii), which we established earlier, it follows that $\mathcal{F}, \mathcal{G}$ are respectively v-conjugate and p-conjugate to ratio scale families. We obtain in particular for each $f \in \mathcal{F}$, the existence of constants $\xi_f, \beta_f > 0$ such that

$$
v[f(a)] = \xi_f v(a),
$$

$$
u[f(a)] = \beta_f u(a),
$$

which yields

$$
v^{-1}[\xi_f v(a)] = u^{-1}[\beta_f u(a)]
$$

with $\xi_{\iota_A} = \beta_{\iota_A} = 1$. Or, letting $u(a) = s$ and noticing that $\beta_f \mapsto \xi_f$ is a strictly increasing continuous function,

$$
(v \circ u^{-1})(\beta s) = \xi(\beta)(v \circ u^{-1})(s)
$$

for all positive β. Using the homogeneity of $\mathcal{F}$ and the fact that the functions $v \circ u^{-1}$ and $\beta \mapsto \xi(\beta)$ are strictly increasing and defined on an interval containing 1, we get

$$
(v \circ u^{-1})(s) = \tau s^\theta
$$

that is

$$
v(a) = \tau u^\theta(a) \tag{63}
$$

for some constant $\tau, \delta > 0$. A similar argument, applied to the scale family $\mathcal{G}$ yields the equation

$$
p(x) = \tau^* h^\delta(x), \tag{64}
$$

with $\tau^*, \delta \neq 0$. Substituting v, p in (25) by their expression in terms of u, h in (63), (64), we obtain

$$M(a,x) = F[\tau u^\theta(a)\tau^* h^\delta(x)]$$
$$= G[u^\theta(a)h^\delta(x)],$$

with

$$G(t) = F(\tau\tau^* t).$$

This completes the proof of Theorem 14.24. ■

Theorem 14.17 follows as an application of the case "(i), (iii) imply (ii)" in Theorem 14.24, in which u, h are identity functions.

We now turn to the proof of Theorem 14.19, which considers a case in which a family $\mathcal{M} = \{M_{f,g}\}$ of numerical codes involves identical scales for the two components; that is, $M_{f,g} \subset \mathcal{M}$ implies $f = g$.

14.25. Proof of Theorem 14.19.   Let $\mathcal{F}, \mathcal{M}$ be as in the hypothesis of the theorem, and let (u, h) be a multiplicative representation of $\mathcal{M}$. Since $\mathcal{M}$ is dimensionally invariant, whether in Case (i), (ii), or (iii) of the theorem to be proved, we have

$$M(\lambda a, \lambda b) = K_\lambda[M(a,b)], \tag{65}$$

for some strictly increasing, continuous function K_λ. Note that λ varies in an interval containing 1, since $\mathcal{F}$ contains the identity scale. In turn (65) gives, using multiplicativity,

$$H[u(\lambda a)h(\lambda b)] = (K_\lambda \circ H)[u(a)h(b)], \tag{66}$$

with H strictly increasing and continuous. Setting $s = u(a)$, $t = h(b)$, we rewrite (66) as

$$u[\lambda u^{-1}(s)]h[\lambda h^{-1}(t)] = (H^{-1} \circ K_\lambda \circ H)(st).$$

Fixing λ and using familiar functional equation arguments, this leads to

$$u[\lambda u^{-1}(s)] = \beta(\lambda)s^{\alpha(\lambda)},$$
$$h[\lambda h^{-1}(s)] = \gamma(\lambda)s^{\alpha(\lambda)},$$

with

$$\alpha(\lambda), \beta(\lambda), \gamma(\lambda) > 0.$$

These functional equations are well known, and have two solutions (cf. 3.10(v).)

Case 1. α is constant; thus $\alpha(\lambda) = 1$ for all λ. Then

$$u(a) = \tau a^\theta \qquad \theta, \tau > 0$$
$$h(a) = \xi a^\delta \qquad \xi > 0, \delta \neq 0$$

yielding

$$M(a,b) = H(\tau a^\theta \xi b^\delta)$$
$$= F(a^\theta b^\delta)$$

with

$$F(c) = H(\tau\xi c).$$

Case 2. α is not constant. Then we obtain the forms

$$u(a) = \tau^* \exp(\tau a^\theta),$$

$$h(a) = \xi^* \exp(\xi a^\delta),$$

yielding

$$M(a,b) = H[\tau^* \exp(\tau a^\theta)\xi^* \exp(\xi b^\delta)]$$

$$= F(\tau a^\theta + \xi b^\delta).$$

Using (65), we obtain

$$\tau(\lambda a)^\theta + \xi(\lambda b)^\delta = (F^{-1} \circ K_\lambda \circ F)(\tau a^\theta + \xi b^\delta),$$

that is, with $s = \tau a^\theta$, $t = \xi b^\delta$ and $F_\lambda = F^{-1} \circ K_\lambda \circ F$,

$$\lambda^\theta s + \lambda^\delta t = F_\lambda(s + t) = F_\lambda(t + s) = \lambda^\theta t + \lambda^\delta s.$$

Thus,

$$s(\lambda^\theta - \lambda^\delta) = t(\lambda^\theta - \lambda^\delta),$$

yielding $\theta = \delta$, and (31) follows. On the other hand, it is easy to check that (30), (31) are compatible with the hypotheses of the theorem, in particular, $\mathscr{F}$ is a ratio scale family.

Equation 30 is also compatible with the assumption that $\mathscr{F}$ is a log interval scale, but (31) is not. Indeed, using the above argument, we would have, with obvious notation, the form

$$\tau(\lambda a^\gamma)^\theta + \xi(\lambda b^\gamma)^\theta = F_{\lambda,\gamma}(\tau a^\theta + \xi b^\theta),$$

which leads easily to $\gamma = 1$.

Finally, in the case where $\mathscr{F}$ is an interval scale family, Equation 30 is easy to eliminate, while (31), again with the same argument, leads to

$$\tau(\lambda a + \gamma)^\theta + \xi(\lambda b + \gamma)^\theta = F_{\lambda,\gamma}(\tau a^\theta + \xi b^\theta),$$

yielding $\theta = 1$ without difficulty. ∎

EXERCISES

1. Show that (19) cannot hold for all $a, b, c, d, \lambda, \gamma > 0$.
2. Is the ratio scale family a subfamily of the interval scale family?
3. Complete the proof given in 14.11 that the family of numerical codes, defined by

$$P_\lambda(s,t) = F_\lambda[s^{\beta(\lambda)} - t^{\beta'(\lambda)}],$$

with F_λ strictly increasing, is not meaningful.

4. Prove that the model defined by (13) is meaningful if and only if δ is constant.
5. Provide three counterexamples, different from those given in the text of the chapter, showing that isotonicity, meaningfulness, and dimensional invariance are independent properties. (This is a part of the proof of Theorem 14.16.)
6. Find a nonmeaningful model satisfying dimensional invariance in the form of Equation 27.
7. Find a condition on the Weber functions Δ_π, which is equivalent to dimensional invariance as specified in Equation 33.
8. For each of the following expressions, check whether meaningfulness, isotonicity, and dimensional invariance are satisfied. In each case, the variables a and x are measured in distinct ratio scales.

   (a) $M(a,x) = a + \delta ax + a^2$
   (b) $M(a,x) = a^x$
   (c) $M(a,x) = a + x$
   (d) $M(a,x) = \log a + x$

9. Provide a counterexample showing that multiplicativity cannot be dropped in Theorem 14.19. In other words, when only one scale family is involved in a numerical code, then meaningfulness, ratio scalability, and dimensional invariance do not imply multiplicativity.

References

Aczél, J. *Lectures on functional equations and their applications*. New York: Academic Press, 1966.

Aczél, J., Belousov, V. D., & Hosszu, M. Generalized associativity and bisymmetry on quasigroups. *Acta Math. Acad. Sci. Hungar.* 1960, *11*, 127–136.

Adams, E. W. Elements of a theory of inexact measurement. *Philosophy of Science*, 1965, *32*, 205–228.

Alpern, M., Rushton, W. A. H., & Tori, S. The size of rod signals. *Journal of Physiology*, 1970, *206*, 193–208. (a)

Alpern, M., Rushton, W. A. H., & Tori, S. The attenuation of rod signals by backgrounds, *Journal of Physiology*, 1970, *206*, 209–227. (b)

Alpern, M., Rushton, W. A. H., & Tori, S. The signals from cones, *Journal of Physiology*, 1970, *207*, 463–475. (c)

Andersen, E. B. A goodness of fit test for the Rasch model. *Psychometrika*, 1973, *38*, 123–140.

Anderson, N. H. Functional measurement and psychophysical judgement. *Psychological Review*, 1970, *77*, 153–170. (a)

Anderson, N. H. Averaging model applied to the size-weight illusion. *Perception & Psychophysics*, 1970, *8*, 1–4. (b)

Anderson, N. H. Information integration theory: A brief survey. In D. H. Krantz, R. C. Atkinson, R. D. Luce, & P. Suppes (Eds.), *Contemporary developments in mathematical psychology, vol. II. Measurement psychophysics and neural information processing*. San Francisco: W. H. Freeman, 1974.

Anderson, N. H. Integration theory, functional measurement, and the psychophysical law, In H.-G. Geissler & Yu. M. Zubrodin (Eds.), *Advances in psychophysics*. Berlin: VEB Deutscher Verlag, 1976.

Anderson, N. H. *Foundation of information integration theory*. New York: Academic Press, 1981.

Anderson, T. W., McCarthy, P. I., & Tukey, J. W. Staircase methods of sensitivity testing. *NAVORD Rep.*, 1946, March 21, 46–65.

Baird, J. C. *Psychophysical analysis of visual space*. Oxford: Pergamon Press, 1970.

Baird, J. C., Green, D. M., & Luce, R. D. Variability and sequential effects in cross-modality matching of area and loudness. *Journal of Experimental Psychology: Human Perception and Performance*, 1980, *6*, 277–289.

Baird, J. C. Psychophysical theory: On the avoidance of contradiction. A commentary to R. M. Warren, Measurement of sensory intensity. *The Behavioral and Brain Sciences*, 1981, *4*, 175–223.

Bamber, D. The area above the ordinal dominance graph and the area below the receiver operating characteristic graph. *Journal of Mathematical Psychology*, 1975, *12*, 387–415.

Barlow, R. E., Bartholomew, D. J., Bremner, J. M., & Brunk, H. D. *Statistical Inference Under Order Restrictions*. New York: Wiley, 1972.

Becker, G. M., DeGroot, M. H., & Marschak, J. Stochastic models of choice behavior. *Behavioral Science*, 1963, *8*, 41–55.

Berliner, J. E., & Durlach, N. I. Intensity perception. IV. Resolution in roving-level discrimination. *Journal of the Acoustical Society of America*, 1973, *53*, 1270–1287.

Berliner, J. E., Durlach, N. I., & Braida, L. D. Intensity perception VII. Further data on roving-level discrimination and the resolution and bias edge effects. *Journal of the Acoustical Society of America*, 1977, *61*, 1577–1585.

Birkhoff, G. *Lattice theory*. Providence, R. I.: American Mathematical Society Colloquium Publication No. XXV, 1967.

Birnbaum, M. H. Controversies in psychological measurement. In B. Wegener (Ed.), *Social attitudes and psychophysical measurement*. Hillsdale, N.J.: Lawrence Erlbaum Associates, 1982.

Blake, R., & Fox, R. The psychophysical inquiry into binocular summation, *Perception and Psychophysics*, 1973, *14*, 161–185.

Blaschke, W., & Bol, G. *Geometrie der Gewebe*. Berlin: Springer, 1938.

Block, H. D., & Marschak, J. Random orderings and stochastic theories of responses. In I. Olkin, S. Ghurye, W. Hoeffding, W. Madow, & H. Mann (Eds.), *Contributions to probability and statistics*. Stanford: Stanford University Press, 1960.

Bock, R. D., & Jones, L. V. *The measurement and prediction of judgement and choice*. San Francisco: Holden-Day, 1968.

Boring, E. G., *A history of experimental psychology* (2nd ed.) New York: Appleton-Century-Crofts, 1950.

Boring, E. G., Langfeld, H. S., & Weld, H. P. *Foundations of psychology*. New York: Wiley, 1948.

Bouchet, A. Etude combinatoire des ordonnés finis. Applications. Thèse. Université scientifique et médicale de Grenoble, 1971.

Bradley, R. A., Incomplete block rank analysis: On the appropriateness of the model for a method of paired comparisons. *Biometrics*, 1954, *10*, 375–390. (a)

Bradley, R. A., Rank analysis of incomplete block designs. II. Additional tables for the method of paired comparisons. *Biometrika*, 1954, *41*, 502–537. (b)

Bradley, R. A. Rank analysis of incomplete block designs. III. Some large sample results on estimation and power for a method of paired comparisons. *Biometrika*, 1955, *42*, 450–470.

Bradley, R. A., & Terry, M. E. Rank analysis of incomplete block designs I. The method of paired comparisons. *Biometrika*, 1952, *39*, 324–345.

Braida, L. D., & Durlach, N. I. Intensity perception. II. Resolution in one-interval paradigms. *Journal of the Acoustical Society of America*, 1972, *51*, 482–502.

Broadbent, D. E., & Gregory, M., Vigilance considered as a statistical decision. *British Journal of Psychology*, 1963, *54*, 309–323. (a)

Brown, J., & Cane, V. R. An analysis of the limiting method. *British Journal of Statistical Psychology*, 1959, *12*, 119–126.

Burt, P., & Sperling, G. Time, distance and feature trade-offs in visual apparent motion. *Psychological Review*, 1981, *82*(2), 171–195.

Campbell, F. W., & Robson, J. G. Application of Fourier analysis to the visibility of gratings. *Journal of Physiology*, 1968, *197*, 551–566.

Campbell, N. R. *Foundations of science: The philosophy of theory and experiment*. New York: Dover, 1957.

Cantor, G. Beitrage zur Begrundung der transfiniten Mengenlehre. *Math. Ann.* 1895, *46*, 481–512.

Causey, R. L. Derived measurement, dimensions, and dimensional analysis. *Philosophy of Sciences*, 1965, *36*, 252–270.

Chernoff, H. On the distribution of the likelihood ratio. *Annals of Mathematical Statistics*, 1954, *25*, 573–578.

Choquet, G. *Topology*. New York: Academic Press, 1966.

Cliff, N., Cudeck, R., & McCormick, D. Evaluation of implied orders as a basis for tailored testing with simulation data. *Applied Psychological Measurement*, 1979, *3*(4), 495–514.

Cogis, O. Determination d'un preordre total contenant un preordre et contneu dans une relation de Ferrers lorsque leur domaine commun est fini. *Compte Rendus de l'Academie des Sciences de Paris*, 1976, *283*, Serie A, 1007–1009.

Cogis, O. Sur la dimension d'un graphe orienté. *Compte Rendus de l'Académie des Sciences de Paris*, 1979, *288*, Serie A, 639–641.

Cogis, O. *La dimension Ferrers des graphes orientés*. Unpublished doctoral dissertation, Université Pierre et Marie Curie, 1980.

Cogis, O. Ferrers digraphs and threshold graphs. *Discrete Mathematics*, 1982, *38*, 33–46. (a)

Cogis, O. On the Ferrers dimension of a digraph. *Discrete Mathematics*, 1982, *38*, 47–52. (b)

Cohen, M., & Falmagne J.-C. Random scale representation of binary choice probabilities: A counterexample to a conjecture of Marschak. *New York University, Mathematical Studies in Perception & Cognition*, 1978, *3*.

Cohen, M., & Narens, L. Fundamental unit structures in the theory of measurement. *Journal of Mathematical Psychology*, 1979.

Coombs, C. H., Dawes, R. M., & Tversky, A. *Mathematical psychology: An elementary introduction*. Englewood Cliffs, N.J.: Prentice-Hall, 1970.

Coombs, C. H. *A theory of data*. New York: Wiley, 1969.

Cornsweet, T. N., & Pinsker, H. M. Luminance discrimination of brief flashes under various conditions of adaptation. *Journal of Physiology* (London), 1965, *176*, 294–310.

Cramér, H. *Mathematical methods of statistics*. Princeton, N.J.: Princeton University Press, 1963.

Cross, D. V. An application of mean value theory to psychological measurement. Progress Report No. 6, Report Number 05613-3-P. Ann Arbor: The Behavioral Analysis Laboratory, University of Michigan, 1965.

Debreu, G. Topological methods in cardinal utility theory. In S. Karlin & P. Suppes (Eds.), *Mathematical methods in the social sciences, 1959*. Stanford: Stanford University Press, 1960.

Derman, C. Non-parametric up-and-down experimentation. Annals of Mathematical Statistics, 1957, *28*, 795–797.

Doignon, J.-P., & Falmagne, J.-C. Difference measurement and simple scalability with restricted solvability. *Journal of Mathematical Psychology*, 1974, *11*(4), 473–499.

Doignon, J.-P., Ducamp, A., & Falmagne, J.-C. Biorders and bidimension of a relation. *Journal of Mathematical Psychology*, in press.

Ducamp, A. Sur la dimension d'un ordre partiel. In *Theory of graphs*. New York: Gordon & Breach, 1967.

Ducamp, A., & Falmagne, J.-C. Composite measurement. *Journal of Mathematical Psychology*, 1969, *6*(3), 359–390.

Durlach, N. I., & Braida, L. D. Intensity perception. I. Preliminary theory of intensity resolution. *Journal of the Acoustical Society of America*, 1969, *46*, 372–383.

Egan, J. P. *Signal detection theory and ROC analysis*. New York: Academic Press, 1975.

Ekman, G. Subjective power functions and the method of fractionation. *Report from the Psychological Laboratory*, University of Stockholm, 1956, No. 34.

Ekman, G. Methodological note on scales of gustatory intensity. *Scandinavian Journal of Psychology*, 1961, *2*, 185–190.

Ellis, B. *Basic concepts of measurement*. London: Cambridge University Press, 1966.

Engen, T. *Psychophysics: Discrimination and detection*. In J. W. Kling & L. A. Riggs (Eds.), *Experimental psychology*. New York: Holt, Rinehart and Winston, 1971.

Erdös, P. On the distribution function of additive functions. *Annals of Mathematics*, 1946, *47*, 1–20.

Fagot, R. F. On the psychophysical law and estimation procedures in psychophysical scaling. *Psychometrika*, 1963, *28*, 145–160.

Falmagne, J.-C. Note on a simple property of binary mixtures. *British Journal of Mathematical & Statistical Psychology*, 1968, *21*(1), 131–132.

Falmagne, J.-C. Bounded versions of Hölder's Theorem with application to extensive measurement. *Journal of Mathematical Psychology*, 1971, *8*, 495–507. (a)

Falmagne, J.-C. The generalized Fechner problem and discrimination. *Journal of Mathematical Psychology*, 1971, *8*, 22–43. (b)

Falmagne, J.-C. Foundations of Fechnerian psychophysics. In D. H. Krantz, R. C. Atkinson, R. D. Luce, & P. Suppes (Eds.), *Contemporary developments in mathematical psychology. Vol. 2. Measurement, psychophysics, and neural information processing*. San Francisco: Freeman, 1974.

Falmagne, J.-C. A set of independent axioms for positive Hölder systems. *Philosophy of Science*, 1975, *42*, 137–151.

Falmagne, J.-C., Random conjoint measurement and loudness summation. *Psychological Review*, 1976, *83*, 65–79.

Falmagne, J.-C. Note: Weber's inequality and Fechner's problem. *Journal of Mathematical Psychology*, 1977, *16*(3), 267–271.

Falmagne, J.-C. A representation theorem for finite random scale systems. *Journal of Mathematical Psychology*, 1978, *18*(1), 52–72.

Falmagne, J.-C. On a class of probabilities conjoint measurement models: Some diagnostic properties. *Journal of Mathematical Psychology*, 1979, *19*, 73–88.

Falmagne, J.-C. A probabilistic theory of extensive measurement. *Journal of Philosophy of Science*, 1980, *47*(2), 277–296.

Falmagne, J.-C. On a recurrent misuse of a classic functional equation result. *Journal of Mathematical Psychology*, 1981, *23*, 190–193.

Falmagne, J.-C. Psychometric functions theory. *Journal of Mathematical Psychology*, 1982, *25*(1), 1–50.

Falmagne, J.-C., & Narens, L. Scales and meaningfulness of quantitative laws. *Synthese*, 1983, *55*, 287–325.

Falmagne, J.-C., & Iverson, G. Conjoint Weber laws and additivity. *Journal of Mathematical Psychology*, 1979, *20*(2), 164–183.

Falmagne, J.-C., Iverson, G., & Marcovici, S. Binaural "loudness" summation: Probabilistic theory and data. *Psychological Review*, 1979, *86*(1), 25–43.

Faverge, J. M. *Methodes statistiques en psychologie appliquee*. Vendome, France: Presses Universitaires de France, 1965.

Fechner, G. T. *Elements of psychophysics*. In D. H. Howes & E. C. Boring, (Eds.), H. E. Adler, trans. New York: Holt, Rinehart and Winston, 1966. (Originally published, 1860.)

Feller, W. *An introduction to probability theory and its applications*. (3rd ed.) New York: Wiley, 1968. (Vol. 1; 1950, 1957, 1968; Vol. 2: 1966.)

Fishburn, P. C. *Utility theory for decision making*. New York: Wiley, 1970. (a)

Fishburn, P. C. Intransitive indifference in preference theory: A survey. *Operations Research*, 1970, *18*, 207–228. (b)

Fishburn, P. C. Intransitive indifference with unequal indifference intervals. *Journal of Mathematical Psychology*, 1970, *7*, 144–149. (c)

Fisher, R. A., & Tippett, L. H. C. Limiting forms of the frequency distributions of the largest or smallest member of a sample. *Proceedings of the Cambridge Philosophical Society*, 1928, *24*, 180–190.

Frank, P. *Between physics and philosophy*. Cambridge, Mass.: Harvard University Press, 1941.

Fréchet, M. Sur la loi de probabilite de l'ecart maximum. *Annales de la Societe Polonaise de Mathematiques* (Cracow), 1927, *6*, 93.

Galambos, J. *The asymptotic theory of extreme order statistics*. New York: Wiley, 1978.

Galanter, E., & Messick, S. The relation between category and magnitude scales of loudness. *Psychological Review*, 1961, *68*, 363–372.

Garner, W. R. An informational analysis of absolute judgements of loudness. *Journal of Experimental Psychology*, 1953, *46*, 373–380.

Garner, W. R. *Uncertainty and structure as psychological concepts*. New York: Wiley, 1962.

Gigerenzer, G., & Strube, G. Are there limits to binaural additivity of loudness? *Journal of Experimental Psychology: Human Perception and Performance*, 1983, *9*(1), 126–136.

Gnedenko, B. V. Sur la distribution limite du terme maximum d'une serie aleatoire. *Annals of Mathematics*, 1943, *44*, 423–453.

Graham, H. C., Bartlett, N. R., Brown, J. L., Hsia, Y., Mueller, C. G., & Riggs, L. A. (Eds.), *Vision and visual perception*. New York: Wiley, 1965.

Gravetter, F., & Lockhead, G. R. Criterial range as a frame of reference for stimulus judgements. *Psychological Review*, 1973, *80, 203–216*.

Gray, D. E. (Ed.) *American Institute Of Physics handbook*. New York: McGraw-Hill, 1957.

Green, D. M. *An introduction to hearing*. Hillsdale, N. J.: Lawrence Erlbaum Associates, 1978.

Green, D. M., & Luce, R. D. Counting and timing mechanisms in auditory discrimination and reaction time. In D. H. Krantz, R. C. Atkinson, R. D. Luce, & P. Suppes (Eds.), *Contemporary developments in mathematical psychology*. Vol. 2. *Measurement, psychophysics, and neural information processing*. San Francisco: Freeman, 1974. (a)

Green, D. M., & Luce, R. D. Variability of magnitude estimates: A timing theory analysis. *Perception & Psychophysics*, 1974, *15*, 291–300. (b)

Green, D. M., & Luce, R. D. Parallel psychometric functions from a set independent detectors. *Psychological Bulletin*, 1975, *82*, 483–486.

Green, D. M., & Luce, R. D. Parallel psychometric functions from a set of independent detectors. *Psychological Bulletin*, 1975, *82*, 483–486.

Green, D. M., & Swets, J. A. *Signal detection theory and psychophysics*. New York: Robert E. Krieger Publishing Co., 1974.

Guilbaud, G. Sur une difficulté de la théorie durisque. *Colloques Internationaux du Centre National de la Recherche Scientifique (Econométrie)*, 1953, *40*, 19–25.

Guilford, J. P. *Psychometric methods*. (2nd ed.) New York: Macmillan, 1954.

Gulick, W. L. *Hearing: Physiology and psychophysics*. New York: Oxford University Press, 1971.

Gumbel, E. G. *Statistics of extremes*. New York: Columbia University Press, 1958.

Guttman, L. A basis for scaling qualitative data. *American Sociological Review, 9*, 1944, 139–150.

Hecht, S., Shlaer, S., & Pirenne, M. H. Energy, quanta, and vision. *Journal of General Physiology*, 1942, *23*, 819–840.

Helmholtz, H. V. Zahlen und Messen erkenntnis-theoretisch betrachtet, Philosophische Aufsutze Eduard Zeller gewidmet, Leipzig, 1887. (Reprinted in Gesammelte Abhandl.), *3*, 1895, 356–391. English Translation by C. L. Bryan, *Counting and measuring*, Princeton, N.J.: Van Nostrand, 1930.

Hölder, O. Die axiome der quantitat und die lehre von mass. *Berichte uber die Verhandlungen der Koniglichen, Sachsischen Gesellschaft der Wissenschaften zu Leipzig, Mathematische-Physysische Classe*, 1901, *53*, 1–64.

Holland, M. K., & Lockhead, G. R. Sequential effects in absolute judgements of loudness. *Perception & Psychophysics*, 1968, *3*, 409–414.

Holman, E. W. Extensive measurement without an order relation. *Philosophy of Science*, 1974, *41*, 361–373.

Holway, A. H., & Pratt, C. C. The Weber-ratio for intensive discrimination. *Psychological Review*, 1936, *43*, 322–340.

Irtel, H., & Schmalhofer, F. Psychodiagnostik auf Ordinalskalenniveau: MeBtheoretische Grundlagen, Modelltest und Parameterschatzung. *Archiv fur Psychologie*, 1982, *134*(3), 197–218.

Iverson, G. J. Note: Conditions under which Thurstone Case III representations for binary choice probabilities are also Fechnerian. *Journal of Mathematical Psychology*, 1979, *20*(3), 263–271.

Iverson, G. J. Weber's Inequality and asymptotic representations of binary choice probabilities. Unpublished manuscript, 1983.

Iverson, G. J., & Falmagne, J.-C. Statistical issues in measurement. Accepted for publication in *Mathematical Social Sciences*, 1985.

Iverson, G. J., & Pavel, M. Invariant properties of masking phenomena in psycho-acoustics and their theoretic consequences. *SIAM-AMS Proceeding*, 1980, *13*, 17–24.

Iverson, G. J., & Pavel, M. On the functional form of partial masking functions in psychoacoustics. *Journal of Mathematical Psychology*, 1981, *24*, 1–20.

James, W. *The principles of psychology*. Vol. I. New York: Holt, 1890. (Dover, 1950.)

Jesteadt, W., & Bilger, R. C. Intensity and frequency discrimination in one and two-interval paradigms. *Journal of the Acoustical Society of America*, 1974, *55*, 1266–1276.

Jesteadt, W., & Sims, S. L. Decision processes in frequency discrimination. *Journal of the Acoustical Society of America*, 1975, *57*, 1161–1168.

Jesteadt, W., Wier, C. C., & Green, D. M. Intensity discrimination as a function of frequency and sensation level. *Journal of the Acoustical Society of America*, 1977, *61*, 169–177.

Johnson, N. I., & Kotz, S. *Distributions in statistics: Discrete distributions*. Boston: Houghton Mifflin, 1969.

Johnson, N. I., & Kotz, S. *Distributions in statistics: Continuous univariate distributions*. Vols. 1 & 2. Boston: Houghton Mifflin, 1970.

Johnson, N. I., & Kotz, S. *Distributions in statistics: Continuous multivariate distributions*. New York: Wiley, 1972.

Junge, K. *Some problems of measurement in psychophysics*. Universitetsforlaget, 1966.

Junge, K. The Garner-Attneave theory of ratio scaling. *Scandinavian Journal of Psychology*, 1967, *8*, 7–10.

Kaufman, L. Sight and mind. New York: Oxford University Press, 1974.

Kesten, H. Accelerated stochastic approximation, *Annals of Mathematical Statistics*, 1958, *29*, 41–59.

Kling, J. W., & Riggs, L. A. *Experimental psychology*. (3rd ed.) New York: Holt, Rinehart and Winston, 1971.

Krantz, D. H. The scaling of small and large color differences. Unpublished doctoral dissertation, University of Pennsylvania, 1964.

Krantz, D. H. Extensive measurement in semiorders. *Philosophy of Science*, 1967, *34*, 348–362.

Krantz, D. H. A survey of measurement theory. In G. B. Dantzig & A. F. Veinott, Jr. (Eds.), *Mathematics of the decision sciences: Part 2. Lectures in applied mathematics*. Providence, R.I.: American Mathematical Society, 1968.

Krantz, D. H. Threshold theories of signal detection. *Psychology Review*, 1969, *76*, 308–324.

Krantz, D. H. Personal communication, 1969.

Krantz, D. H. Integration of just noticeable differences. *Journal of Mathematical Psychology*, 1971, *8*, 591–599.

Krantz, D. H. A theory of magnitude estimation and cross-modality matching. *Journal of Mathematical Psychology*, 1972, *9*, 168–199. (a)

Krantz, D. H. Visual scaling. In D. Jameson & L. M. Hurvitch (Eds.), *Handbook of sensory physiology: Visual psychophysics*. New York: Springer-Verlag, 1972. (b)

Krantz, D. H. Personnal communication, 1978.

Krantz, D. H. Note: A comment on the development of "direct" psychophysics. *Journal of Mathematical Psychology*, 1983, *27*, 325.

Krantz, D. H., Luce, R. D., Suppes, P., & Tversky, A. *Foundations of Measurement*. Vol. 1. New York: Academic Press, 1971.

Krantz, D. H., Luce, R. D., Suppes, P., & Tversky, A. *Foundations of Measurement*. Vol. 2. New York: Academic Press, in preparation.

Kristofferson, A. B., & Dember, W. N. Detectability of targets consisting of multiple small points of light. University of Michigan: Vision Research Laboratories, Technical Report No. 2144-298-T, 1958.

Kruskal, J. B. Nonmetric multidimensional scaling: A numerical method. *Psychometrika*, 1964, *29*, 115–129.

Kuhn, H. W., & Tucker, A. W. (Eds.) Linear inequalities and related systems. *Annals of Mathematics Studies*, 1956, *38*.

Laming, D. R. J. Differential coupling of sensory discriminations inferred from a survey of stable decision models for Weber's Law. *British Journal of Mathematical and Statistical Psychology*, 1982, *35*, 129–161.

Laming, D. R. J. Sensory analysis. Unpublished monograph, University of Cambridge, Department of Experimental Psychology, 1983, 1–329.

Levelt, W. J. M., Riemersma, J. B., & Bunt, A. A. Binaural additivity in loudness. *British Journal of Mathematical and Statistical Psychology*, 1972, *25*, 1–68.

Levin, M. V. Transformations that render curves parallel. *Journal of Mathematical Psychology*, 1971, *7*, 410–444.

Levine, M. V. Transforming curves into curves with the same shape. *Journal of Mathematical Psychology*, 1972, *9*, 1.

Levine, M. V. Geometric interpretations of some psychophysical results. In D. H. Krantz, R. C. Atkinson, R. D. Luce, & P. Suppes (Eds.), *Contemporary developments in mathematical psychology. Vol. 2. Measurement, psychophysics, & neural information processing*. San Francisco: Freeman, 1974.

Levine, M. V. Additive measurement with short segments of curves. *Journal of Mathematical Psychology*, 1975, *12*, 212–224.

Levitt, H. Transformed up-down methods in psychoacoustics. *The Journal of the Acoustical Society of America*, 1970, *49*, 467–476.

Levitt, H. Decision theory, signal detection theory and psychophysics. In E. E. David & P. D. Denas (Eds.), *Human communication: A unified view*. New York: McGraw-Hill, 1972.

Lim, J. S., Rabinowitz, W. M., Braida, L. D., & Durlach, N. I. Intensity perception. VIII: Loudness comparisons between different types of stimuli. *Journal of the Acoustical Society of America*, 1977, *62*, 1256–1267.

Lippman, R. P., Braida, L. D. & Durlach, N. I. Intensity perception. V: Effect of payoff matrix on absolute identification. *Journal of the Acoustical Society of America*, 1976, *59*, 121–134.

Lochner, J. P., & Burger, J. F. Form of the loudness function in the presence of masking noise. *The Journal of the Acoustical Society of America*, 1961, *33*, 1705–1707.

Luce, R. D. Semiorders and a theory of utility discrimination. *Econometrika*, 1956, *24*, 178–191.

Luce, R. D. *Individual choice behavior: A theoretical analysis*. New York: Wiley, 1959. (a)

Luce, R. D. On the possible psychophysical laws. *Psychological Review*, 1959, *66*(2), 81–95. (b)

Luce, R. D. Detection thresholds: A problem reconsidered. *Science*, 1960, *132*, 1495.

Luce, R. D. Comments on Rozeboom's criticism of "On the possible psychophysical laws." *Psychological Review*, 1962, *69*(6), 548–551.

Luce, R. D. A threshold theory for simple detection experiments. *Psychological Review*, 1963, *70*, 61–79. (a)

Luce, R. D. Detection and Recognition. In R. D. Luce, R. R. Bush, & E. Galanter (Eds.), *Handbook of mathematical psychology*. Vol. 2. New York: Wiley, 1963. (b)

Luce, R. D. Three axiom systems for additive semiordered structures. *SIAM Journal of Applied Mathematics*, 1973, *25*, 41–53.

Luce, R. D. Thurstone discriminal processes fifty years later. *Psychometrika*, 1977, *42*(4), 461–498. (a)

Luce, R. D. The choice axiom after twenty years. *Journal of Mathematical Psychology*, 1977, *15*, 215–233. (b)

Luce, R. D. Dimensionally invariant numerical laws correspond to meaningful qualitative relations. *Philosophy of Science* 1978, *45*, 1–16.

Luce, R. D., Bush, R. R., & Galanter, E. (Eds.) *Handbook of mathematical psychology*. Vol. 1. New York: Wiley, 1963.

Luce, R. D., & Edwards, W. The derivation of subjective scales from just noticeable differences. *Psychological Review*, 1958, *65*, 227–237.

Luce, R. D., & Galanter, E. Detection and recognition. In R. D. Luce, R. R. Bush, & E. Galanter (Eds.), *Handbook of mathematical psychology*. Vol. 1. New York: Wiley, 1963. (a)

Luce, R. D., & Galanter, E. Discrimination. In R. D. Luce, R. R. Bush, & E. Galanter (Eds.), *Handbook of mathematical psychology*. Vol. 1. New York: Wiley, 1963. (b)

Luce, R. D., & Green, D. M. A neural timing theory for response times and the psychophysics of intensity. *Psychological Review*, 1972, *79*, 14–57.

Luce, R. D., & Green, D. M. Neural coding and psychophysical discrimination data. *Journal of the Acoustical Society of America*, 1974, *56*, 1554–1564.

Luce, R. D., Green, D. M., & Weber, D. M. Attention bands in absolute identification. *Perception & Psychophysics*, 1976, *20*, 49–54.

Luce, R. D., & Marley, A. A. J. Extensive measurement when concatenation is restricted and maximal elements may exist. In S. Morgenbesser, P. Suppes, & M. G. White (Eds.), *Philosophy, science, and method: Essays in honor of Ernest Nagel*. New York: St. Martin's Press, 1969.

Luce, R. D., & Suppes, P. Preference, utility and subjective probability. In R. D. Luce, R. R. Bush, & E. Galanter (Eds.), *Handbook of mathematical psychology*. Vol. 3. New York: Wiley, 1965.

Manski, C. F. The structure of random utility models. In G. L. Eberlain, W. Kroeber-Reil, W. Leinfellner, & F. Schick (Eds.), *Theory and decision*. Dordrecht, Holland: D. Reidel, 1977.

Marks, L. E. On scales of sensation: Prolegomena to any future psychophysics that will be able to come forth as science. *Perception & Psychophysics*, 1974, *16*, 358–376. (a)

Marks, L. E. *Sensory processes*. New York: Academic Press, 1974. (b)

Marschak, J. Binary choice constraints and random utility indicators. In K. E. Arrow, S. Karlin, & P. Suppes (Eds.), *Proceedings of the first Stanford symposium on mathematical methods in the social sciences*. Stanford: Stanford University Press, 1960.

Mashour, M., & Hosman, J. On the new "psychophysical law": A validation study. *Perception & Psychophysics*, 1968, *3*, 367–375.

McCormick, D. TAILOR-APL: An interactive computer program for individual Tailored testing. Tech. Report (5). Department of Psychology, University of Southern California, 1978.

McFadden, D. Quantal choice analysis: A survey. *Annals of Economic and Social Measurement*, 1976, *5*(4).

McFadden, D., & Richter, M. K. Revealed stochastic preference. Unpublished manuscript, University of California, 1970.

McFadden, D., & Richter, M. K. On the extension of a set function to a probability on the Boolean generated by a family of events, with applications. Unpublished manuscript, University of California, Berkeley, 1971.

McGill, W. J., & Goldberg, J. P. Pure-tone intensity discrimination and energy detection. *Journal of the Acoustical Society of America*, 1968, *44*, 576–581.

Miller, G. A. What is information measurement? *American Psychologist*, 1953, *8*, 3–11.

Miller, G. A. The magical number seven, plus or minus two: Some limits on our capacity for processing information. *Psychological Review*, 1956, *63*, 81–97.

Mills, A. W. Auditory localization. In J. V. Tobias (Ed.), *Foundations of modern auditory theory*. Vol. 2. New York: Academic Press, 1972.

Nachmias, J. On the psychometric function for contrast detection. *Vision Research*, 1981, *21*, 215–224.

Nachmias, J., & Steinman, R. M. Study of absolute visual detection by the rating-scale method. *Journal of the Optical Society of America*, 1963, *53*, 1206–1213.

Nachmias, J. On the psychometric function for contrast detection. *Vision Research*, 1981, *21*, 215–224.

Naka, K. I., & Rushton, W. A. H. S-potentials from colour units in the retina of fish (Cyprinidae). *Journal of Physiology, London*, 1966, *185*, 536–555. (a)

Naka, K. I., & Rushton, W. A. H. An attempt to analyse color perception by electrophysiology. *Journal of Physiology, London*, 1966, *185*, 556–586. (b)

Naka, K. I., & Rushton, W. A. H. S-potentials from luminosity units in the retina of fish (Cyprinidae). *Journal of Physiology, London*, 1966, *185*, 587–599. (c)

Narens, L. A general theory of ratio scalability with remarks about measurement-theoretic concept of meaningfulness. *Theory and Decision*, 1981, *13*, 1–70. (a)

Narens, L. On the scales of measurement. *Journal of Mathematical Psychology*, 1981, *24*(3), 249–275. (b)

Narens, L., & Luce, R. D. The algebra of measurement. *Journal of Pure and Applied Algebra*, 1976, *8*, 197–233.

Neyman, J., & Pearson, E. S. On the problem of the most efficient tests of statistical hypotheses (Phil. Trans.). *Royal Society of London*, Series A, 1933.

Norman, M. F. *Markov processes and learning models.* New York: Academic Press, 1972.

Ore, O. *Theory of graphs.* Providence, R. I.: American Mathematical Society, 1962.

Parducci, A. Range frequency compromise in judgement. *Psychological Monographs*, 1963, *77*(2, Whole No. 565).

Parducci, A. Category judgement: A range frequency model. *Psychological Review*, 1965, *72*, 407–418.

Parducci, A. Contextual effects: A range frequency analysis. In E. C. Carterette & M. P. Friedman (Eds.), *Handbook of perception.* Vol. II. New York: Academic Press, 1974.

Parducci, A., & Perrett, L. F. Category rating scales: Effects of relative spacing and frequency of stimulus values. *Journal of Experimental Psychology*, 1971, *89*, 427–452.

Parker, S., & Schneider, B. Loudness and loudness discrimination. *Perception and Psychophysics*, 1980, *28*(5), 398–406.

Parzen, E. *Stochastic processes.* San Francisco: Holden-Day, 1962.

Pavel, M. Homogeneity in complete and partial masking. Unpublished doctoral dissertation, New York University, 1980.

Pavel, M. Personal communication, 1982.

Pavel, M., & Iverson, G. J. Invariant characteristics of partial masking: Implications for mathematical models. *Journal of the Acoustical Society of America*, 1981, *69*(4), 1126–1131.

Peterson, W. W., Birdsall, T. L., & Fox, W. C. The theory of signal detectability (Trans.). *IRE Prof. Group on Info. Theory*, PGIT-4, 1954, 171–212.

Pfanzagl, J. *Theory of measurement.* (2nd ed.) New York: Wiley, 1971.

Pirenne, M. H. Binocular and uniocular thresholds for vision. *Nature*, 1943, *153*, 698–699.

Piéron, H. *La sensation.* Presses Universitaires de France: Paris 1967.

Plateau, M. J. Sur la measure des sensations physiques, et sur la loi qui lie l'intensité de ces sensations à l'intensité de la cause excitante. *Bulletin de l'Académie Royale des Sciences, des Lettres et des Beaux Arts de Belgique*, 1872, *33*, 376–388.

Pollack, I. Information in elementary auditory displays. *Journal of the Acoustical Society of America*, 1952, *24*, 745–750.

Poulton, E. C. The new psychophysics: Six models for magnitude estimation. *Psychological Bulletin*, 1968, *69*, 1–19.

Polya, G., & Szego, G. *Problems and theory in analysis.* Vol. 1. New York: Springer-Verlag, 1972.

Pratt, J. W. Robustness of some procedures for the two-sample location problem. *Journal of the American Statistical Association*, 1964, *59*, 665–680.

Purks, S. R., Callaghan, D. J., Braida, L. D., & Durlach, N. I. Intensity perception. X. Effect of preceding stimulus on identification performance. *Journal of the Acoustical Society of America*, 1980, *67*, 634–637.

Pynn, C. T., Braida, L. D., & Durlach, N. I. Intensity perception. III. Resolution in small-range identification. *Journal of the Acoustical Society of America*, 1972, *51*, 559–566.

Quick, R. F. A vector magnitude model of contrast detection. *Kybernetic*, 1974, *16*, 65–67.

Rabinowitz, W. M., Lim, J. S., Braida, L. D. & Durlach, N. I. Intensity Perception. VI. Summary of recent data derivations from Weber's law for 1000–IIz tone pulses. *Journal of the Acoustical Society of America*, 1976, *59*, 1506–1509.

Rasch, G. *Probabilistic models for some intelligence and attainment tests.* Copenhagen: The Danish Institute of Educational Research, 1960.

Riguet, J. Les relations de Ferrers. *Comptes Rendus de l'Académie des Sciences de Paris.* 1951, *232*, 1729–1730.

Robbins, H., & Monro, S. A stochastic approximation method. *The Annals of Mathematical Statistics,* 1951, *22*, 400–407.

Roberts, F. S. On nontransitive indifference. *Journal of Mathematical Psychology,* 1970, *1*, 243–258.

Roberts, F. S. Measurement theory. In Gian-Carlo Rota (Ed.), *Encyclopedia of mathematics and its applications.* Vol. 7. *Mathematics and the social sciences.* Reading, Mass.: Addison-Wesley, 1979.

Roberts, F. S., & Luce, R. D. Axiomatic thermodynamics and extensive measurement. *Synthese,* 1968, *18*, 311–326.

Robinson, G. H. Biasing power law exponents by magnitude estimation instructions. *Perception & Psychophysics,* 1976, *19*, 80–84.

Rozeboom, W. W. The untenability of Luce's principle. *Psychological Review,* 1962, *69*, 542–547.

Rudin, W. *Principles of mathematical analysis.* 2nd. ed. New York: McGraw-Hill, 1964.

Sakitt, B. Counting every quantum. *Journal of Physiology,* 1972, *233*, 131–150.

Savage, C. W. Introspectionist and behaviorist interpretations of ratio scales of perceptual magnitudes. *Psychological Monographs,* 1966, *80*(19).

Savage, C. W. *The measurement of sensation.* Berkeley: University of California Press, 1970.

Scharf, B. In E. C. Carterette & M. P. Friedman (Eds.), *Handbook of perception.* Vol. 4. *Hearing.* New York: Academic Press, 1978.

Scott, D. Measurement models and linear inequalities. *Journal of Mathematical Psychology,* 1964, *1*, 233–247.

Scott, D., & Suppes, P. Foundational aspects of theories of measurement. *Journal of Symbolic Logic,* 1958, *23*, 113–128.

Shepard, R. N. Psychophysical relations and psychophysical scales: On the status of "direct" psychophysical measurement. *Journal of Mathematical Psychology,* 1981, *24*, 21–57.

Sincov, D. M. Notes sur la calcul fonctionnel (Russ.). *Bull. Soc. Phys. Math.,* 1903, *13*, 48–72. (a)

Sincov, D. M. Uber eine funktionalgleichung. *Arch. Math. Phys.,* 1903, *6*, 216–217. (b)

Sirovich, L., & Abramov, I. Photopigments and pseudo-pigments. *Vision Research,* 1977, *17*, 5–16.

Skitlovič, V. P. *Izvestia Acad. Nauk SSSR,* 1954, *18*, 185–200.

Stevens, J. C. Brightness function: Binocular versus monocular stimulation. *Perception & Psychophysics,* 1967, *2*, 189–192.

Stevens, S. S. On the psychophysical law. *Psychological Review,* 1957, *64*, 153–181.

Stevens, S. S. Cross-modality validation of subjective scales for loudness, vibration, and electric shock. *Journal of Experimental Psychology,* 1959, *57*, 201–209. (a)

Stevens, S. S. Review of L. L. Thurstone "The measurement of values." *Contemporary Psychology,* 1959, *4*, 388–389. (b)

Stevens, S. S. Procedure for calculating loudness: Mark VI. *Journal of the Acoustical Society of America,* 1961, *33*, 1577–1585. (a)

Stevens, S. S. The psychophysics of sensory function. In W. A. Rosenblith, (Ed.), *Sensory communication.* New York: Wiley, 1961. (b)

Stevens, S. S. To honor Fechner and repeal his law. *Science*, 1961, *133*, 80–86. (c)

Stevens, S. S. The surprising simplicity of sensory metrics. *American Psychologist*, 1962, *50*, 23–29.

Stevens, S. S. Matching functions between loudness and ten other continua. *Perception & Psychophysics*, 1966, *1*, 5–8. (a)

Stevens, S. S. A metric for the social consensus. *Science*, 1966, *151*, 530–541. (b)

Stevens, S. S. *Psychophysics: Introduction to its perceptual neural, and social prospects.* New York: Wiley, 1975.

Stevens, S. S., & Greenbaum, H. B. Regression effect in psychophysical judgement. *Perception & Psychophysics*, 1966, *1*, 439–446.

Stevens, S. S., & Guirao, M. Loudness functions under inhibition. *Perception & Psychophysics*, 1967, *2*, 459–465.

Stouffer, S. A., Guttman, L., Schuman, E. A., Lazarsfeld, P., Starr, S. A., & Clausen, J. A. *Measurement and prediction.* Princeton, N.J.: Princeton University Press, 1950.

Strackee, G., & van der Gon, J. J. D. The frequency distribution of the difference between two Poisson variables. *Statistica Neerlandica*, 1962, *16*, 17–23.

Suppes, P. *Introduction to logic.* Princeton, N.J.: Van Nostrand, 1957.

Suppes, P. Measurement, empirical meaningfulness, and three-valued logic in C. W. Churchman & P. Ratoosh (Eds.), *Measurement: Definitions and theories.* N.Y.: Wiley, 1959.

Suppes, P. *Axiomatic set theory.* Princeton, N.J.: Van Nostrand, 1960.

Suppes, P., & Zinnes, J. Basic measurement theory. In R. D. Luce, R. R. Bush, & E. Galanter (Eds.), *Handbook of mathematical psychology.* Vol. 1. New York: Wiley, 1963.

Swets, J. A. Detection theory and psychophysics: A review. *Psychometrika*, 1961, *26*, 49–63.

Swets, J. A., *Signal detection and recognition by human observers: Contemporary readings.* New York: Wiley, 1964.

Szpilrajn, E. Sur l'extension de l'ordre partiel. *Fundamenta Mathematicae*, 1930, *16*, 386–389.

Tanner, W. P., Jr., & Swets, J. A. A new theory of visual detection, Technical Report, University of Michigan: Electric Defense Group, No. 18, 1953.

Tanner, W. P., Jr., & Swets, J. A. The human use of information: I. Signal detection for the case of the signal known exactly (Trans.). *IRE Prof. Group on Info Theory*, PGIT-4, 1954, 23–221. (a)

Tanner, W. P., Jr., & Swets, J. A. A decision-making theory of visual detection. *Psychological Review*, 1954, *61*, 401–409. (b)

Teghtsoonian, R. On the exponents in Steven's law and the constant in Ekman's law. *Psychological Review*, 1971, *78*, 71–80.

Thompson, W. A., Jr., & Singh, J. The use of limit theorems in paired comparison model-building. *Psychometrika*, 1967, *32*, 255–264.

Thurstone, L. L. A law of comparative judgement. *Psychophysical Review*, 1927, *34*, 273–286. (a)

Thurstone, L. L. Psychological analysis. *American Journal of Psychology*, 1927, *38*, 368–389. (b)

Thurstone, L. L. *The measurement of values.* Chicago: The University of Chicago Press, 1959.

Tumarkin, A. A biologist looks at psycho-acoustics. *Journal of Sound and Vibration*, 1972, *21*, 115–126.

Tumarkin, A. A biologist looks at psychoacoustics. A commentary to R. M. Warren, Measurement of sensory intensity. *The Behavioral and Brain Sciences*, 1981, *4*, 175–223.

Tversky, A. Finite additive structures. Technical report MMPP, 64–6. University of Michigan, Michigan Mathematical Psychology Program, 1964.

Tversky, A., & Russo, J. E. Substitutability and similarity in binary choices. *Journal of Mathematical Psychology*, 1969, *6*, 1–12.

Urban, F. M. On the method of just perceptible differences. *Psychological Review*, 1907, *14*, 244–253.

van Meter, D., & Middleton, D. Modern statistical approaches to reception in communication theory (Trans.). *IRE Prof. Group on Info. theory.* PGIT-4, 1954, 119–141.

von Bekesy, G. *Experiments in hearing.* New York: McGraw-Hill, 1960.

von Mises, R. La distribution de la plus grande de n valeurs. *Revue mathematique de l'union interbalkanique*, 1939, *I*, (1), 141–160. (Reprinted in *Selected papers II.*) Amer. Math. Soc., Providence, R.I. 1954, 271–224.

Vorberg, D. Personal communication, 1982.

Wald, A. *Sequential analysis.* New York: Wiley, 1947.

Wald, A. *Statistical decision functions.* New York: Wiley, 1950.

Wandell, B., & Luce, R. D. Pooling peripheral information: Average vs. extreme values. *Journal of Mathematical Psychology*, 1978, *17*(3), 220–235.

Ward, L. M., & Lockhead, G. R. Sequential effects and memory in category judgements. *Journal of Experimental Psychology*, 1970, *84*, 27–34.

Ward, L. M., & Lockhead, G. R. Response system processes in absolute judgement. *Perception & Psychophysics*, 1971, *9*, 73–78.

Warren, R. M. Measurement of sensory intensity. *The Behavioral and Brain Sciences*, 1981, *4*, 175–223.

Wasan, M. T. *Cambridge tracts in mathematics and mathematical physics (58): Stochastic approximation.* Cambridge: Cambridge University Press, 1969.

Watson, C. S. Visual sensitivity to changes over time. In K. R. Boff, L. Kaufman, & J. Thomas (Eds.), *Handbook of human perception and performance*, in press, 1985.

Watson, C. S., Rilling, M. E., & Bourbon, W. T. Receiver-operating characteristics determined by a mechanical analog to the rating scale. *Journal of the Acoustical Society of America*, 1964, *36*, 283–288.

Weber, D. L., Green, D. M., & Luce, R. D. Effects of practice and distribution of auditory signals on absolute identification. *Perception & Psychophysics*, 1977, *22*, 223–231.

Weiss, D. J. Quantifying private events: A functional measurement analysis of equisection. *Perception & Psychophysics*, 1975, *17*, 351–357.

Wetherill, G. B. Sequential estimation of quantal response curves. *Journal of Royal Statistical Society*, 1963, *B25*, 1–48.

Wetherill, G. B., Chen, H., & Vasudeva, R. B. Sequential estimation of quantal response curves: A new method of estimation. *Biometrika*, 1966, *53*, 439–454.

Wilks, S. S. *Mathematical statistics.* New York: Wiley, 1962.

Yellott, J. I., Jr. The relationship between Luce's choice axiom, Thurstone's theory of comparative judgement, and the double exponential distribution. *Journal of Mathematical Psychology*, 1977, *15*, 109–144.

Zuriff, G. E. A behavioral interpretation of psychophysical scaling. *Behaviorism*, 1972, *1*, 118–133.

Answers or Hints
to Selected Exercises

CHAPTER 1

3. $\mathscr{D}(R_1 - R_2) = \{a,b\}$
6. $R_2 = \{(c,c),(a,c),(a,a)\}$
11. $R = \{(c,a)\}$

17.

	a	d	b	c	e
a	—	—	R	R	R
b	—	—	—	R	R
c	—	—	—	—	R
d	—	—	—	—	R
e	—	—	—	—	—

Thus, aRb, bRc but neither aRd nor dRc. Could you construct a similar example with $A = \{a,b,c,d\}$?

20. *Hint.* Let $\mathbf{a}^+, \mathbf{a}^-$ be the maximal and minimal elements of $\mathbf{A}$, if these exist; let $\mathbf{B} = \{\mathbf{b}|\mathbf{b} = \mathbf{a} \cap B \neq \varnothing, \mathbf{a} \in \mathbf{A}\}$. Using the fact that

$$C = \mathbf{B} \cup \mathscr{F} \; (\|) \cup \{\mathbf{a}^+, \mathbf{a}^-\}$$

is countable, assert the existence of a real-valued function $\check{h}$ satisfying $\check{h}(a) \leqslant \check{h}(b)$ iff $a \lesssim b$ whenever $a \in \mathbf{a}, b \in \mathbf{b}$, for some $\mathbf{a},\mathbf{b} \in C$. Construct an extension h of $\check{h}$ by

$$h(a) = \sup\{\check{h}(b)|b \lesssim a, b \in \mathbf{b} \in C\}, \text{ etc.}$$

22. In 1.43(iv), consider the case $R = \{(a,c),(a,d)\}$, $S = \{(c,b)\}$, $T = \{(d,b)\}$.

26. We say that (A,P) satisfies *strong stochastic transitivity* (s.s.t.) iff for all $a,b,c \in A$,

$$\max\{P_{a,b}, P_{b,c}\} \leqslant \tfrac{1}{2} \text{ implies } P_{a,c} \leqslant \min\{P_{a,b}, P_{b,c}\},$$

with a strict inequality holding in the conclusion whenever $\min\{P_{a,b}, P_{b,c}\} < \tfrac{1}{2}$. We say that (A,P) satisfies *order-independence* iff

$$P_{a,c} \leqslant P_{b,c} \quad \text{iff} \quad P_{a,d} \leqslant P_{b,d}$$

for a, b, c, $d \in A$. Either of strong stochastic transitivity or order-independence is necessary and sufficient for the existence of a representation $P_{a,b} = F[u(a),u(h)]$, with u,F as in Exercise 26. Prove these facts (see Tversky and Russo, 1969).

28. Use Theorem 1.23 to solve this exercise.

29. Prove first the equivalence of the following two conditions.

(i) For all $a,b \in A$ and $x,y \in X$,

$$P_{a,x} \leqslant P_{b,x} \qquad \text{iff} \qquad P_{a,y} \leqslant P_{b,y}$$

and

$$P_{a,x} \leqslant P_{a,y} \qquad \text{iff} \qquad P_{b,x} \leqslant P_{b,y}.$$

(ii) For all a, b, $c \in A$ and x, y, $z \in X$,

$$\text{if} \qquad P_{a,z} \leqslant P_{b,z} \qquad \text{and} \qquad P_{c,x} \leqslant P_{c,y}, \qquad \text{then} \qquad P_{a,x} \leqslant P_{b,y}.$$

Next, fix $a_0 \in A$ and $x_0 \in X$, and define

$$u(a) = P_{a,x_0}, \quad g(x) = 1 - P_{a_0,x}, \quad F[u(a),g(x)] = P_{a,x}.$$

Using the equivalence between (i) and (ii), prove that F is a well-defined function, satisfying the required condition. It is easy to show that (i) and (ii) are necessary.

CHAPTER 2

1. $\frac{1}{3}$

4. (ii) Formula 9 yields $-(p_{18}/p'_{18})(p'_{18} + 1)^{-1} < \gamma_{18} < (p'_{18})^{-1}$. Since $2^{17} * w_{18} \precsim w_1 \precsim y$ and $x \precsim y$, we have $2^{17} \leqslant p'_{18}$ and $(p_{18}/p'_{18}) \leqslant 1$. We conclude that $-(p'_{18} + 1)^{-1} < \gamma_{18} < (p'_{18})^{-1}$, $|\gamma_{18}| \leqslant p'_{18}{}^{-1} \leqslant 2^{-17}$.

8. (i) Assume that $xy \prec y$. Suppose that $y \precsim x$. Using Axiom 3 we obtain $yy \in X$, $yy \precsim xy \prec y$, and Axiom 2 yields $yy \prec y$, contradicting Axiom 4. Thus, by Axiom 2 again, $x \prec y$. We use Axiom 5 to assert that $xz \sim y$ for some $z \in X$. By Axiom 3, $xz \sim y$, $x \sim x$, and $xy \in X$ imply that $xxz \sim xy \prec y \sim xz$. We have thus $xxz \prec xz$. Using Axioms 2 and 4, we have $z \precsim z$, $x \prec xx$, which gives us $xz \precsim xxz$, a contradiction.

11. Axiom 3.

14. Axiom 6.

24. Computing $\psi'(s)/\psi'(t)$ and setting $t = 0$ yields, with $\psi'(0) = \gamma$, $\psi'(s) = \gamma(1 - s^2)^{1/2}$. By integration, we obtain $\psi(s) = \gamma \sin^{-1} s + \beta$, and it follows easily that $\beta = 0$. Replacing ψ by $\sin^{-1}$ in the equation indicates that the function $\psi(s) = \sin^{-1} s$ is indeed a solution, and so is $\psi(s) = \gamma \sin^{-1} s$ for any constant γ. We have thus, for any rod a, $\psi[\ell(a)] = \gamma \sin^{-1}\ell(a) = \zeta f(a)$, where $\zeta > 0$ is as in the preceding exercise, and $\gamma > 0$ follows. With $\alpha = \zeta/\gamma$, we conclude that $\ell(a) = \sin[\alpha f(a)]$, as asserted.

25. (i) Suppose that $\ell(x) = r$, $\ell(y) = s$, and $\ell(z) = t$. We have $x \prec z$ since $\ell > 0$ and $\ell(x) + \ell(y) \leqslant \ell(z)$. Thus, there exists $w \in X$ satisfying $xw \sim z$, $\ell(x) + \ell(w) = \ell(z)$. This yields $y \precsim w$. (Indeed, if $w \prec y$, then $\ell(z) = \ell(x) + \ell(w) < \ell(x) + \ell(y)$.) We have thus $y \precsim w$, $x \precsim x$ and $xw \in X$. Axiom 3 gives $xy \in X$, with $\ell(xy) = \ell(x) + \ell(y)$.

27. Axiom 3.

CHAPTER 3

4. *Sketch of the proof.*

$$\mathbb{P}\{\mathbf{T} > s + t \,|\, \mathbf{T} > t\} = \frac{\mathbb{P}\{\mathbf{T} > s + t, \mathbf{T} > t\}}{\mathbb{P}\{\mathbf{T} > t\}} = \frac{\mathbb{P}\{\mathbf{T} > s + t\}}{\mathbb{P}\{\mathbf{T} > t\}} = g(s).$$

Writing $h(t) = \mathbb{P}\{\mathbf{T} > t\}$, we get $h(s + t) = g(s)h(t)$, with $h(0) = 1$; thus, $g(s + t) = g(s)g(t)$, and the result follows from 3.3 (or Table 3.9 (ii)).

6. (vi) $v_3(t) = e^{-\lambda t}\left[\dfrac{(\alpha_1 t)^3}{3!} + \alpha_1\alpha_2 t^2 + \alpha_3 t\right]$

$$= e^{\lambda t} \sum_{r_1 + 2r_2 + 3r_3 = 3} \prod_{i=1}^{3} \frac{(\alpha_i t)^{r_i}}{r_i!}.$$

8. We define a function f on the open interval $(2,5)$ by

$$f(a) = \begin{cases} .5a + 1 & \text{if} \quad 2 < a \leqslant 3 \\ 1.5a - 2 & \text{if} \quad 3 < a \leqslant 4 \\ .5a + 2 & \text{if} \quad 4 < a < 5 \end{cases}$$

Then f is continuous, strictly increasing, and if $2 < a < 5$, $2 < b < 5$, we have $2 < a + b < 5$ only if $a,b \leqslant 3$, in which Case $4 < a + b < 5$; thus: $f(a) + f(b) = .5a + 1 + .5b + 1 = .5(a + b) + 2 = f(a + b)$ (cf. Falmagne, 1981).

9. *Sketch of the proof.* Suppose that $I = (0,\zeta)$. Take c, $0 < 2c < \zeta$ and notice that $0 \in I_c = (-c, \zeta - 2c)$. For a, b, $a + b \in I_c$, $h(a + b + 2c) = v(a + c) + k(a + c)g(b + c)$, which we write $h_c(a + b) = v_c(a) + k_c(a)g_c(b)$. Since $0 \in I_c$, the theorem holds for the functions h_c, v_c, k_c, g_c in virtue of the first part of the proof; the parameters in the equations might, however, depend on c. The result follows from the fact that $h_c(a) = h(a + 2c) = v(2c) + k(2c)g(a)$. The proof in the case $I = (\zeta',0)$ is similar.

10. *Sketch of proof of Theorem 3.7.* Let r be a continuous or strictly increasing function defined on an open interval I having 0 as a limit point, and satisfying

$$r(\alpha s + \alpha' t) = \alpha r(s) + \alpha' r(t). \tag{*}$$

Assume $0 \in I$. Setting successively $s = 0$ and $t = 0$ in (*), we obtain $r(\alpha' t) = \alpha r(0) + \alpha' r(t), r(\alpha s) = \alpha r(s) + \alpha' r(0)$, yielding

$$r(\alpha s + \alpha' t) = r(\alpha s) + r(\alpha' t) - r(0)(\alpha + \alpha'). \tag{**}$$

Defining

$$f(a) = r(a) - r(0)(\alpha + \alpha'), \qquad \alpha s = a, \qquad \alpha't = b,$$

(**) becomes

$$f(a + b) = f(a) + f(b),$$

and it can be shown without much difficulty that the conditions of Theorem 3.2 are satisfied. The result follows. If $0 \notin I$, define $r(0) = \lim_{s\to 0} r(s)$, or $r(0) = \inf\{r(s)|s \in I\}$, etc.

17. The transformation $2\mathbf{X}_a - \mathbf{X}_b = \mathbf{Y}_1, \frac{1}{3}\mathbf{X}_a + \frac{2}{3}\mathbf{X}_b = \mathbf{Y}_2$ has an inverse $\mathbf{X}_a = \frac{1}{5}(2\mathbf{Y}_1 + 3\mathbf{Y}_2), \mathbf{X}_b = \frac{1}{5}(6\mathbf{Y}_2 - \mathbf{Y}_1)$. Since $\Delta = (\frac{2}{5})(\frac{6}{5}) - (\frac{3}{5})(-\frac{1}{5}) = \frac{3}{5} > 0$,

$$(y_1, y_2) \mapsto [\tfrac{1}{5}(2y_1 + 3y_2), \tfrac{1}{5}(6y_2 - y_1)]$$

is a 1-1 mapping of the plane onto itself. Notice that such linear transformation changes a bivariate normal into another bivariate normal (e.g., Feller, 1966, Chapter III). Let f, f_a, f_b, ψ be the densities of $(\mathbf{X}_a, \mathbf{X}_b)$, $\mathbf{X}_a, \mathbf{X}_b$, $(\mathbf{Y}_1, \mathbf{Y}_2)$, respectively. Let σ^2 be the common variance of $\mathbf{X}_a, \mathbf{X}_b$; let m_a, m_b be the expectations of $\mathbf{X}_a, \mathbf{X}_b$.

$$\psi(y_1, y_2) = f[\tfrac{1}{5}(2y_1 + 3y_2), \tfrac{1}{5}(6y_2 - y_1)] \cdot \Delta$$

$$= f_a[\tfrac{1}{5}(2y_1 + 3y_2)]f_b[\tfrac{1}{5}(6y_2 - y_1)] \cdot \Delta$$

$$= \frac{1}{2\pi\sigma^2} \exp\left\{-\frac{1}{2\sigma^2}\left\{[\tfrac{1}{5}(2y_1 + 3y_2) - m_a]^2 \right.\right.$$

$$\left.\left. + [\tfrac{1}{5}(6y_2 - y_1) - m_b]^2\right\}\right\} \cdot \Delta$$

$$= \frac{1}{\sqrt{2\pi} \cdot \sqrt{5}\sigma} \exp\left\{-\frac{1}{2 \times (5\sigma^2)}[y_1 - (2m_a - m_b)]^2\right\}$$

$$\times \frac{1}{\sqrt{2\pi}(\sqrt{5/3})\sigma} \exp\left\{-\frac{1}{2(5/9)\sigma^2}\left[y_2 - \left(\frac{1}{3}m_a + \frac{2}{3}m_b\right)\right]^2\right\}$$

21. 100.

24. (*Hint.* Prove the existence of a collection $\{f_\alpha\}$ of functions satisfying (i) $f_\alpha(s,t) = G(s\alpha, t)$; (ii) $f_\alpha \circ f_{\alpha'} = f_{\alpha\alpha'}$.)

CHAPTER 4

3. Differentiate (*) with respect to a on one hand, with respect to b on the other hand, take ratios and simplify. Set $b = sa$, and simplify again. Apply functional equation arguments.

4. No. *Proof:* If such functions u, F exist, then $u(a) - u(d) = F^{-1}(.8) = u(b) - u(e)$. But $u(a) - u(d) = [u(a) - u(c)] + [u(c) - u(d)] = F^{-1}(.75) + F^{-1}(.6) > F^{-1}(.75) + F^{-1}(.55) = [u(b) - u(d)] + [u(d) - u(e)] = u(b) - u(e)$, a contradiction.

6. No.
9. Balance.

CHAPTER 5

3. It is clear that (v) implies (ii). The converse implication also holds, since any case of (v) corresponds to a case of (ii) or takes a form such as

$$P_{a,b} + P_{b,a} + \min\{P_{c,a}, P_{c,b}\} \geqslant 1.$$

4. Let n_{st} be the number of choices of s over t in the course of N trials. For large N, $n_{ac} - n_{ab} - n_{bc}$ is distributed very nearly normally, with expectation $N(P_{a,c} - P_{a,b} - P_{b,c})$. Use a one-tailed t test of the null hypothesis: $P_{a,c} \leqslant P_{a,b} + P_{b,c}$.

6. *Hint.* $P_{a,b} = \Phi\left\{\dfrac{u(a) - u(b)}{[\Phi^{-1}(P_{a,b})]^2}\right\}.$

(See Krantz, personnel communication, 1969.)

12. *Hint.* You may try to use Exercises 5 and 6 here.

CHAPTER 6

* 3. *Sketch of proof.* If $\mathscr{F}^*$ is Fechnerian, then $p_b^*(a) = G[u(a) - u(b)]$, which leads to the functional equation

$$F[u(\xi a) - u(\xi b)] = \xi^\delta F[u(a) - u(b)],$$

with $F = \Phi^{-1} \circ G$, $\delta = \eta - \mu$. With $u(a) = s$, $u(b) = t$ we obtain

$$F(s - t) = \xi^{-\delta} F\{u[\xi u^{-1}(s)] - u[\xi u^{-1}(t)]\}$$
$$= H_\xi[g_\xi(s) - g_\xi(t)].$$

Thus g_ξ is linear, $g_\xi(s) = \alpha(\xi)s + \beta(\xi)$ or equivalently $u(\xi a) = \alpha(\xi)u(a) + \beta(\xi)$. Apply 3.10 (iv).

8. Using symmetry and balance, we get

$$p_b(b + \delta) + p_b(b - \delta) = 1$$
$$p_{b-\delta}(b) + p_b(b - \delta) = 1$$

yielding

$$p_b(b + \delta) = p_{b-\delta}(b)$$

or, with $b = a + \delta$,

$$p_a(a + \delta) = p_{a+\delta}(a + 2\delta).$$

The result follows by induction.

9. Suppose that $\mathscr{F}$ is not parallel, say

$$p_b(b + \delta) < p_c(c + \delta)$$

with $b < c$. Then, we must have

$$p_b(b + \delta) = p_{b+n\delta}[b + (n + 1)\delta] < p_c(c + \delta)$$

for some $n \in \mathbb{N}$ such that $b < c \leqslant b + n\delta$, which shows that the functions $p_a(a + \delta)$ are not monotonic in a.

CHAPTER 7

1. A proof is obtained by a slight generalization of 4.14.
8. $(\text{Log}, 1/\mu)$, where $1/\mu$ denotes the function $a \mapsto a/\mu$.
13. Generalize the proof of Theorem 7.27 and use 5.3(iv).
14. *Sketch of proof.* Suppose that $\mathscr{F} \overset{u}{\longmapsto} \mathscr{F}^*$. This implies $p_a(b) = F[u(a) - u(b)]$, with u, F strictly increasing and continuous, and $F(\delta) + F(-\delta) = 1$, if $\mathscr{F}$ is symmetric and centered. We obtain

$$F[u(b) - u(b + \delta)] + F[u(b) - u(b - \delta)] = 1$$

yielding

$$u(b) - u(b - \delta) = u(b + \delta) - u(b).$$

Conclude by using Theorem 3.14. (It can be assumed without loss of generality that $0 \in I$.) The converse is obvious.

CHAPTER 8

2. Weber's law implies, by 8.13(2), that $p_b(a) = G(\log a - \log b)$ for some strictly increasing, continuous function G. We obtain

$$\frac{\mu(a) - \mu(b)}{[\sigma(a)^2 + \sigma(b)^2]^{1/2}} = (\Phi^{-1} \circ G)(\log a - \log b).$$

Theorem 5.16 can be applied, to yield the two solutions: (i) $\sigma > 0$ is constant and $\mu(a) = \alpha \log a + \beta$, in which $\alpha > 0$ and β are constants; (ii) $\mu(a) = \alpha\sigma(a) + \beta$ and $\sigma(a) = \theta a^\gamma$, with α, θ, $\gamma > 0$, and β constants (cf. 5.7).
5. h is defined on an open, real interval.
8. The condition corresponding to (weak) bicancellation is as follows: for all probabilities π_1, π_2, π_3, π_3' whenever $(\xi_{\pi_3} \circ \xi_{\pi_2} \circ \xi_{\pi_1})(a) = a$ and $(\xi_{\pi_3'} \circ \xi_{\pi_2} \circ \xi_{\pi_1})(a') = a'$ for some a, a', then $\pi_3 = \pi_3'$.

CHAPTER 9

1. *Hint.* Compare the two models specified by (15) and (16).
3. Equation (15) leads to

$$\Delta_\pi(a) = [\Phi^{-1}(\pi) + \alpha(a)]^{1/\beta(a)} - \alpha(a)^{1/\beta(a)}.$$

while (16) yields

$$\Delta_\pi(a) = \Phi^{-1}(\pi)^{1/\beta(a)}.$$

Note that the last equation does not depend on the parameter $\alpha(a)$.

4. We recall (cf. 8.15) that a real-valued function f defined on an open interval J is called convex iff for every point $q = (x, f(x))$ of its graph there is a straight line L containing q such that the graph of f lies on or above L.

In symbols,

$$f(z) \geqslant f(x) + k(z - x) = L(z) \tag{*}$$

for all $z \in J$, with k the slope of L (see figure). The function f is strictly convex iff the equality in (*) is strict; it is concave (respectively strictly concave) iff $-f$ is convex (resp. strictly convex), or equivalently iff the inequality (resp.

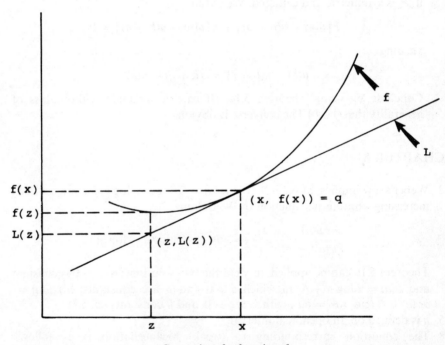

Convexity of a function f.

strict inequality) is reversed in (*). Let $p_a = f$, a function that is strictly convex on some open interval in which the mass of $\mathbf{X}_\infty$ is concentrated. Taking expectations in (*), we obtain

$$E[p_a(\mathbf{X}_\infty)] > E[p_a(x)] + k[E(\mathbf{X}_\infty) - x]$$
$$= p_a[E(\mathbf{X}_\infty)].$$

if we choose $x = E(\mathbf{X}_\infty)$ (cf. Feller, 1966). For example, if p_a is the distribution function of a normal random variable, using the approximation (8) involves no bias, since p_a is then, to a very good approximation, linear at the point $[\xi, p_a^{-1}(\xi)]$, with $\xi = \xi_{.5}(a)$. But if p_a is concave, say exponential, of the form

$$p_a(x) = \begin{cases} 1 - e^{-\lambda(a)[x - \alpha(a)]}, & x \geqslant \alpha(a); \\ 0, & 0 \leqslant x < \alpha(a); \end{cases}$$

then the above argument leads to a positive bias, $E[p_a(\mathbf{X}_\infty)] < p_a[E(\mathbf{X}_\infty)]$.

8. $\xi_{.794\ldots}(a)$ is estimated by $n = 3$.

CHAPTER 10

2. For $\mathbf{S} = s,n$ we write $F_\mathbf{S}$ and $F_\mathbf{S}^*$, for the distribution functions of the random variables $\mathbf{U_S}$ and $\mathbf{U_S^*} = g(\mathbf{U_S})$, respectively. We have

$$F_\mathbf{S}^*(x) = \mathbb{P}\{g(\mathbf{U_S}) \leqslant x\} = \mathbb{P}\{\mathbf{U_S} \leqslant g^{-1}(x)\} = F_\mathbf{S}[g^{-1}(x)].$$

Thus, $\mathbf{U_S^*}$ has a density function if $F_\mathbf{S}^* = F_\mathbf{S} \circ g^{-1}$ is differentiable. This occurs if g^{-1} is differentiable, which in turn implies that g must be differentiable, with $g' > 0$. (Note in passing that the fact that g is strictly increasing does not imply $g' > 0$: consider the case $g(x) = x^3$.) We conclude that $\mathscr{U}^*$ is differentiable if g is differentiable with $g' > 0$. Notice that in such a case, $[g^{-1}]' > 0$. Under these assumptions, we have for $\mathbf{S} = s,n$

$$f_\mathbf{S}^*(x) = (F_\mathbf{S}^*)'(x) = (F_\mathbf{S} \circ g^{-1})'(x) = f_\mathbf{S}[g^{-1}(x)](g^{-1})'(x),$$

yielding, in particular, $f_n^* > 0$. For the likelihood function, we obtain

$$\begin{aligned} \ell^*(x) &= f_s^*(x)/f_n^*(x) \\ &= f_s[g^{-1}(x)]/f_n[g^{-1}(x)] \\ &= \ell[g^{-1}(x)], \end{aligned}$$

and the rationality of $\mathscr{U}^*$ follows from the rationality of $\mathscr{U}$ and the fact that g^{-1} is strictly increasing and continuous.

5. By definition, $\mathscr{U}$ is rational iff the likelihood ratio

$$\ell(x) = f_s(x)/f_n(x)$$

is strictly increasing. Replacing the density functions by their Gaussian expressions as specified in the exercise, it follows after simplification that $\ell(x)$ is strictly increasing with

$$[(x - \mu_n)/\sigma_n]^2 - [(x - \mu_s)/\sigma_s]^2.$$

This function is strictly increasing in x iff the quadratic terms vanish, that is, $\sigma_s = \sigma_n$ and $\mu_s > \mu_n$.

7.   (i) $\beta_\theta = \frac{1}{6}$.
    (ii) $\lambda_\theta \approx -1.29$.
    (iii) $p_s(\theta) \approx .989$; $p_n(\theta) \approx .901$.

CHAPTER 11

4. $p_{12}(p) = \gamma p + (1 - \gamma)$, with $\gamma = \dfrac{(1 - p_{1,a})(1 - p_{2,x})}{(1 - p_{1,n})(1 - p_{2,n'})}$.

6. $(m_{xy} \circ m_{zw})(a) = f^{-1}\{g(x) - g(y) + f[m_{zw}(a)]\}$

$= f^{-1}\{g(x) - g(y) + (f \circ f^{-1})[g(z) - g(w) + f(a)]\}$

$= f^{-1}[g(x) - g(y) + g(z) - g(w) + f(a)]$

$= (m_{zw} \circ m_{xy})(a)$.

10. Suppose that the medians are defined by $m_{xy}(a) = \dfrac{x}{y} + a$. Then

$$(m_{xy} \circ m_{zw})(a) = \frac{x}{y} + m_{zw}(a)$$

$$= \frac{x}{y} + \frac{z}{w} + a$$

$$= (m_{zw} \circ m_{xy})(a).$$

Thus, the commutativity rule is satisfied. It is easy to check that the cancellation rule does not hold.

12. Take $\mu_{1,a} = 8, \mu_{2,x} = 2$, and $\mu_{1,n} = \mu_{2,n'} = 1$. Then $d'_{12} = 4 < d'_{1} = 7/\sqrt{2}$ and thus $\Phi(d'_{12}) < \Phi(d'_{1})$, contradicting Equation 4.

CHAPTER 12

1. Applying G^{-1} on both sides of the equation, gives

$$a^{\alpha}b^{\beta}c^{\gamma} = G^{-1}[M(a,b,c)] = g,$$

the last equation defining the variable g. Solving for a, we obtain

$$a(b,c,g) = (b^{-\beta}c^{-\gamma}g)^{1/\alpha},$$

which, in turn, yields

$$a(\lambda b, \lambda c, \lambda g) = [(\lambda b)^{-\beta}(\lambda c)^{-\gamma}(\lambda g)]^{1/\alpha} = \lambda^{(1 - \beta - \gamma)/\alpha}a(b,c,g).$$

Thus, a is homogeneous of degree $(1 - \beta - \gamma)/\alpha$. Obviously, we could have solved for another variable, with similar results.

6. To show that Q_2 is well defined, suppose that $ay/bx = a'y'/b'x'$. Define

$$\xi = yb'x'/y'bx, \qquad \theta = a'y'x/ayx', \qquad \gamma = ax'/a'x;$$

then

$$\xi a = a', \qquad \theta b = b', \qquad \gamma \xi x = x', \qquad \gamma \theta y = y'.$$

Notice, moreover, that by appropriate multiplications we can make a, x, b, y small enough to ensure that each of ξa, ξx, θb, θy, $\gamma\xi x$, $\gamma\theta y \in I$. Thus

$$Q_2(ax/by) = P_{ax,by} \qquad \text{(by definition)},$$
$$= P_{(\xi a)(\xi x),(\theta b)(\theta y)} \qquad \text{(SCWI)},$$
$$= P_{(\xi a)(\gamma\xi x),(\theta b)(\gamma\theta y)} \qquad \text{(SCWII)},$$
$$= Q_2[(\xi a)(\gamma\theta y)/(\theta b)(\gamma\xi x) \qquad \text{(by definition)},$$
$$= Q_2(a'y'/b'x').$$

Hence, Q_2 is well defined, and also strictly increasing, since p is strictly increasing in the first variable.

11. There are shift invariant functions η that are not consistent with a gain control representation. Iverson and Pavel (1981) give the example $\eta(x,y) = x[1 + \ln(\beta x/y)]$, with $0 < y < \beta x$. It suffices to notice that this form is not consistent with either (36) or (37). On the other hand, $\eta(x,y) = (x + x^{1/2})/(y + y^2)$ is a gain control representation, but is not shift invariant.

CHAPTER 13

7. (i) Define $M(a,b) = a + b$. This function is homogeneous of degree one. If we assume that $u(a + b) = [u(a)u(b)]^{1/2}$, we obtain $u(2a) = u(a)$, contradicting the assumption that u is a one-to-one function.

   (ii) With $u(a) = a + 1$ and $M(a,b) = [(a + 1)(b + 1)]^{1/2} - 1$, the function M satisfies (13) but is not homogeneous of degree one.

CHAPTER 14

2. No.
3. With H_λ as in 14.11, and $B = \beta(1)$ and $B' = \beta'(1)$, we have

$$H_\lambda(a^B - b^{B'}) = (\lambda a)^{\beta(\lambda)} - (\lambda b)^{\beta'(\lambda)}.$$

Setting $a^B - b^{B'} = 1$, leads to

$$H_\lambda(1) = \lambda^{\beta(\lambda)}(1 + b^{B'})^{\beta(\lambda)/B} - \lambda^{\beta'(\lambda)}b^{\beta'(\lambda)}$$

Show that the right member varies with b except if β and β' are constant, a case treated earlier.

9. $\mathcal{M} = \{M_\lambda \mid M_\lambda(a,b) = F_\lambda[a + b + (ab)^{1/2}]; a, b, \lambda > 0\}$.

Author Index

Subject Index

(A page number in boldface indicates a definition.)

DATE DUE